Changing Food Habits

Food in History and Culture

A series edited by *Carole M. Counihan*, Dept. of Anthropology, Millersville University, Millersville, Pennsylvania and *Steven L. Kaplan*, Dept. of History, Cornell University, Ithaca, New York

Food in History and Culture examines the history of food, food consumption and food-based rituals in order to provide a greater understanding of culture and society.

Changing Food Habits

Case Studies from Africa, South America and Europe

Edited by

Carola Lentz

*Institut für Historische Ethnologie
der Johann Wolfgang Goethe–Universität
Frankfurt am Main, Germany*

harwood academic publishers

Australia Canada China France Germany India
Japan Luxembourg Malaysia The Netherlands
Russia Singapore Switzerland

Amsteldijk 166
1st Floor
1079 LH Amsterdam
The Netherlands

Versions of chapters 2, 4, 5, 6 and 8 were published previously in the journal *Food and Foodways*, 5(1).

Chapter 1 originally appeared in German in a different form in *Kulturthema Essen*, copyright © 1993 Akademie Verlag, Berlin, Germany.

A version of chapter 3 was printed under another title in *African Encounters in Domesticity*, copyright © 1992 Rutgers University Press, New Brunswick, New Jersey, USA.

Chapter 11 was first published in *Marketing in a Multicultural World: Ethnicity, Nationalism and Cultural Identity*, copyright © 1995 Sage Publications, Thousand Oaks, California, USA.

All are reprinted with permission.

British Library Cataloguing in Publication Data

Changing food habits : case studies from Africa, South
America and Europe. – (Food in history and culture ; v. 2 –
ISSN   1028-2653)
1. Food habits – Africa – Case studies 2. Food habits –
Europe – Case studies 3. Food habits – South America – Case
studies 4. Diet – Social aspects – Africa – Case studies
5. Diet – Social aspects – Europe – Case studies 6. Diet –
Social aspects – South America – Case studies
I. Lentz, Carola
641.3

ISBN   90-5702-564-7

CONTENTS

INTRODUCTION TO THE SERIES

Food in History and Culture seeks to examine and illuminate the role of food in various cultures and throughout history, in order to provide a greater understanding of civilization and society. Food contributes to the creation of people's lives—socially, economically, politically, morally and nutritionally—in powerful but often subtle ways. This series explores the history of food production, distribution and consumption, as well as the role of food in rituals. In their analyses, the authors included in *Food in History and Culture* are committed to the idea of food as a matter of social, as much as biological, importance.

Carole Counihan
Steve Kaplan

INTRODUCTION—CHANGING FOOD HABITS: AN INTRODUCTION

Carola Lentz

Institut fuer Historische Ethnologie, University of Frankfurt, Germany

The flood of publications on food and food habits makes it necessary to begin by stating what this book is *not*: it is not a comprehensive and theoretically homogeneous volume on processes of change in food habits. It intends to add, however, its share of interesting case studies, most of them based on original field work and devoted to processes of change in African, South American and European countries. And the cases presented here suggest alternative readings of some established models of change in food habits and contribute to a more comprehensive theory of dietary transformations.[1]

The case studies presented in the following articles are quite diverse, as are the nature and scope of changes considered. They cover rural as well as urban modes of food consumption and patterns of drinking. They discuss dietary change in different societal contexts, ranging from crisis-ridden African societies with fuzzy class boundaries and without a highly differentiated cuisine, to South American states such as Ecuador and Peru with deeply entrenched ethnic-cum-social hierarchies, and finally to European countries that passed from class-structured food cultures to post-war "mass consumption," cultivating a plurality of tastes and individual food styles. Although most of the case studies analyze changing food habits (and patterns of alcohol consumption) as an integral part of ongoing ecological, economic, political and social transformations, some research into dietary change resulting from directed, applied interventions by persons and agencies is included, hence, the deliberately ambiguous title of this book, "Changing Food Habits," which allows for both notions of "change."

But despite such diversity of cases which furnish ample material for innovative comparisons, all chapters were written from an implicitly "antistructuralist" anthropological or sociological perspective and privilege a historical approach to food studies. All chapters share the conviction that studying processes of change provides an excellent laboratory for the discovery of the complex factors that shape people's food habits. And despite the wide range of geographical areas and time spans covered, some common themes seem to emerge that deserve closer attention: the relationship between agricultural production and changing food habits, patterns of urban and market-dependent food and alcohol consumption, aspects of food security, the role of household structures and gender in dietary transformations, and the symbolic mediations of changing patterns of food and alcohol consumption. This introduction, then, intends to draw the reader's attention to these topics, to underline some of the articles' explicit arguments and to offer a personal reading of some of the more implicit ideas.[2]

FOOD PRODUCTION AND DIETARY PATTERNS

Many chapters in this book address food habits of peasant populations, which produce at least part of the foodstuffs they consume. Gerd Spittler's provocative praise of the "simple, but perfect meal" of African pastoralists and peasants draws attention to the close links among agricultural subsistence production, limiting the diversity of available foodstuffs, and the persistence of local notions of good taste centered on a simple everyday dish of grain or root-crop porridge with a sauce. Consequently, changes in agricultural production are highly relevant to the development of patterns of food consumption. This becomes particularly evident in Achim von Oppen's analysis of the introduction of cassava in northwestern Zambia. In this case, the dynamics of peasant production are at the source of dietary innovation. The clear advantages of cassava with regard to food security (its adaptability to difficult ecological conditions, high yields relative to caloric energy produced per area, long and secure storability) motivated the peasants to adopt it first as a supplement, then as a substitute for the grain crops that they traditionally cultivated. This happened despite ambivalent and often negative indigenous evaluations of the new staple ("poor food"). Of course, more than two centuries passed from the first introduction of cassava by the Portuguese to the almost complete displacement of millets, and individual producer-consumers might not have been fully aware of the scope of the ongoing change. Furthermore, the composition of the peasants' customary meals—porridge and relish or, to use Mintz' terms (1987: 35–9), complex carbohydrate center and protein-rich aromatic periphery—facilitated the incorporation of cassava with little modification of the structure of the dish, much like potatoes easily found their way into north German stews (Wiegelmann 1967: 87–111). Nevertheless, the fact that close neighbors continued to prefer millet and, more recently, introduced maize, must have kept alive notions of the differences between grain and root-crop porridges. More important than considerations of taste and nutritional value were the advantages that cassava offered as a reliable foodstuff and as a commodity: it provided access to the market (and thus to a wide range of desired goods such as cloth and salt) and it enhanced the social position of groups as diverse as women, elders and chiefs.

The complex issues of gender and time economy involved in the adoption of cassava will be discussed later. What I want to stress here is that in von Oppen's case study, the factors responsible for dietary change are clearly to be sought in the sphere of peasants' economic strategies. Similarly, Elisabeth Meyer-Renschhausen's example of the displacement of millet porridge in central Europe during the course of the nineteenth century shows that, apart from the ideological connotations involved in the spread of coffee-sugar-and-bread morning meals, it was mainly for economic reasons that millet virtually disappeared from peasant production (and hence diet). Millet required labor-intensive cultivation, which an increased tax burden and falling prices for raw produce made increasingly impractical. In addition, the costly obligation to process one's grain at state-licensed mills made it cheaper and more convenient for peasants to obtain the necessary starch from purchased flour or bread rather than from home-grown and pounded millet.

Similar considerations seem to have motivated the Sudanese peasants described by Joachim Theis, who analyzes how over the past three decades purchased sorghum has partially replaced home-grown millet. Central Kordofan peasant producers have found it more advantageous to expand the production of sesame and groundnuts and to use income from these cash crops to buy cheap sorghum than to engage in subsistence production of millet. Much as in von Oppen's case, sorghum can replace millet in the customary porridge-and-sauce meals with little change in the structure of the dish, and it requires even less innovation in cooking techniques than cassava. This would suggest, then, that peasants more readily implement economically rational changes if the corresponding dietary innovations fit in easily with the dominant composition of meals. The peasants whom Theis observed, however, maintained that millet porridge was definitely more palatable than preparations from sorghum and was the proper food to eat during periods of hard labor, for which they always tried to reserve some of the coveted grain. Interestingly, the same line of argument—that porridge prepared from millet was the most satisfying and tasty while

sorghum was the ideal grain from which to brew beer—was repeatedly reported by villagers whom I interviewed in northwestern Ghana.
Similar patterns of preserving the displaced but still highly valued foodstuffs can be discovered in the South American case studies and in Meyer-
Renschhausen's examples: frequently, foods for special occasions continue
to be prepared from "traditional" ingredients. By contrast, new staples (or
manufactured foodstuffs purchased in order to supplement an insufficient
agricultural production) seem to be quickly incorporated into the everyday
diet, where considerations of taste and symbolic ranking become secondary
to harsh economic realities.

The issue of economic rationality behind dietary change is, of course,
complex, and I wish to point out that the authors' case studies should not
be read as illustrations of Marvin Harris's "cultural materialist" paradigm
and his, in my view, rather simplistic approach to the evolution of food
habits (Harris 1987). Joachim Theis's study, like that of von Oppen, for
instance, raises the question of the "unintended consequences" of rational
behavior: what was once introduced as a sensible response to new marketing
opportunities has since developed into an element of environmental degradation, and in the long run become a factor leading to undernourishment
(or even famines) when additional strains like a severe drought intervene.
But before I go further into the issues of food security, I want to briefly
mention the role of economic change in my own case study, which com-
pares the production and consumption of beer in Ghana and Ecuador, and
in the two case studies of dietary transformations in Andean villages of
Peru and Ecuador.

Economic change is clearly among the central factors responsible for
changing patterns of alcohol production and consumption in northwestern
Ghana and highland Ecuador. In the case of northern Ghana, the increasing
availability of sorghum on local and regional markets allowed a growing
number of women to purchase the ingredients necessary for brewing beer
independently, instead of having to rely solely, as they did before, on the
grain made available to them by their husbands and fathers. In addition,
the greater variety of goods, such as cloth, manufactured soap, and enamel
pots, which gradually began to appear in local markets from the 1950s
onward, became an incentive for the women actually to engage in beer-
brewing activities in order to generate the income necessary to purchase
these attractive goods. Finally, the demand for beer and, more important,
the ability to purchase the desirable liquid, increased along with the ever-
larger numbers of young men migrating seasonally to the south and returning to their homes with some cash. Here, then, it is not so much the item
of consumption itself which has changed, but the amount of consumption

and the range of consumers, which expanded far beyond the scope of the elders traditionally in a position to purchase and drink beer.

In highland Ecuador, on the other hand, the income from Indian labor migration was spent on beer brewed not by the Indian village women, but by Mestizo entrepreneurs in the parish centers. Since the 1950s, village- and home-brewed beer, both the ordinary beer made from barley and the festive beer made from maize, were produced less often and in lesser quantities, due mainly to the diminishing size of agricultural plots and meager harvests, resulting in a shortage of grain available for brewing. Moreover, male labor migration shifted an increasing workload to the village women, making them less willing to engage in the time-consuming pro- cess of brewing. And, different from northern Ghana, home-brewed beer was and is never paid for by the male consumers, thus brewing was not an attractive source of income for the village women. Consequently, the Indian demand for beer was satisfied by Mestizo brewers. These commer- cial brewers were not only able to accumulate considerable riches, reduc- ing the costs of production to a minimum by partly replacing grain by ammoniac and sugar, but also involved the Indian villagers in networks of debts which had to be paid off by free labor. In this context, it was a change in the drink itself, more specifically, the replacement of the Mestizo-brewed beer by manufactured, bottled beer and sugar cane liquor, often purchased on the coast, which, among other factors, enabled the Indian villagers to break away from the Mestizo control over their alcohol con- sumption. Here, then, changes in the pattern of drink are intertwined not only with changes in the agricultural production, but also with the transfor- mation of the political economy of interethnic relations.

The pattern of dietary change observed by Leticia Delgado and Mary Weismantel does not seem to be one in which one staple crop replaces another (be it home-grown or purchased), but rather one in which industri- ally processed foodstuffs are introduced to complement poor harvests and make up for land shortage. Historically, however, barley, which today is the main staple in Weismantel's parish and is of some importance in Delgado's village as well, was introduced by the Spaniards and subse- quently adopted by the indigenous peasants in much the same way as cassava became the dominant crop in northwestern Zambia. In the more recent transformations of Andean diets and unlike the African cases, the role of social differentiation, to a high degree dependent on the size and quality of the land owned, becomes immediately apparent. Delgado shows that it is precisely the better-off peasant commodity producers who adhere more closely to a "traditional" diet from their own products, with fewer manufactured supplements (but more meat) than the poorer strata of the community, who are forced to hire out their labor force in an unequal exchange for cash or kind. The latter arrangement is usually organized under the cover of traditional relations of reciprocity (*minga*), a good part of the retribution being returned not in the customary form of typical Andean produce but in the form of manufactured products which the employers have often received via Food Aid programs. Despite the differences in the amount of commercially produced foodstuffs used, however, both wealthier and poorer households seem to incorporate the new food items into old dishes in a way similar to African peasants (Orlove 1987: 493–7).

Mary Weismantel's impoverished Indian parish in highland Ecuador, finally, forms no exception to what can be seen in the other case studies: it is changes in the economic strategies of survival that most profoundly affect dietary patterns. Particularly in younger families, land is of poor quality and not sufficient to allow for food self-reliance or the generation of monetary income. Consequently, the men have to migrate as wage laborers while the women remain in the village as subsistence farmers, complementing the meager harvests of barley, fava beans and potatoes with oats, wheat flour, noodles, and other foodstuffs that their husbands bring from the city. In this case then, dietary innovation seems to be governed basically by poverty, although there are some new items and dishes of prestige.

URBAN FOOD CONSUMPTION

In the urban context, straightforward economic factors such as levels of income, availability and prices of foodstuffs are no less important for urban consumers' dietary choices than for food-producing peasants. Karen Hansen's study of colonial and post-colonial cooking practices in urban Zambia provides a particularly clear case in point. Not only gendered notions of cooking and domestic work (see below), but also severe economic constraints such as prohibitive food expenses and unaffordable kitchen technology prevented the new skills of European cuisine that African male cooks had acquired in colonial domestic service from transforming the standard porridge-and-sauce meal in the servants' own homes. The economic crisis of the 1980s even forced many affluent households to return to the charcoal brazier and, hence, to the porridge-and-sauce diet more easily prepared than European-style individual dishes, which had begun to mark their elite status through a differentiated cuisine, featuring "non-traditional" ingredients and cooking techniques. With the exception of very few really wealthy Zambians who can still afford such a "cuisine of luxury," the strained economy with severe cutbacks in income and bottle-necks in the availability of foodstuffs leveled the emerging class-related differentiation of food habits. Thus today, the everyday standard meals of both poor and relatively rich urbanites are prepared in like manner and share the same basic ingredients—a "cooking of necessity."

In the same vein, Michael Wildt's research into changes in food consumption in postwar Germany shows that only substantial raises in real income and the comforting certitude of long-lasting affluence made the gradual transformation of the "taste for necessities" (Bourdieu 1979) into patterns of consumption emphasizing plurality of taste, freedom of choice and individuality possible. The first decade after the war was still governed by previous experiences of scarcity, of having to make much out of little. Besides replacing durable goods that were lost or destroyed during the war, West German working-class families used their increased incomes primarily to purchase larger quantities of accustomed and highly cherished foodstuffs such as meat, butter and coffee that they had badly missed. Not before the 1950s and then throughout the 1960s, with wages still on the increase, did these households incorporate more and more new products and tastes into their diet, including tropical fruit, condensed milk, and many readymade articles such as dehydrated potato dumplings or pancakes, biscuits and cookies as well as canned food. Of course, changing discourses on food—propagated through newspapers, women's magazines, radio programs or posters—that associated "modernity" and "health" with light, low calorie meals and privileged "international" dishes helped to promote new desires, tastes and styles of cooking. But Wildt points to the sound economic and material prerequisites of such innovations, for instance, new forms of marketing through self-service shops and new technologies of storage and cooking such as refrigerators, deep-freezers, electric stoves and kitchen machines that the majority of households could afford only from the 1960s onward.

Economic factors also played a crucial role in the spread of *döner kebab,* a Turkish fast food consisting of slices of roasted meat served in a piece of flat bread, in Berlin and more generally in Germany. Highlighting the economic strategies of the producers and marketeers of *döner kebab*, Ayse Çaglar's article traces the beginnings of this ethnic fast food business to the early 1970s when new recruitments of Turkish "guest workers" for industrial jobs were stopped, but the permitted "family reunification" nevertheless resulted in a drastic increase in the number of Turks living in Germany. The unemployment of the new arrivals and the earlier immigrants' willingness to invest their savings into businesses contributed toward the establishment of an increasing number of Turkish grocery stores and fast food stalls offering *döner kebab*. That *döner* rapidly attracted many German customers, without any advertising campaign, and is able to hold its own with, and even surpass, accustomed local fast food varieties such as *Bockwurst* or *Curry Wurst* (different types of sausage) seems to be mainly due to its tangible advantages over other fast foods: *döner* consists of starches (bread), meat and vegetables, and thus makes for a complete and filling meal at a reasonable price. This is not to deny that other factors such as aesthetic attractiveness, compatibility with the dominant discourse on healthy, low-fat nourishment and connotations of Mediterranean ambience also contribute to *döner kebab*'s success in Germany. But the basis of *döner*'s triumphant advance was laid by sound economic calculations, of both producers and consumers, embedded, of course, in a dominant way of work and life that makes snacks and fast food indispensable to broad sectors of the population (see Mintz 1987, chapter 5).

Jakob Tanner's chapter on wartime food policy in Switzerland presents perhaps the most extreme case of economic-cum-political determination of (or encroachment on) food habits from above. Nutritional scientists and politicians not only defined standards of an adequate diet, but also made them effective by enforcing a strict food rationing system. At the same time, however, Tanner's case provides a particularly clear example of the tenacity with which people cling to their own ideas about taste and good food. Wherever and on whatever scale possible, they resorted to the black market or their own garden products or at least particular skills of preparation in order to transform official food rations into acceptable meals, far removed from nutrional science's notions of a "healthy" diet that would ensure maximum output and performance in the war economy. But here again, economic factors such as income and class-differentiated access to black market networks played an important role in determining the extent to which consumers were capable of dodging the constraints imposed by official food policies.

FOOD SECURITY

The conclusion that profound changes in food habits and patterns of drink are normally a consequence of transformations in the economic strategies of survival or accumulation might seem too commonplace to elaborate. In view of a substantial literature on symbolic dimensions of foodways (see, for example, Douglas 1984; Manderson 1986), however, the more obvious and profane aspects of food habits need to be called to mind from time to time. Much less trivial is the question of how the changes in food habits relate to food security, particularly in the Third World cases presented here. It seems to me that none of the case studies argues a monocausal link between changes in food production, dietary habits and food security. Much depends, of course, on how food security is defined—as regular and quantitatively sufficient food supplies or with regard to quality of diet, for instance. As Elisabeth Meyer-Renschhausen aptly shows in her analysis of changing popular and scientific evaluations of grain porridge, these definitions are themselves historically variable and an issue of controversy. The debate among Swiss nutritional scientists presented in Tanner's chapter, who regarded the war as a "mass experiment in nutrition" and attempted to define quantitatively and qualitatively adequate standards of daily caloric intake, provides another clear example of contested definitions of food security, as does Spittler's well-argued critique of the conflation of indigenous evaluations of periodic scarcity with an Eurocentric diagnosis of "hunger".

Gretel and Pertti Pelto's (1983) model of general trends in dietary change and food security and Richard Franke's arguments (1987) are a useful starting point here. They suggest that it is mainly a trend of increasing "delocalization" of food production and distribution that characterizes the worldwide transformations in food use and food habits during the last two centuries and, at an accelerated rate, since World War II. Varieties of foods, methods of production, and patterns of consumption are disseminated throughout the world, intensifying socioeconomic and political interdependency with respect to food security. In the industrialized countries especially, an ever-increasing number of daily consumed foodstuffs come from distant places through commercial channels. In general, the delocalization processes seem to produce opposite effects in the First and Third World. In industrialized countries, diets have improved as a result of the increased diversity of available foods and of expanded food supplies. In the developing countries, on the other hand, the same process of delocalization has normally meant a growing involvement in the production of some of the food needs of the industrialized countries. As a result, resource competition for export and for domestic use has increased. Frequently, this has led to a growing dependence of national food systems on the importation of grains and other foodstuffs from industrialized nations. One of the effects of this new dependence has been the substitution of more monotonous foods of inferior nutritional value for the diversified traditional diets. And, as the Peltos and Franke conclude, with the exception of a small elite, delocalization in the Third World involves a decrease in the diversity of available foods, in nutritional status, and in food security in general (see also Messer 1984: 233–7).

At a first reading, the African and South American case studies in this book corroborate to a certain extent the hypothesis of the largely negative effects of increasing (world-) market integration on Third World food security: all processes of change described here seem to result in dietary situations worse than before. Today, Weismantel's Indians consume more and more noodles, white breads, and sugar; in other words foods much poorer in proteins, vitamins, and minerals than the formerly dominant potatoes, maize, beans, and barley. Theis's peasant cash-crop producers are no longer able to complement their porridge with nutritionally valuable fresh or sour milk. The 1983–85 drought nearly brought about a collapse of their already vulnerable economy, making relief food their only resource. The austere economic recovery program that the World Bank imposes in Zambia results in severe bottlenecks of food availability and in prohibitive prices for protein-rich sauce ingredients. The list of examples could be continued, but a closer examination reveals a more complicated picture.

There is a tendency among some Marxist anthropologists to see increasing market integration and capitalist transformation *per se* at the source of a general Third World economic, social, and moral decline and to idealize the precapitalist past (e.g., Scott 1976; Hyden 1980). But Theis, for example, points out that the great famines (and wars) toward the end of the past century nearly depopulated the Kordofan. Thus, he seems to suggest that drought affected people in a much more severe way when communications and infrastructure were less developed and when obtaining food supplies from less affected areas was much more difficult than is the case today. Spittler (1989) has convincingly shown for an area of Niger that has been severely affected by recent droughts that twentieth-century economic and political transformations, rather than resulting in an inevitable general decrease of food security, have probably contributed to its increase. Similarly, I agree with Weismantel that the present diet of poor Andean peasants is far from being satisfactory from a nutritional point of view. Nevertheless, I would argue that, with limited market integration and hence greater sensitivity to harvest failures under the hacienda system, these peasants were unlikely to have been much better nourished in the past than they are today (Lentz 1988: 44–66, 186–90).

Von Oppen's chapter illustrates how ambiguous and historically variable the links between market integration and food security can be. Cassava was introduced as a hedge against famine and provided definitively more food security than millet. A protein-rich relish, made from ingredients such as fish and game, which were obtained through well-organized regional trade links, could compensate for the lower nutritional value of cassava porridge. The cultivation of cassava shifted the bulk of labor to women, and hence allowed men to participate more fully in pre-colonial long-distance trade. Later, under colonial rule, cassava cultivation in the hands of women cushioned the effects of male labor migration, which resulted in food insecurity in neighboring areas. It is only recently that rapidly spreading plant pests reveal the vulnerability the predominance of cassava cultivation produces and that the increasing scarcity of fish and game may lead to dietary insufficiency. On the whole, however, cassava made possible market integration without an overall decrease of food security. The problems the peasants now face are due to a complex inter-play of different factors, the "poor food" cassava being only one of them.

HOUSEHOLD, GENDER, AND CHANGING FOOD HABITS

New economic opportunities/constraints and changing strategies of sur-vival provide the general context for the transformation of food habits. As a rule, however, dietary innovation has to be effected within the household and, more concretely, has to be implemented by those primarily concerned with the preparation and serving of meals, namely, women. In order to better understand the dynamics of change in food consumption, it is essential to pay attention to property rights, to the division of labor, to sex and age roles within the household (or, to use a more precise term, within the cooking group or unit of consumption because these, in Africa, do not always coincide with residency), and, particularly, to the interests and strategies of women.

This is not always easy, of course, especially in studies of past dietary transformations for which scholars have to draw on historical, written sources that are usually silent about the female role in cooking and cuisine. But as von Oppen demonstrates by carefully interpolating from the scanty historical evidence available and from more detailed studies of present-day situations, it is possible to highlight, for instance, the central role women played in the adoption of cassava. Von Oppen shows that cassava is attractive for women because it renders them less dependent on unreli-able male support for bush clearing and the provision of tools and grain stores. This does not mitigate the fact that the cultivation of cassava requires more female labor than customary millets and hence allows men to invest more time in commercial activities. However, women also profit in another way. Traditionally, northwest Zambesian women are entitled to the surplus produced on their own fields (and to half of the surplus produced

on fields jointly owned with their husbands) that remains after all family
food needs have been satisfied. By adopting cassava, the women are able
to augment this surplus and to participate more fully in village networks of
exchange (cassava for labor assistance or male products like dried fish)
and regional markets. A similar dynamic is at work in the case of the
northern Ghanaian beer brewers who greatly increased their brewing activities in order to enhance their monetary income and hence purchasing power.
Similarly, in Joachim Theis's study, it is the peasant women's interest in
devoting more time to the cultivation of their own land and in increasing
their income that leads them to incorporate a certain amount of what could
be termed fast foods such as white bread or wheat flour doughnuts into the
daily diet. Spittler points to comparable developments among Tuareg
women in Niger, whose arduous tasks of fetching firewood and water and
of pounding and grinding millet is the indispensable basis of the "simple,
but perfect meal," namely the tasty and satisfying *ashin* (millet porridge).
To ease their heavy workload women resort to mills, wherever possible,
or, particularly in the towns, use rice or other food products that require
less time to prepare.

Women's time economy also played a role in the nineteenth-century
displacement of grain porridge in central Europe discussed by Meyer-
Renschhausen. At a first reading, it seems as though the dietary transformation clearly resulted in an overall decrease of time spent on food
preparation and allowed females to participate more substantially in extra-
domestic employment (see also Mintz 1987: 158–61). A closer examination, however, reveals that the argument of time economy, which is often
invoked to substantiate why commercially milled flour and bread have
rapidly replaced home-pounded cereals, is at least partially misleading.
As Meyer-Renschhausen shows, the moistening, drying/roasting, and
pounding of the grain in fact required much labor. But because of the long
shelf-life of the grain thus processed, these activities had to be carried out
only occasionally and, more important, the actual preparation of the daily
porridge demanded much less time than most "modern" dishes. Similar
considerations of time economy, in addition to prohibitive food prices and
unavailable kitchen technology, could also have been among the reasons
why in Hansen's Zambian example women have continued to prepare
porridge-and-sauce meals, regularly dodging the European-style cooking
and general housekeeping instructions imparted to them by church or state
organized homecraft courses.

In order to compare meaningfully women's workloads "before" and
"after" the disappearance of grain porridge from the diets of European rural
(and urban) populations, one would, of course, need to take into account

many geographic and historical variables. Teuteberg and Wiegelmann's research on the development of food habits in Germany during the period of industrialization suggests, for instance, that the early nineteenth-century coffee-potato and coffee-bread-butter-marmalade meals of the poorest strata of the population reduced female time spent on food preparation (1972: 276–87, 296–98). However, growing incomes and the spread of urban bourgeois patterns of food consumption (the use of individual plates and forks, more varied dishes and complex methods for preparing meat, potatos and so forth) among workers and peasants toward the end of the past century contributed to a considerable increase in women's domestic chores. Wildt quotes postwar opinion polls among German housewives praising the time-saving properties of canned foods and new kitchen machines. But at the same time, these women insisted that for the sake of quality, certain tasks like peeling potatoes or scouring vegetables needed to be performed by hand. They also continued to bake cakes and to prepare their own fruit and vegetable preserves because homemade foods were regarded as a visible proof of desirable housewifely skills and were believed to taste unmistakably better than manufactured products. It remains to be seen, then, whether in Theis's Kordofan case, for instance, the time and energy women can save by using certain new food items will be eventually swallowed up by the introduction of dishes that require more complicated cooking procedures.

It would also be fascinating to collect more detailed information on potential inner-household conflicts over new foods. Such conflicts could, for instance, develop between Kordofan male peasants who insist on being served what they consider "real food" for hard-working people (namely millet or sorghum porridge, which require tedious preparation) and their wives who want to maintain marital peace, but who also wish to allocate their time more profitably. Theis's data suggest that the women avoid this dilemma by selecting foodstuffs that not only suit their time economy but that are also valued as "modern," urban and, hence, desirable foods by the men who have often come into closer contact with non-peasant food habits during periods of labor migration.

Many papers in this book point to the active role women play in the introduction of new food items. But they also frequently act as "gatekeepers" who reject foodstuffs that are considered unpalatable, too difficult to prepare, or generally undesirable such as, for instance, the egg powder, ersatz coffee and synthetic grape honey in Swiss wartime food rations or the green peas and canned pork of Food Aid distributions in Peru. From Delgado's evidence it appears that the decision to incorporate the Food Aid foodstuffs into everyday dishes, feed them to animals, exchange them for *minga* labor, or simply return them to the aid agency ultimately rests with the village women. In the same vein, Tanner's study points to the crucial part that ordinary women's decisions and culinary skills played in the adaptation or modification of the wartime diet designed by male nutritional experts and politicians.

Karen Hansen's Zambian case and Mary Weismantel's study of food in highland Ecuador offer the most explicit discussion of the role of gender in changing food habits. In Weismantel's case, cooking and food are one of the arenas where conflicts that result from an increasing differentiation between male migrant proletarians and female subsistence farmers are acted out not only materially, but also on a symbolic level. Before going further into the intricacies of gendered Indian food terminology, let me briefly mention the impact of age roles within the household on dietary innovation. It is interesting that women's position as "gatekeepers" mentioned above is not only challenged by their husbands, but evidently also and with more success by their children. Weismantel (1988: 154–9) illustrates how young Indian children struggle to redefine bread that had been an occasional luxury food into a necessary part of the morning meal, although parents can hardly afford to buy this new staple on a regular basis and certainly prefer the customary *máchica*, finely ground toasted barley, for their own breakfast. Similar evidence on the crucial role of children in dietary innovation and particularly in the proliferation of white bread is presented by Goody (1982: 180–2) for Ghana and by Theis for his Sudanese peasants. Although it might seem a bit far fetched, I would also call to mind the enormous importance fast-food companies like McDonalds attach to children in their advertisement strategies (Grefe et al. 1985: 266–75). Children seem to be a strong resource in undermining adult dietary conservatism, especially with respect to daily diet and "in-between" meals, whereas special occasion foods more closely reflect standards of prestige and decency defined within wider communities.

It is, of course, not only children and parents who quarrel about foods and meal times but also husbands and wives and elders and young couples who, as in Weismantel's village, often still live under one roof and develop quite different notions of proper conduct (see also Lentz 1988: 73–80). Foodstuffs consumed within impoverished Ecuadorian Indian households come from a variety of markedly gender-specific origins: foods contributed by men became synonymous with commercially produced purchased items while women provide foods from subsistence economy. Foods that are consumed daily and that derive from the female agricultural sphere (mainly barley and its derivates) are symbolically referred to as *mishqui* (sweet, tasty), whereas "luxury" foods like hot peppers, tobacco and sugar cane liquor from the lowlands are called *jayaj* (strong, hot or bitter) and belong to the sphere of prestige and inter-household exchange. To provide the *jayaj* items is a male task while cooking remains, of course, the quintessential female task. The third important category of foods is *wanlla*, a term that could be translated as "snacks" or "treats" and refers to formalized gifts between spouses or, more often, between households. Indigenous etiquette prescribes that *wanlla* forms a necessary part of social interaction but not of the everyday maintenance of households in an economic sense. It is highly significant, then, that commercial foodstuffs purchased through male wage labor are consistently defined as mere *wanlla*, despite the fact that they have become indispensable elements of the family's daily alimentation. On the one hand, the idea of male-provided foods as voluntary gifts entails numerous conflicts between the spouses, who do not pool their properties at marriage but continue to own certain individual resources and "exchange" labor and products within the household. Women cannot oblige their men to contribute food on a regular basis. On the other hand, as Weismantel stresses, the definition of purchased basic foodstuffs as "luxury" items not only reinforces an "Indian-farmer" identity and reflects the experience that urban wages are insufficient, but also stresses indigenous concepts of the autonomy and equality of women as producers. Similar tensions govern the time economy of cooking and consuming meals, which has to straddle two contrasting temporal orders, agrarian and metropolitan (Weismantel 1996).

In many Third World countries and particularly in Africa, but also in European history, the everyday "simple, but perfect meal" seems to be intimately connected with the work of women while any trend toward the emergence of haute cuisine regularly implies the professionalization of cooking by male specialists (Goody 1982: 191–4; Mennell 1985: 201–4). Spittler notes that when forced to prepare their own meals, Tuareg men regularly cook much worse than women, and he asks why women should take so much more time and trouble to prepare tasty daily food than men. Part of the answer seems to lie in gendered notions of desirable talents, linking a girl's marriageability with her cooking skills, as Spittler points out with reference to an Igbo example. Karen Hansen's analysis of skills learned in colonial domestic service in Zambia and their non-application to the servants' own households takes this analysis a step further. Domestic service, and particularly the task of a cook, was and continues to be regarded as skilled wage labor, as men's work. Colonial whites imposed their own conceptions of Africans' gender-specific abilities. They preferred to employ women, whom they considered lazy, slow and dull, only as nannies, while African men were assumed to be capable of learning etiquette and of being trained as cooks who could prepare a differentiated, European-style cuisine. But cooking as a "job of work," as paid labor, of which the servants could be proud, ended at the doorstep of the latter's own households where women were expected to unquestioningly perform the unpaid work of feeding the family. And, as mentioned above, women obviously developed little interest in abandoning the daily starch-and-relish meal format. Thus, besides economic constraints, it was mainly the dominant gender relations that prevented the newly acquired "male" cooking skills from spreading to ordinary African households.

FOOD, DRINK AND THE SYMBOLIC MEDIATION OF CHANGE

The assumption that foods (and drink) are not only good to eat (and drink) but also good to think guides—to a greater or lesser extent—all articles in this book. Food and drink are strong markers of social boundaries, be they constructed with respect to gender, ethnicity, regional origin, profession, or class. Because food and alcohol play an important part in intra-group relations, they also provide a potent means of expressing the relations between groups. The discourses in which food and alcohol are embedded and their symbolic connotations are, of course, historically (and culturally) variable, in much the same way as changes in food habits and patterns of drink are closely related to transformations of ideologies and symbolic frameworks.

Spittler's comparison of African and European food cultures with their different notions of taste and of what makes a "perfect" meal provides a good starting point. Among the Tuareg nomads as well as among African peasants (and, I would add, also among most of the African urban population), the simple meal consisting of a single dish prepared from few ingredients, namely a grain or root-crop porridge and a sauce, is idealized as perfect food that without much variation, can be eaten day after day. What a Eurocentric perspective would consider as a primitive, poor and monotonous diet is praised as satisfying, health-giving, digestible, and tasteful by indigenous African judgments. Differentiation of taste relates not to large varieties of diverse foodstuffs and dishes, but to the differing quality and the intrinsic flavor of the few ingredients of the simple meal. Although they place higher demands on quality and quantity, for instance, of sauce ingredients such as meat, even affluent African consumers, who could afford completely new food styles, regularly prefer the accustomed porridge-and-sauce diet. They do not regard the enormous variety of foodstuffs, the three-(or more) course meals and the daily variation of dishes which characterize European food ideals as superior. It seems to be this satisfaction with, and even pride in, the indigenous simple but perfect meal that accounts for the amazing persistence of food habits in the cases described by Hansen, von Oppen and Theis, inspite of some modifications of ingredients as a result of economic constraints (or inducements).

Because kin networks and marriage ties continue to bridge the widening gaps between educated and illiterate, affluent and poor, urbanites and villagers, social stratification in Africa has not been marked by the development of a class-specific cuisine, and the simple meal is highly valued by all. It is interesting to note, however, that this conservatism does not seem to apply to the consumption of alcoholic beverages. In the Ghanaian case which I have studied, the consumption of factory-produced bottled beer was regularly used as a marker of social status. Even though middle-class educated northern Ghanaians may still enjoy, from time to time, the customary taste of sorghum beer, they rarely consume the traditional beer when sharing drinks with their co-equals. Further distinctions of prestige can be attained by offering whisky or other expensive strong alcoholics, alongside with or instead of bottled beer. That middle and upper class sociability is connected with factory produced drinks rather than with locally-brewed beer has, of course, much to do with the setting in which sorghum beer is normally consumed. Popular beer "bars" in villages, market squares and the urban peripheries, consist normally of just a few benches under the open sky, outside the brewer's hut, which invite passers-by to sit down and quench their thirst in a fairly public atmosphere—a setting which is rather adverse to the desire of most better-off consumers to drink with their companions in a more intimate environment. If middle class consumers wish to drink sorghum beer, they often buy it in a plastic container and then drink it at home, not in the popular beer bar. But however much sorghum beer may be cherished because of its taste and nutritious qualities, bottled beer is regarded as the appropriate drink for the educated salary-earning middle class. Even illiterate and less well-off peasants will purchase and consume small quantities bottled beer and even whisky on special occasions, such as weddings and funerals, and particularly when having to entertain higher status visitors. However, in Ghana as in most African societies, this social grammar of drink has not extended into the realm of food.

By contrast, social stratification in European history resulted in the emergence of haute cuisine (produced by professionalized male cooks) and the gradual devaluation of the simple meal. This becomes particularly clear in Meyer-Renschhausen's article on the history of popular, as well as scientific discourses, about grain porridge in central Europe. Here, early nineteenth-century rural diets and agricultural rituals continued to feature porridge and gruels of home-pounded grains, and peasants maintained that these tasted much better than dishes prepared from commercially milled products. At the same time, the higher class of urban society had banned porridge from their tables, and economically less prosperous groups followed suit. These town dwellers generally associated porridge with poverty and rural backwardness, a view that contemporary scientists, who considered porridge unsatisfactory from a nutritional point of view, corroborated. By the late nineteenth century and in interaction with dramatic changes in peasant strategies of production, these urban tastes had influenced rural foodways, and porridge was consumed regularly only in a few poor Alpine valleys and other economically depressed areas. It seems to be no coincidence that a revalorization of the nutritional properties of grain porridge did not occur among the ranks of established nutritionists. While the latter preferred to debate the importance of animal proteins for a balanced diet, early activists of "alternative" movements like the *Lebensreformbewegung* (movement for the reform of life style) propagated vegetarianism for a variety of ethical and political reasons. Grain porridge and, more commonly, "muesli" have since regained some importance as morning meals, but consumption has been restricted mainly to urban middle-class groups and still serves as an indication of "ecologist" views. (see also Wirz 1993). As Tanner shows, Swiss nutritional scientists agreed that the more vegetable-based diet forced upon households by war-related food shortages and the rationing system was indeed healthier than the previous emphasis on fat and protein-rich foodstuffs. But popular tastes—bad habits in the experts' eyes—were far removed from scientific recommendations, and as soon as food supplies improved, people were eager to return to normalcy, namely to a fat- and meat-centered consumption pattern. Wildt's article points to the subsequent developments in postwar Germany: the increasing internationalization of tastes and, most important, individualization of food styles gradually supplanted more rigidly class-related food habits and the lower class's "taste for necessities" (Bourdieu 1979). Only within this context did the "slim line" and "healthy nutrition" discourse regain ground.

The fact that the symbolic value of food changes over time and according to context is clearly borne out by Çaglar's analysis of the construction of *döner kebab* as Turkish fast food in Germany. In urban Turkey, *döner*, served in a sandwich bread and garnished with a pickle or ketchup, never gained much popularity. Introduced on the German fast food market by Turkish migrants, *döner kebab* was completely refashioned, with *pide* (Turkish flat bread) replacing the sandwich bun, and salad, cucumber and tomato, topped with garlic yoghurt dressing, supplanting the pickle and ketchup garnishing. Inspite of the fact that the Germany version of *döner kebab* bears only vague resemblance to the Turkish "original", it is strongly associated with "Turkishness". The word *döner* even came to stand as a synonym for Turks and Turkish culture. Interestingly, in order to conquer new markets and reach groups of customers little susceptible to Mediterranean folklore, some of the Turkish entrepreneurs currently work hard at disconnecting *döner kebab* from its ethnic connotations and at renewing its image according to the model of American fast food chains. At the same time, the fact that *pide*, which traditionally was only baked during Ramadan and bore religious connotations, is now produced on a massive scale throughout the year, forced the Turkish immigrant community in Germany to refashion their Ramadan bread in order to differentiate it clearly from the fast food context.

Weismantel's observations on the use of foodstuffs as ethnic markers, too, point to historically conditioned transformations of the symbolic value of food. Introduced by the Spaniards, barley was once a "white" food crop, but it has since developed into a core element of "Indianness." Respect toward Indian *compadres* (godparents) is expressed by serving lavish meals of barley and *cuy* (guinea pig), whereas white or mestizo *compadres* are honored with dishes of chicken and white rice, the food that Indian villagers most closely associate with urban, white foodways. To offer white rice to Indian kin and friends, for instance during a baptism or wedding celebration, is to assert one's knowledge and fluency with the ways of the outside world (Weismantel 1988: 159–66). What had been introduced in this manner as prestigious foodstuff can, however, develop into an item of everyday consumption and lose its symbolic value. Much of this process (including the evolution of new ethnic markers) can be observed in other Ecuadorian highland villages and seems to be due mainly to the further weakening of subsistence agriculture and to the concomitant increase of purchased foodstuffs (Lentz 1988: chapters 7–9). In addition, the political economy of interethnic relations plays an important role, as can be gathered from my case study of drinking patterns in an Ecuadorian Indian village. Here, the once ritually so important and cherished *chicha* (maize beer) was more or less abandoned in favor of bottled beer and *aguardiente* not only because of the scarcity of raw material and questions of prestige, but also because the Mestizo entrepreneurs had managed to convert *chicha* into a means of exploitation from which the Indians now wished to escape.

The dynamic at work in the case of the Indian adoption of white rice seems to be the one Wiegelmann (1974) once described as *sinkendes Kulturgut* (sinking cultural values): a new food item is first adopted by the

highest level of society to set off their wealth and prestige, is then incorporated into highly valued special occasion meals by the lower classes, and is
finally popularized and consumed as part of the daily diet. This evolution
from an element of conspicious consumption into a sine qua non of everyday nourishment cannot be explained by any cyclical self-perpetuating
movement from innovation and diffusion (via imitation and social competition) to devaluation and new innovation. Such processes have also to be
viewed in the context of changing economic and class relations, as Mintz
insists (1987: 183–220). In Theis's Sudanese example, for example, some
new dishes and foodstuffs such as rice and lentils or bread enjoy among
Kordofan peasants the high prestige associated with urban, "civilized"
ways of life. Therefore, they are readily adopted, but equally quickly
dropped from the menu when ingredients are not easily available or are
too expensive. Similarly, Hansen describes for urban Zambia that foodstuffs associated with "modernity" and European-style dishes are served as
special occasion food, but hardly incorporated into the everyday diet. This
fact is not to be explained by a lack of symbolic value on the part of the
new foreign or urban produced foodstuffs, nor by the absence of social
classes to trigger off the dynamics of imitation and social competition, as
Goody's analysis of the lack of a high cuisine in African food systems
would suggest (1982: 204ff). Rather, Theis's example points to the vital
role subsistence agriculture continues to play for the peasants' strategies of
survival and, hence, for their diets, as well as for indigenous notions of
basic foodstuffs. Similarly, Hansen highlights that in the cities, too, a radical departure from the starch-and-sauce meal format is prevented not only
by severe economic constraints, but also by pervasive gender-related
notions of the simple meal as satisfying, tasteful food.

Von Oppen's cassava case reveals a relation between the transformation of
symbols and changes in food reality that seems to run somehow in
a direction opposite to that described by Weismantel, Theis and Hansen. In
northwestern Zambia, the new staple had evidently not been introduced as
a prestigious food, but as a stronghold against famines, regardless of the
peasants' reservations about taste and nutritional properties. The history of
cassava in Zambia, then, seems to have run parallel to the European proliferation of potatos, which had been introduced as poor man's food or even
animal feed and which only much later found their way into more prestigious
uses—a process that Wiegelmann (1974) has termed "poverty innovation" or
"rising cultural values" (*aufsteigendes Kulturgut*). Nevertheless, cassava
was eventually incoporated into the symbolic system and today plays
a prominent role in girls' initiation rituals. While the case studies of food
consumption address the religious meanings of certain foodstuffs only

implicitly, if at all, this dimension becomes much more evident in the chapter on the consumption of alcohol. This is perhaps so because alcohol's capacity to produce altered states of mind may lead many societies to see in drink (more than in food) a substance apt to carry ritual–religious meaning. In northwestern Ghana, for instance, the pouring of sorghum beer, together with the necessary incantations, is believed to invoke the presence of the ancestors. Beer is a necessary ingredient of all sacrifices at the family shrines as well as at the villages' earth shrines. While industrially processed liquor has made its way into all ritual and religious contexts in highland Ecuador (and has more or less replaced the traditional *chicha*), this is not the case in northwestern Ghana. Here, libation must be poured with home-brewed sorghum beer. Although liquor can be allowed as an addition, bottled beer may never be used in ritual contexts. From oral history it appears that up until the proliferation of brewing from the 1950s onwards, sorghum beer was nearly exclusively produced for ritual purposes. For funerals, and various annual festivities, elders gave out some of the coveted grain to their wives to prepare beer, and invited family members and friends to witness the libation and afterwards share in the communal drinking. At least in theory, beer brewed from grain purchased on the market should not be used for sacrifices; vice versa, any left-over ritual beer should never be sold to customers. Thus different from Ecuador, the sphere of commercial transactions is, as much as possible, kept outside of the sphere of ritual activities. While in many other cases, ritual and non-ritual settings are distinguished by the use of different products, here the same item of consumption, namely sorghum beer, takes on different meanings according to the circumstances of its production.

Theis's and Delgado's studies of relief food as an important and somewhat peculiar stimulus of change in Third World countries, and Tanner's research into wartime food policies in Europe provide additional insights into the role of ideological and symbolic aspects of changing food habits. The recipients have little influence on the composition of food aid (or wartime food) rations, and one would normally expect that dire need leads them to accept whatever is being offered. This is not, however, the case: even where, as in Theis's case, famine forced peasants to depart from customary meal patterns, part of the aid foodstuffs were sold in order to buy more coveted grains. Relief food was conceived of as emergency foods of low prestige and used in much the same manner as the wild seeds gathered during past famines. Consequently, it did not leave a lasting impression on the peasants' food habits. Tanner points to the considerable ideological efforts with which nutritional experts and politicians attempted to propagate their food rationing policies designed to maximize the efficiency and output of workers in the war economy. Potential discontent and resistance to a graded rationing system was to be obviated by a discourse that emphasized fair distribution and drew on pseudobiological metaphors, projecting the Swiss people as a united "body" whose "organs" that bore a heavier load had to receive privileged rations in order to ensure the survival of the whole community. In practice, however, ration coupons for certain foodstuffs such as millet, legumes or egg powder remained unused.

Similarly, Delgado argues that peasants readily accepted only those food aid foodstuffs that already enjoyed a certain prestige. Much the same as in Theis's case, however, more traditional dishes, which were more closely related to past agricultural patterns of self-sufficiency, continued to occupy top ranks in the food hierarchy. Furthermore, Delgado shows that it is not only the food items *per se* that villagers evaluate, but also the channels of distribution. Wheat flour, for instance, purchased on the market or at the village retailer is more easily accepted than the same product handed out by the Food Aid agency, whose flour is suspected to be "old" and harmful. In my Ecuadorian experience, I encountered rumors about food aid foodstuffs having added contraceptives or other undesirable ingredients. On a more general level, this suggests that foods are inscribed with meanings derived from the social relations that surround them, the same food item can acquire different meanings in different social contexts and can be accepted, rejected, or subverted accordingly. I would argue that the cases presented in this book—and particularly the historical sequence of Meyer-Renschhausen's, Tanner's, Wildt's and Çaglar's studies that document the recent shift in Europe from a "taste for necessities" to the dominance of "fine differences" and "multiculturalism" illustrate convincingly that an adequate analysis of these contexts has to go beyond the family or the village level and also has to take into consideration larger networks of power.

* * *

In conclusion, I would like to reiterate some of the central issues and methodological points the articles suggest. All the chapters seem to insist that it is only by stressing the complex interplay of productive patterns in agriculture and market-related factors of food availability, strategies of survival and accumulation, and local perceptions of foodways that changes in food habits and patterns of drink can be explained. The emergence of new tastes and appetites, the incorporation of new food items into the daily diet, or even the evolution of completely new meal patterns are processes which involve a symbolic level and that are embedded in (often competing) ideological discourses at the village, parish, and national level.

At the same time, the modification of food habits is mediated by changes in household strategies of production and reproduction. The introduction of new foods covers a whole spectrum of situations, from forced imposition accelerated by extreme crisis such as war, drought and famine to voluntary appropriation resulting from the dynamics of prestige and imitation. Either way, household processes of acquisition, preparation and consumption of food and drink with all their dimensions of symbolic action and conflict constitute something like the missing link between the basic transformations of land-tenure systems, methods of production, new urban income opportunities, and new food habits. Of course, in order to understand local change fully, the wider networks of economic and political power and broader, long-term trends in dietary change also have to be taken into account. But I would insist that people are not mere victims of world-market strategies nor of national elites promoting new tastes. People's patterns of consumption have their own, potentially oppositional, logic. Given the present state of the discipline, more actor-oriented research into the intermediate level of household-related and gender-specific food strategies is needed.

Likewise, the notion of change needs to be more thoroughly discussed. A war or hunger-crisis imposition of certain ersatz-products or the rapid popularization of specific "modern" food items, for instance, may very well prove to be a transitory fashion, followed by a durable return to more traditional meal patterns at a later stage. Some patterns of change may involve only single food items, leaving the meal formats relatively intact; such is the case, for instance, with the substitution in porridges of sorghum or cassava for millet. Even the study of South American Indian foodways and their strong reliance on commercial ingredients reveals that meals still obey traditional rules of composition, of preparation, and serving. Goody's observations about dietary "diglossia" in modern Ghana, which the Zambian, Ghanaian and Sudanese examples in this book corroborate and which I feel apply to many other cases as well, suggest that traditional meals can coexist with modern dishes in the same family over a long period of time without one cuisine displacing the other (1982: 184ff). It seems to be an open question, then, which aspect deserves more scholarly attention: the overall continuity and amazing tenacity of customary meal formats and tastes, or the often hidden, but nevertheless significant, innovations in available food items and drinks as well as in food acquisition and preparation.

As past studies have pointed out, basic and profound transformations of food habits and patterns of drink normally occur at a very slow pace. This underlines the undeniable importance of long-term historical studies.

However, in order to complement long-term analyses, we also need to employ anthropological approaches that enable us to understand actors' perceptions, material strategies, and patterns of symbolic ordering, which are not easily accessible through the study of conventional historical sources. In any case, the focus on change constitutes a fine challenge to conventional approaches that reduce foodways to mere matters of symbolic structure or, conversely, view food purely in economic or nutritional terms.

NOTES

1. The theme of this book developed thanks to the European Society for Rural Sociology which helped organize a theme-section on "Changing Food Habits and the Problems of Food Security" at the 1988 World Congress of Rural Sociology in Bologna/Italy. Many of the articles reproduced here were originally presented at the Bologna conference and are influenced by other contributors and discussants of that theme section, namely Jean-Marie Apovo, Thomas Bierschenk, the late Jae-Hyeon Choe, Peter Heine and Klaus-Peter Henn. I also wish to thank Steven Kaplan for his useful advice to the editor and his initiative to develop the conference papers into a special issue of *Food and Foodways* (and ultimately into the present, more comprehensive collection).
2. A full discussion of recently published studies on food cultures is beyond the scope of this introduction, but there are some useful overviews of the state of the art in anthropological food studies: see, for instance, Goody 1982: 10–39; Messer 1984; Mennell 1985: 1–19 and Harris 1987.

REFERENCES

Bourdieu, Pierre, 1979. *La distinction. Critique sociale du jugement.* Paris: Editions de Minuit.
Douglas, Mary, ed. 1984. *Food in the Social Order: Studies of Food and Festivities in three American Communities.* New York: Russell Sage Foundation.
Franke, Richard W. 1987. "The Effects of Colonialism and Neocolonialism on the Gastronomic Patterns of the Third World". In *Food and Evolution. Toward a Theory of Human Food Habits*, ed. Marvin Harris and Eric Ross, pp. 455–479. Philadelphia: Temple University Press.
Goody, Jack, 1982. *Cooking, Cuisine and Class. A Study in Comparative Sociology.* Cambridge: Cambridge University Press.
Grefe, Christiane, et al., 1985. *Das Brot des Siegers. Das Hackfleisch-Imperium.* Bornheim-Merten: Lamuv Verlag.
Harris, Marvin, 1987. "Foodways: Historical Overview and Theoretical Prologomenon". In *Food and Evolution. Toward a Theory of Human Food Habits*, ed. Marvin Harris and Eric Ross, pp. 57–90. Philadelphia: Temple University Press.
Hyden, Goran, 1980. *Beyond Ujamaa in Tanzania: Underdevelopment and an Uncaptured Peasantry.* Berkeley: University of California Press.
Lentz, Carola, 1988. *"Von seiner Heimat kann man nicht lassen." Migration in einer Dorfgemeinde in Ecuador.* Frankfurt: Campus. (Spanish edition: Migración e identidad étnica: la transformación de una Canvnidad lndigena en la Sierra icuatoriana. Quito: Abyayala, 1997).

Manderson, Lenore, ed. 1986. *Shared Wealth and Symbol. Food, Culture and Society in Oceania and Southeast Asia.* Cambridge: Cambridge University Press.

Mennell, Steven, 1985. *All Manners of Food. Eating and Taste in England and France from the Middle Ages to the Present.* Oxford: Blackwell.

Messer, Ellen, 1984. "Anthropological Perspectives on Diet". *Annual Review of Anthropology*, 13: 205–249.

Mintz, Sidney W. 1987. *Die süße Macht. Kulturgeschichte des Zuckers.* Frankfurt: Campus (Originally published as *Sweetness and Power. The Place of Sugar in Modern History.* New York: Viking Press, 1985).

Orlove, Benjamin, 1987. "Stability and Change in Highland Andean Dietary Patterns". In *Food and Evolution. Toward a Theory of Human Food Habits*, ed. Marvin Harris and Eric Ross, pp. 481–515. Philadelphia: Temple University Press.

Pelto, Gretel, and Pertti Pelto, 1983. "Diet and Delocalization: Dietary Changes since 1750". *Journal of Interdisciplinary History*, 14: 507–528.

Scott, James, 1976. *The Moral Economy of the Peasant. Rebellion and Subsistence in Southeast Asia.* New Haven: Yale University Press.

Spittler, Gerd, 1989. *Dürren, Krieg und Hungerkrisen bei den Kel Ewey (1900–1985).* Wiesbaden: Franz Steiner

Teuteberg, Hans J. and Günter Wiegelmann, 1972. *Der Wandel der Nahrungsgewohnheiten unter dem Einfluß der Industrialisierung.* Göttingen: Vandenhoeck & Ruprecht.

Weismantel, Mary, 1988. *Food, Gender and Poverty in the Ecuadorian Andes.* Philadelphia: University of Pennsylvania Press.

Weismantel, Mary, 1996. "Children and Soup, Men and Bulls: Meals and Time for Zumbagua Women", *Food and Foodways*, 6: 307–327.

Wiegelmann, Günter, 1967. *Alltags- und Festspeisen—Wandel und gegenwärtige Stellung.* Marburg: Elwert.

Wiegelmann, Günter, 1974. "Innovation in Food and Meals". *Folk Life. A Journal of Ethnological Studies*, 12: 20–30.

Wirz, Albert, 1993. Die Moral auf dem Teller. Zürich: Chronos Verlag.

1. IN PRAISE OF THE SIMPLE MEAL: AFRICAN AND EUROPEAN FOOD CULTURE COMPARED*

Gerd Spittler
University of Bayreuth, Germany

In contrast to our meals, which are characterized by many ingredients and frequently varied dishes, meals in an agricultural society (except those of the upper social groups) are very simple and do not change from day to day. For us it therefore follows that such meals are insipid and monotonous. But are the taste stimuli and perpetual variety that we demand an anthropological constant or are these needs subject to historical and cultural change? Is variety in food the norm and the simple and unchanging a phenomenon requiring explanation? Or, on the contrary, is it our need for alternating tastes that calls for investigation?

Research into the Kel Ewey Tuareg shows that in Africa a simple meal that does not vary from day to day is regarded as perfect. This prompts the question of whether Europeans think differently and, if so, why.

THE SIMPLE MEAL AMONG THE KEL EWEY

The everyday diet of the nomadic Kel Ewey Tuareg, who live in the Aïr Mountains of south central Sahara in Niger,[1] is very simple and always the same. For breakfast they drink *eghale*, a mixture of millet, cheese and dates stirred in water. At midday and in the evening they eat a cooked meal called *ashin*, which is a solid mass rather than a gruel: what used to

---

*This article is a translation from *Lob des einfachen Mahles. Afrikanische und europäische Esskultur in Vergleich*. In: Alois Wierlacher et al. (eds.), *Kulturthema Essen*. Berlin 1993, 193–210.

be called a dumpling or, in Italy, is known as polenta. This millet polenta is sprinkled with soured camel or goat's milk and served in a wooden bowl. *Eghale* and *ashin* are eaten every day throughout the year. There is no weekly festive meal, but special dishes of rice or wheat are served to mark family celebrations and major Islamic festivals. Such occasions are also marked by the slaughter of a goat or a sheep.

Ashin and *eghale* have a long tradition. The German traveller in Africa Henry Barth, the first European to visit the Kel Ewey in the middle of the 19th century, mentions the same dishes. Barth strongly favoured the diet of the Kel Ewey and always breakfasted on *eghale*, which he described as "palatable" (Barth 1890: 1,120). However, this opinion is not widely shared. Most Europeans, then as now, saw little to attract them in these dishes, which they found insipid and monotonous: for them the qualities either of a poor man's food or of a primitive, underdeveloped cuisine.

Anthropology begins when an attempt is made to break free from ethnocentric perspectives and understand the stranger in his otherness instead of measuring him by one's own yardstick. How do the Kel Ewey Tuareg themselves describe and rate their own food? To begin with the conclusion: they consider that simple food is a sign neither of poverty nor of barbarism, but is in every respect excellent.

Let us look first at millet, milk, cheese and dates. Certainly there is no great variety here, but in the eyes of the Kel Ewey these foods are distinguished by a special quality. Millet is superior to any other cereal in its ability to satisfy hunger and its nutritional value, health-giving qualities and taste. Millet is the king of foods. The Kel Ewey buy their millet from the Hausa. Other foods are from Aïr itself. Goat's milk is principally used to make cheese, of which the Kel Ewey are especially proud. The high meadows of Aïr with their wide variety of trees provide the basis of a specific type of grazing that gives "Kel Ewey cheese", also known as "mountain cheese" or "tree cheese", its flavour and spiciness. The smell of the cheese alone distinguishes it from the cheese of the plains, where the goats eat grass rather than leaves and the cheese is often mixed with sheep's cheese. Of course, the difference consists in more than just taste and smell. The mountain cheese contains more strength and health. It is considered a preventive and curative means in various diseases.

The goat's cheese from Aïr has long been known well beyond Aïr. In 1850 Barth wrote: "We were anxious to buy some of the famous Aïr cheese, for which we had been longing the whole way of the dreary desert, and had kept our spirits with the prospect of soon indulging in this luxury" (Barth 1890: 1,135).

The Kel Ewey of Timia are proud of their dates as well as of their cheese. Long before the oases were planted with cereals and vegetables there were date palms, which were famous even in the 19th century. Barth himself did not visit the area in 1850 but passed nearby; his Kel Ewey companion pointed it out to him. "Near the foot of the extensive mountain called Ajuri, there are some very favoured spots, especially a valley called Chimmia, ornamented with a fine date-grove, which produces fruit of excellent quality" (Barth 1890: 1,167). Today Timia produces dozens of different kinds of dates, some of which are particularly renowned for their flavour.

The quality of the ingredients is a prerequisite for the perfect dish, but its preparation is just as important. In making millet polenta preparation rather than cooking constitutes the main work. Theoretically, preparation consists only in separating out the bran and grinding the grain to produce meal. However, to achieve this a complex process is required in which the millet is pounded five times in a mortar and winnowed ten times. The millet is wetted with water four times to make the process easier. The first task is to clean out sand and other contaminants, after which the bran and the grain are separated. Then the grain must be converted into meal in a series of steps. The preparation of a kilogram of millet, which will make a dish to feed five adults, takes an hour. The actual cooking, during which the pot is constantly stirred, as when cooking polenta, takes a further thirty minutes.

Millet for the drink *eghale* is prepared in similar manner except that the millet is not boiled. The dates and cheese are also pounded in a mortar. The dry mixture of millet, cheese and dates can then be stored for weeks, shaken with water as required and drunk from a calabash with a ladle. When *eghale* is prepared in the right proportions—with lots of cheese and dates—it becomes, in the eyes of the Kel Ewey, a unique dish that satisfies hunger, relieves thirst, gives health and strength and tastes good. This dish can only be an object of envy to others: for example, other Tuareg, with whom the Kel Ewey come into contact during their caravan journeys but who lack this superlative food. When told that *eghale* does not exist in Germany, they reply that life there cannot be much fun. To the objection that, when offered to tourists, the dish has enjoyed little success, the Kel Ewey respond: "They just don't know what tastes good". And once again one hears the story of a French colonial officer who at first was very cautious and only tasted the *eghale*, but who liked the taste so much that afterwards he drank it every day.

The Kel Ewey praise their *eghale* not least because, despite its simple composition, it is perfect and can be drunk every day. The perfection of a dish is greater if no costly ingredients are required. They are no less positive in their opinion of *ashin*, which is made of nothing more than millet, water and milk: "You need no spice, no salt and no oil. You eat *ashin* with milk, followed by a gulp of water, rise and are satisfied". That is true not for one day but for every day, month after month, year after year. These dishes are perfect in that they are appetizing every day and do good. A wheat or a rice dish on feast days, spiced with a good sauce, certainly make a pleasant change, but for the Kel Ewey they would be inconceivable as everyday meals. The Kel Ewey would certainly not consider it desirable to make a feastday meal into an everyday dish. In fact, *ashin* and *eghale* also form part of the festive board, while a banquet prepared for a guest should also include them.

It is the simple rather than the complex, the everyday rather than the feastday dish that forms the perfect meal. Perfect means that few ingredients are required, since the intrinsic value of the foods is so high that all the criteria according to which food is positively judged are fulfilled (ability to satisfy hunger, health-giving qualities, good taste, digestibility) and the dish can be eaten day after day. Significantly, most of the remarks that have been quoted concerning *ashin* and *eghale* were made not by poor people, making a virtue of necessity and wishing to endow their meagre food with lofty qualities, but by the richest man in Timia. He is able, if he wishes, to eat rice and gravy prepared with meat and oil and also knows the dishes of the Europeans. If he speaks with such pride of *ashin* and *eghale* this is an expression not of deficit as ideology but of the ideal of the simple as the perfect.

The food of the Kel Ewey may be poor measured by our standards, but it is not so by their own. They value their dishes highly and do not envy Europeans their diet. They consume few foods, but the demands they place on the quality of these are high. For example, they eat their best produce themselves instead of selling it, whereas poor people throughout the world sell what is valuable and expensive and keep what is less valuable. The author's own budgetary investigations also confirm that the Kel Ewey are not poor. In normal years they spend no more than 10 to 20 percent of their income on their staple food, millet: less than is expended on tea and sugar.

Neither is the food of the Kel Ewey primitive in the evolutionary sense. The concept of the primitive is often associated with the raw and coarse. But the dishes of the Kel Ewey are certainly not basic in the sense of being unprepared. The Kel Ewey fundamentally prefer cultivated to wild crops. They rarely eat anything in its raw state and are horrified if, for example, they see Europeans eating uncooked tomatoes. If food products are not already processed, they are preserved: milk is soured if it is not made into cheese, dates are dried. As in the case of millet, however, bringing food to the table is a laborious and complicated process.

Whether the taste of the Kel Ewey can be seen as coarse compared to the highly developed, refined taste of Europeans is very debatable. The Kel Ewey certainly do not enjoy the same variety of foods and luxury dishes that we are familiar with and therefore their taste must also be undeveloped. However, in regard to the foods they do know their sense of taste is highly differentiated. Because they do not use a large number of spices, their awareness of the intrinsic flavour of foods is highly developed and they can distinguish the quality of water, millet, cheese, dates and milk very accurately. Just as a wine expert can tell the origin, variety of grape and year of a wine, the Kel Ewey can make fine distinctions between their food products.

THE SIMPLE MEAL OF THE AFRICAN PEASANT

Let us turn from the foods and dishes of camel-owning nomads to the diet of the African peasant. This has been the subject of a number of studies dealing with anthropological as well as nutritional questions. As early as 1936 a special issue of *Africa* dealt with the African diet. Most of the contributions dealt exclusively with nutritional matters, an exception being an article by the Fortes entitled "Food in the domestic economy of the Tallensi". *Hunger and Work in a Savage Tribe* (1932) and *Land, Labour and Diet in Northern Rhodesia* (1939) by Audrey Richards were pioneering works. But food became a central concern of anthropology only in the 1980s.

Despite the similarity between the diet of nomads and peasants, three important differences exist: (1) the basic food, whether cereals or tubers, is grown by the peasants themselves, while the nomads must buy it; (2) instead of milk the peasants add a sauce to their polenta; (3) the time required to prepare the food is greater, since preparation of the sauce requires as much time as preparation of the polenta.

For the peasants, who grow the millet themselves, the grain usually has a religious quality that is lacking among the nomads. This can be seen, for example, among the Hausa peasants from whom the Kel Ewey buy millet. For the Kel Ewey and the Hausa millet is king. Among the Hausa one must not interrupt the eating of a millet dish even if an important guest arrives, since "on ne fait pas attendre un roi" (Nicolas 1975: 243). But millet is also sacred to the Hausa and its cultivation and use is subject to many ritual prescriptions.

Millet (and sorghum) form the most important food outside the rain forest, where yams often assume pride of place, as millet does in the savannah. Whether millet or yams are used, a similar meal is prepared: a polenta-like pudding. A sauce of vegetables or herbs or possibly meat replaces the milk used by the nomads. This dish, called porridge in English or bouillie or pâte in French, is usually prepared twice a day by the women, day in and day out. Only the ingredients of the sauce vary. In peasant societies, too, cooked food is fundamental and the simple dish is the perfect dish.

Among the Tallensi only cooked food is considered a meal and two hot meals a day (porridge and sauce) are regarded as necessary for daily requirements (see the Fortes 1936: 264). Preparation of food is exclusively a female affair. Fetching firewood and water requires most time and work. The Fortes calculated that no more than an hour was needed to cook and serve a meal for ten people, more than half this time being spent on preparing the sauce (ibid.: 269).[2] Overall, however, preparing a meal (including gathering wood and fetching water) is so time-consuming that it sometimes comes into conflict with the women's agricultural work and is then given a lower priority (ibid.: 264 ff).

The Tallensi vary the sauce they use, "so that they do not tire of eating the same" (ibid.: 266), but they are not bothered by the arrival of millet on the table day after day, since they cannot have enough of it: "When root crops are in season they are cooked instead of porridge, but not because porridge becomes a monotonous diet to the Tallensi, or they wish to vary the diet, it is done in order to make the grain last longer. 'Porridge is food, it makes you strong', and there can never be too much of it in the Tale point of view" (ibid.: 265). The Tallensi do not, therefore, envy Europeans their food. In a footnote the Fortes comment: "A Tale friend enquired what kind of food he would be given in our country, and when told that he would eat meat, fish, bread, and eggs, he exclaimed, 'what no porridge? I call that starvation'" (ibid.: 265).

The same attitude is found thousands of kilometers away among the Bemba of Northern Rhodesia: "Millet porridge is not only necessary, but it is the only constituent of his diet which actually ranks as food" (Richards 1939: 47). In addition, millet plays an important role in many ceremonies (initiation of the young girls, weddings, installation of a chief). The "perfect meal" consists of nothing more than millet porridge and a sauce. The European practice of eating several courses at a meal is not followed by the Bemba: "The Bemba do not like to mix their foods, and despise the European habit of eating a meal composed of two or three kinds of dishes ... It is like a bird first to pick at this and then at that, or like a child who nibbles here and there through the day" (ibid.: 49).

For the Bemba, too, cooking is women's work. Preparing a good meal is time-consuming. The Bemba women combine the tasks of crushing and grinding. Threshing, winnowing, grinding and cooking six pounds of millet, the amount required for the evening meal of a normal family, will take a woman about an hour. Making a good sauce requires a further 30 to 90 minutes, depending on the ingredients, so that the preparation of the evening meal (not counting the fetching of water and firewood) lasts from one and a half to two and a half hours (ibid.: 204).

On the West African coast the daily dish of yams is often called *fufu*: for example, among the Ashanti in Ghana (see Goody 1982: 50) and the Igbo in southern Nigeria (Okere 1983: 212ff.). There the yam is "the king of crops" (ibid.: 112) and *fufu* is considered a "cultural superfood". Once again, this does not signify uniqueness or exoticism: on the contrary, the dish demonstrates its perfection through its "monotonous" daily consumption (ibid.: 212). Whatever other dishes a person has eaten and in whatever amount, there is nevertheless something imperfect about them. Only *fufu* forms the perfect meal (ibid.: 213). And it is yams and *fufu* that enjoy the greatest prestige among the Igbo: "The envied prestigious diet is not that eaten by an elite which is as yet ill differentiated. It is above all the daily diet which is consumed by the ancestors and is based on the staple food, granted by the Supernatural powers, which confers man's condition within a given society" (ibid.: 218). The Igbo, too, prefer a "monotonous" daily diet of *fufu* to Western dishes. This is true even of Igbo students in the United States (ibid.: 212).

THE SIMPLE MEAL AS THE PERFECT MEAL: SOCIAL PREREQUISITES

Throughout Africa the standard meal (polenta with sauce or milk) is simple, consisting of a single dish prepared from a few ingredients. The basis of the polenta varies according to the region (it is usually millet, yams or maize), but differs little within a given society. Sauces show a greater range of variation. The ingredients of a standard meal are accessible to all; except among the nomads, they form the local subsistence crops that each family grows for itself. Preparation of the simple meal is lengthy and laborious: lengthy because it is prepared from raw ingredients, laborious because pounding or grinding is a strenuous task. For each meal the ingredients are freshly prepared.

All African societies also have feast days, for which nonstandard dishes are prepared and eaten. There is no doubt that a feast gives particular pleasure, yet typically the perfect meal is regarded as being the simple daily dish rather than feastday food. Perfect because each individual ingredient testifies to high quality, because the meal is complete with a few ingredients and because all the criteria applied to food are fulfilled: satisfaction of hunger, healthiness, digestibility and good flavour. Perfection is demonstrated by everyday experience inasmuch the meal can be eaten every day without the consumer coming to any harm or suffering any deterioration in health. If the simple meal is declared the perfect meal, this not simply because of shortage or ignorance. Even in comparison to European cuisine Africans praise their own food rather than remaining coyly reticent about it in face of the rich variety of European cooking.

I should like to append two questions to this account:

1. What are the conditions for the predominance of simple food and its idealization as the perfect meal?
2. As a rule, the preparation of a simple meal is not simple, but time-consuming and often complex. What are the circumstances with which this process of preparation is associated?

Let us begin with the first question. Why is the simple daily meal so widespread and why is it regarded as perfect? The obvious explanation is provided by the contrast between the cultures of hunger and affluence. According to this thesis, preindustrial societies are constantly threatened by hunger; day to day existence itself is characterized by shortage. Hunger is substituted for a differentiated taste and it is therefore not surprising that the simple meal is accepted and enjoyed despite its monotony. A taste for a wide variety of food can develop only in the absence of hunger.[3]

Ethnographic descriptions of the simple meal do not conform to this model. All the societies described here experience seasonal deprivation, during which the customary food is in short supply, and sometimes even undergo periodic famines during times of drought. However, the assumption that man's life amounts only to survival and to filling his stomach and that the differentiated judgement of food cannot develop under these conditions is false. All African societies have fully-fledged original theories that classify dishes and their ingredients according to healthiness, digestibility and good flavour as well as the ability to satisfy hunger.

A prerequisite for the dominance of the simple meal is certainly the distinctive subsistence economy of traditional Africa.[4] Where cooking is essentially limited to local produce, opportunities for variety are necessarily more limited than in regional, national or even worldwide markets.[5] Whether market expansion is only the cause or also the consequence of changes in taste remains an open question.

The question of how far taste merely responds to the pressure of circumstances and how far necessity is made a virtue by styling the simple as the perfect meal must be addressed. This is certainly not the case here.

In the African societies described, deficit is seen as such and hunger is not reinterpreted as fasting.

Of course, not everything that we would characterize as deficit is regarded as such in Africa and this is a crucial distinguishing factor. From the point of view of our affluent society, whatever we lack is seen as a deficit. But in the author's opinion the argument is conducted too much from the viewpoint of plenty. If the simple is taken as a yardstick, variety seems superfluity or confusion; thus, the Bemba for example, compare the meals of Europeans with the unselective pecking of a bird.[6]

The same can be said of the accusation, constantly levelled at African cuisine, that since it consists of simple dishes, constantly repeated, containing few ingredients, it is "monotonous". Apart from feastdays, the same simple meal is eaten every day, often more than once. The belief is widespread that this monotony is extremely hard to tolerate and can be explained only by conditions of extreme poverty. However, it is debatable whether eating the same food is really perceived by Africans as monotonous or whether, on the contrary, this conforms to our conceptions, that is, the view of people who demand frequent changes and many stimuli. Even when the additional element (for example, milk) as well as the basic material of the dish (polenta) is unchanged, one does not hear complaints from Africans of the "monotony" of these dishes: on the contrary, their goodness is praised.

Compared to Europe, precolonial Africa was a classless society without stratum-specific cultural practices: that is, without varying eating styles (Goody 1982). Goody stresses the absence of class endogamy in Africa and therefore—above all in the kitchen—the impossibility of differentiation in gastronomic culture. Women of the people who married into the aristocracy continued to cook in the way they had learned at home. The absence of written recipes was also important. This lack of class differentiation was essential to the ideal of the simple as the perfect meal. Whereas the differentiation of taste in a class society tends towards expensive and exotic foods, taste differentiation in a classless food culture reveals itself with respect to a few products: a connoisseur can judge with great subtlety the origin of water, milk, or millet, just as a wine expert can determine the origin and year of wines.

The simple meal is perfect only if it is well prepared. This brings us to our second question: under what conditions is the simple meal created? We have seen that the preparation of simple dishes in Africa is time-consuming. Since the women bring up the children and work on the land and herd cattle as well as cook, they must divide their working day and often have less time at their disposal for cooking than the optimum period for preparing dishes.[7]

Apart from these specific limitations of time, which often vary from season to season, there are more general matters, such as the amount of time the women are ready to devote to cooking and who decides this. Pounding millet in a mortar and grinding it are among the most arduous tasks performed by African women, more arduous than most work performed by men. That the women themselves perceive this work as hard is confirmed by the changes they are making today. In the towns rice, which is easier to prepare, has largely replaced millet, while in country areas the work is at least lightened by the existence of mills, although there, too, other food products are to some extent gaining ground.

But why did women do this work? The exceptions to the rule are indicative. Among the Tuareg the men take a greater part in house work than anywhere else. In some Tuareg groups, for example, the Iforas, they take an equal if not a greater part in the arduous work, such as pounding millet.[8] The high standing of women among the Tuareg has prevented marked inequality in the division of labour. In contrast to haute cuisine, in which professionalization by men leads to the development of an art of cookery, equal rights for men has led in this case to a decline in standards. Meals are taken irregularly and eaten cold and food prepared from ready-made flour displaces the traditional millet dishes.

We have hitherto considered a situation in which both men and women are present in the home. However, among the Tuareg the activities of men and women are often physically separated. The Kel Ewey men are often away with their caravans for half a year while the women remain at home. Camelherds graze their animals far from the home camp. The men must, therefore, prepare their own meals—and regularly do so worse than the women. In the case of the Bilma caravans this is understandable, as a 16–18-hour daily march scarcely leaves time for cooking. However, even the camelherds, who have far more time than the female goatherds, prepare their millet polenta far less carefully or do not cook at all and drink camel milk instead.

When the men are involved in everyday kitchen tasks the results are, again, worse than when the work is done by women alone. Once more the question arises: why do women take so much time and trouble to prepare a simple but perfect meal? Is this expected and demanded by men? Among the Igbo, at least in earlier times, women were especially valued for their cooking skills: "In older days, a woman's cooking was an important qualification for marriage" (Okere 1983: 217). Why this should have been so only "in older days" remains unclear. However, the observation is interesting in itself. The value placed by men upon good cooking is shown by scattered remarks in various studies, but the problem has nowhere been dealt with systematically. The relationship between a girl's cooking skills and her chances of marriage would be a profitable subject for examination. The fact that food preparation not only takes up a great deal of the women's time, but also forms an important subject in their thoughts and conversation, is often noted (Okere 1983: 215; Richards 1939: 46). Conversely, it is an established rule in many societies that men do not talk about food. However, it is often mentioned that the men are anything but indifferent to food and attach importance to good cooking. The consequences of this have not been investigated. A man cannot interfere in his wife's kitchen. It is not clear whether he is entitled to assign praise or blame to the meal as prepared. Among the Tuareg, at least, it would be considered improper for a man to praise or criticize food, even that prepared by his own wife.

It may well be that the food culture of the women is influenced less by the demands and sanctions of the men than by their own traditions. If this is the case, investigation of gender-specific differences in the evaluation of cooking and meals will have to be more specific than hitherto.

THE SIMPLE MEAL IN EUROPE

Is the simple meal something specifically African or was it widespread in Europe, too? One thing can be stated with certainty: the simple meal may have been common in Europe, but it was certainly not considered the perfect meal. Far more typical of Europe was the development of "haute cuisine" with many ingredients and complex preparation. Whereas Africa lacked a class-specific cuisine, the structure of social stratification was crucial to European gastronomic culture. According to the logic of a stratified model, the upper strata develop a "cultivated" style of their own to distance themselves from the lower strata. The lower strata imitate the upper strata, thereby encouraging the latter to develop new patterns to maintain their distinctiveness.

This dynamic has often been described and analysed, greater emphasis being placed sometimes on the need of the upper strata to create boundaries and sometimes on the need of the lower strata to imitate. In his classic study *The Theory of the Leisure Class* (1899), Veblen concentrated on the need of the upper strata to demarcate themselves and the effects of this, while Tarde in his equally classic work *Les lois de l'imitation* (1890) focussed principally on imitation by the lower strata. Both topics have often been addressed since in various forms. The best-known recent contribution to this debate was made by Bourdieu in *La distinction. Critique sociale du jugement* (1979). Goody (1982) exposes the dynamics of the model with especial clarity, contrasting classless (Africa) and class-based (Europe and Asia) societies.

The development of European gastronomic culture was described by Mennell (*All Manners of Food*, 1985) entirely within the framework of a stratified model. Mennell studied the way in which the undifferentiated pleasure in eating of the Middle Ages, the product of hunger and gluttony, gradually developed into a differentiated gastronomic culture. Haute cuisine originated in the culture of the court; after the French Revolution it was shaped by master chefs in restaurants. Through cookery books, restaurant guides and women's periodicals the art of cooking of the grand kitchens, in modified form, also reached the bourgeois kitchen.

Although largely ignored by the master chefs, cookery books and scholarship, the simple meal in the form of purees, gruel and soup continued to predominate for a long time among the "ordinary people": "Until the beginning of the modern 'nutrition revolution' in the 18th century the mass of the population remained in their daily diet in principle dependent on a puree–gruel–soup staple" (Teuteberg 1989: 8; see also Braudel 1979). Together with potatoes, coffee, tea, sugar and bread the "nutrition revolution" of the 18th century brought a "recoining of the Central European dietary system" for the middle and lower classes (Wiegelmann 1982: 149). However, in rural areas gruel and soup still occupied an important place in the 19th century. Mennell, who, as well as the "cultivation of the appetite", occasionally mentions simple food, even considers that soup (and gruel) was the main dish at each meal for the majority of French people into the 20th century (Mennell 1985).

Although, owing to insufficient sources and the lack of interest shown by scholars, we possess few details of puree, gruel and soup meals (Ruf's book *Die sehr bekannte dienliche Löffelspeise* [*The Very Well-Known Useful Spoon Meal*] (1989) is a laudable exception), it is beyond dispute that these simple dishes predominated outside the kitchens of the nobility and the bourgeoisie into the 18th century and in many areas and social groups for a long time after that.

There can be no doubt that a "simple meal" also existed in Europe. However, was this simple meal also the perfect meal, as it is in Africa? In social history adverse judgements predominate. Braudel writes of the insipid and monotonous gruel, puree, soup or bread diet separating the majority of people from the meat eaters (Braudel 1979). Mennell (1985) also stresses the monotony and poverty of peasant cooking in France and England. In a chapter entitled "Social and historical aspects of German cuisine" added to the German edition of his book, Eva Barlösius expressed a similar view of the German situation: "Sources show that peasant cooking was coarse and monotonous. Gruel made of barley or millet boiled with water, milk and salt formed the basis of the daily diet" (Barlösius 1988: 426).

All these statements refer to the everyday diet of middle and lower social groups. Feastday dishes, which lend a glamour even to the peasant kitchen, contrast with the coarse, monotonous everyday menu (see Wiegelmann 1967). Precisely by distinguishing the "feasts that stand out from the daily monotony" (ibid.: 240), the author makes clear the low value placed on everyday dishes.

What are the criteria according to which everyday dishes are judged to be insipid and monotonous? Do modern dietary scholars take their standards from haute cuisine? Or do they rely on the pronouncements of the contemporary upper classes or, at least, the literate, who judged the diet of the people negatively? Since the 18th century puree and gruel have fallen into disrepute (Meyer-Renschhausen 1991). In literature gruel and, still more, soup are usually associated with low social status and poverty (Ehlert 1989).

However, the simple meal is also praised. Von Rumohr, in his renowned book *Geist der Kochkunst* (*The Spirit of Cuisine*), (1882) opposed feasting and delicacies, but devoted a chapter each to soup and gruel. A further chapter is entitled "On the simplicity or variety of dishes". Von Rumohr contrasts Hippocrates as the advocate of simplicity with Aristotle as the apologist of variety. His plea for the simple meal has remained in practice largely ignored, but in German literature it had a strong influence on Stifter, Keller and Fontane (Wierlacher 1987: Chapter 5.2).

Praise of the simple meal is found principally in the work of critics, who condemned feasting and luxury in food. Praise of the simple forms a constant critical undertone accompanying the development of haute cuisine in Europe and Asia (Goody 1982: Chapter 4). But is this only as a counter-movement to luxury—as Goody perceives it—or are older traditions of the simple meal being expressed in a fresh guise? We are confronted by the important question of whether the tradition of the simple as the perfect meal exists in Europe, too. The articles "Gruel", "Groats" and "Soup" in the *Handwörterbuch des deutschen Aberglaubens* (*Dictionary of German Superstition*) (1927–42) contain many indications of old notions of the strength-giving and beneficent effects of these dishes (see Ehlert 1989: 162; Meyer-Renschhausen 1991). Thus, gruel and soup do not appear always to have been associated with coarseness, poverty and monotony.

On the other hand, peasants are certainly influenced by the gastronomic culture of the higher social orders and take over, at least in part, the latter's view of the monotony and poverty of peasant dishes. They see themselves and their dishes through the eyes of the higher orders and imitate their gastronomic culture. If, for reasons of cost, this is not possible in everyday food, they at least attempt to achieve it in feastday meals. Thus, the contrast between everyday and feastday dishes acquires a different significance in a class society from that attached to it in a classless society.

Apart from stratum-specific evaluations, we must also consider that over time the simple meal has steadily lost its perfection and been degraded to the status of the food of the poor. If constant references are made to "thin" or "watery" soup (Ehlert 1989: 161, 174), more than upper social group prejudice is being expressed. Quite often the simple meal is poor because gruel or soup lack the ingredients that used to make them a perfect meal. Not only the ingredients but also the preparation has declined. As Meyer-Renschhausen points out in her article "The Porridge Debate" (1991), the techniques of cereal pounding that are still widely practised in Africa but that survive in Europe only as relics are better adapted to extracting the nutritional value of the grain than milling.

CONCLUSION

The simple meal is not an isolated phenomenon: parallels can be found in clothes and housing.[9] We are dealing here with a system of simple needs, in which people are content with few possessions and a simple pattern of consumption.

Simple needs should not be equated with deficit. Societies with simple needs also experience periods of deficit in which simple needs are not met: for example, seasonal hunger. Such deprivations are often accepted with little complaint as part of life, in which plenty and shortage alternate.

Such shortages should be distinguished conceptually from poverty. Poverty should always be seen in relation to wealth: the poor exist only where there are also the rich. Shortage without poverty presupposes a society that does not compare itself with other, prosperous societies. This is becoming increasingly unlikely and so today shortage and poverty in fact usually coincide.

NOTES

1. The present chapter is partly taken from the author's *Handeln in einer Hungerkrise. Tuaregnomaden und die grosse Dürre von 1984* (*Coping with famine. Tuareg Nomads and the Great Drought of 1984*) (1989). His research into the Kel Ewey of Timia have been supported by the DFG since 1980.

2. It is not clear whether this includes grinding the millet. In view of the time indicated, it seems unlikely.
3. In the European tradition the sensory organs that man shares with the animals occupy a lower place than intelligence, which distinguishes man from the animals. In an evolutionary perspective more developed sensory organs are therefore often attributed to the "savages" as a limiting factor on the intelligence. This applies in particular to taste and smell, which belong to the "lower senses". It is worthy of note that where this can be grasped concretely—in the taste of food—the sense of taste is suddenly denied once more to the "savages"
4. This does not apply to the nomads, who must buy cereals. In their case limited diet can be partially attributed to their mobility: variety serves to complicate life.
5. In this, of course, the great richness of preindustrial plant life should not be underestimated. The use of wild plants in the preparation of sauces is mentioned in most studies and gives more opportunity for experiment than has been described in the present account, which focuses on polenta.
6. It is difficult to find examples of simplicity in our society that compare to variety in others. One is marriage. From the viewpoint of a polygamous society, monogamous marriage is characterized above all by a deficit of wives. Adherents of monogamy will reject this view. They will proceed from the same premise of a numerical requirement—one man marries one woman—but will not regard this as a deficit, stressing instead the intensity and the fulfilment of the relationship. The decisive factor is not the absence of several wives, but the uniqueness of one. Similarly, Moslems and Christians will reject with indignation the argument that their monotheism is characterized by a lack of variety of gods.
7. For details of peasant cooking times, see the Fortes on the Tallensi (1936: 264); for the Bemba, see Richards (1939: 104ff.); for details of the female goatherds of the Kel Ewey, see Spittler (1989: 147).
8. Oral communication by Georg Klute and Ehya ag Sidiyene.
9. With respect to the following, see my article "Armut, Mangel und einfache Bedürfnisse" ("Poverty, deficit and simple needs"), Zeitschrift für Ethnologie, 116, 1991, 65–89.

REFERENCES

Barlösius, Eva (1988). Social and historical aspects of the German cuisine. In: Stephen Mennell, ed, Die Kultivierung des Appetits, Frankfurt, 423–44.
Barth, Henry (1890). Travels and Discoveries in North and Central Africa, 2 volumes, London.
Bourdieu, Pierre (1982). La distinction. Critique sociale du jugement, Paris.
Braudel, Ferdinand (1979). Les structures du quotidien, Paris.
Ehlert, Trude (1989). Puree, gruel and soup in proverb, superstition and literature. In: Fritz Ruf, ed, Die sehr bekannte Löffelspeise, Velbert-Neviges, 159–85.
Fortes, Meyer and Sonia, L. (1936). Food in the domestic economy of the Tallensi. In: Africa 9, 237–76.
Goody, Jack (1982). Cooking, Cuisine and Class. A Study in Comparative Sociology, Cambridge.
Handwörterbuch des deutschen Aberglaubens (1927–42), 10 volumes, Berlin.
Mennell, Stephen (1985). All Manners of Food. Eating and Taste in England and France from the Middle Ages to the Present, Oxford.
Meyer-Renschhausen, Elisabeth (1991). The porridge debate. In: Food and Foodways, 5, 95–120.
Nicolas, Guy (1975). Dynamique sociale et appréhension du Monde au sein d'une société hausa, Paris.
Okere, Linus (1983). Anthropology of Food in Rural Igboland, Nigeria, New York.

Richards, Audrey (1932). *Hunger and Work in a Savage Tribe*. London.
Richards, Audrey (1939). *Land, Labour and Diet in Northern Rhodesia*, London.
Ruf, Fritz, ed (1989) *Die sehr bekannte dienliche Löffelspeise. Mus, Brei und Suppe— kulturgeschichtlich betrachtet*, Velbert-Neviges.
Rumohr, Carl F. von (1822). *Geist der Kochkunst*, Stuttgart.
Spittler, Gerd (1989). *Handeln in einer Hungerkrise. Tuareg-nomaden und die grosse Dürre von 1984*, Opladen.
Spittler, Gerd (1991). Armut, Mangel und einfache Bedürfnisse. *Zeitschrift für Ethnologie*, 116, 65–89.
Spittler, Gerd (1993). *Lob des einfachen Mahles. Afrikanische und europäische Esskultur im Vergleich*. In: Wierlacher, Alois, ed. *Kulturthema Essen*, Berlin.
Tarde, Gabriel (1890). *Les lois de l'imitation*, Paris.
Teuteberg, Hans J. (1989). Preface to Ruf, Fritz, ed, *Die sehr bekannte dienliche Löffelspeise*, Velbert-Neviges.
Veblen, Thorsten (1899). *The Theory of the Leisure Class*, New York.
Wiegelmann, Günter (1967). *Alltags- and Festspeisen. Wandel and gegenwärtige Stellung*, Marburg.
Wiegelmann, Günter (1982). Der Wandel von Speisen- und Tischkultur im 18. Jahrhundert. In: Hinrichs, Ernst and Wiegelmann, Günter, eds, *Sozialer und kultureller Wandel in der ländlichen Welt des 18. Jahrhunderts*, Wolfenbüttel, 149–61.
Wierlacher, Alois (1987). *Vom Essen in der deutschen Literatur*, Stuttgart.

2. CASSAVA, "THE LAZY MAN'S FOOD"? INDIGENOUS AGRICULTURAL INNOVATION AND DIETARY CHANGE IN NORTHWESTERN ZAMBIA (ca. 1650–1970)

Achim von Oppen

Freie Universität Berlin, Institut für Soziologie,
Babelsberger Strasse 14–16, D-1000 Berlin 31, Germany

INTRODUCTION

"They just struggle with their cassava leaves!" This statement typifies the disparaging comments "progressive farmers" and frustrated officials make about the large majority of poorer peasants in the Zambezi and Kabompo districts of northwestern Zambia.[1] They look down on these peasants because their main crop and staple food is cassava (manioc; botanical name, *manihot utilissima*; see Figure 1), of which they eat not only the starchy tubers instead of maize, but often even the leaves, instead of "proper relish" (sauce) such as meat or at least fish. "I don't think we can educate our children with cassava," another "progressive" maize and vegetable farmer declared; and, talking about his wife who is still growing some cassava, he added: "Cassava is only for consumption, that's all, so she is doing our consumption."[2]

In Zambia, "rural development" means first and foremost increasing the output of maize, which is needed for *mealie meal*, the main ingredient of any urban type of diet. Cassava growing, in contrast, is widely considered to be backward, a domain of women, a "traditional" foodstuff that is good at best for villagers' subsistence.

Although cassava now contributes significantly to the diet of over 800 million people, with a still growing importance particularly in tropical

43

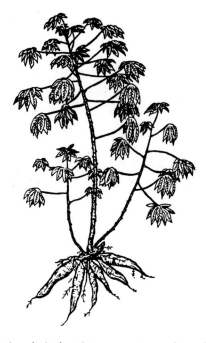

Figure 1   Cassava (manioc) plant (stems grow to maximum height of about 3 m, roots to depth of about 50 cm).

Africa, it has been a very controversial crop among scientists and development planners since the colonial era.[3] In British-dominated central African territories it was seen as at best an anti-famine emergency crop, with high productivity but bad taste, little nutritional value, and negative ecological impact.[4] Because it demanded relatively little male labor, some colonial agricultural officers used to label cassava "the lazy man's crop." After Independence, the accusation of laziness was still used in Zambia against cassava growers, but it referred rather to the failure of peasants to fulfill what was seen as almost a political duty of every rural citizen, the growing of sufficient maize *to feed the nation*. In the neighboring former Belgo-Portuguese sphere, in contrast, cassava has always been more highly valued and was sometimes even celebrated as the "manna of Central Africa,"[5] There, cassava has been a basis of food policy up to the present day.

Such controversies resulted in sometimes contradictory policies towards this crop. But they also reflected contradictory views among central African cultivators themselves as to whether cassava is "proper food" or not. In Zambia, a majority of peasants keep to their conviction that a good meal is based on a porridge (*nshima*) of grains (traditionally millet or sorghum, but increasingly maize), although in periods of hunger they may rely reluctantly on cassava as a secondary staple.[6] Through neighboring Zaire, northern Angola, and adjacent states, however, stretches a vast, circular belt of land in which peasants consider porridge made purely from cassava (or mixed with some grain flour) definitely palatable and far from a famine food (see Figure 2).[7] Among the Luunda, in what is now western Shaba Province (Zaire), for example, the term for cassava is equivalent to "food", and a neighboring group calls itself simply *Bena Kalundwe*, literally. "cassava people."[8] This cassava belt extends into Zambian territory, namely, to the Luapula Lunda in the north, and to a group of closely related peoples in the extreme northwestern corner of the country: the Southern Lunda, Luvale, Chokwe, Luchazi, and Mbunda in the Zambezi and Kabompo districts (see Figure 3).

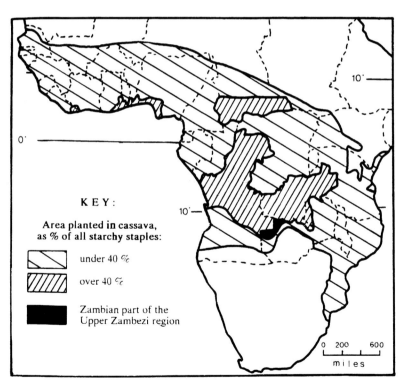

Figure 2 Cassava in Africa (ca. 1950). Adapted from W. O. Jones, *Manioc in Africa* (Stanford: Stanford University Press, 1959), pp. 56, 58.

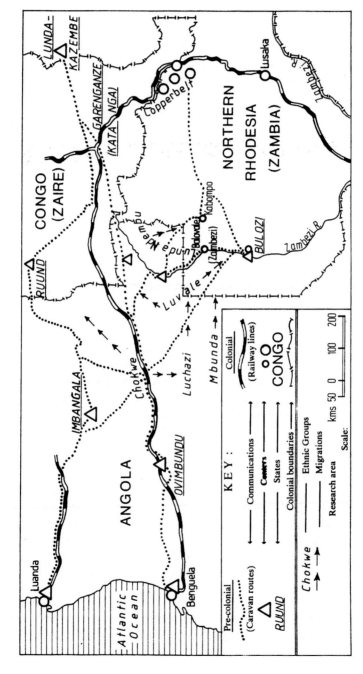

Figure 3   West-central Africa in the nineteenth and twentieth centuries.

This latter group of "cassava eaters" (another derogatory term used by local officials) around the Upper Zambezi, an area that historically includes the neighboring part of Angola, will be the focus of this article. The importance of cassava in their land use systems and diet is unusual even by central African standards. And yet, the traditional staple here as elsewhere in central Africa was not cassava but varieties of millet. The local population itself recalls that long ago bulrush millet was grown for *nshima* (porridge) and finger millet for beer. Only later did cassava replace bulrush millet, which in turn replaced finger millet as the main ingredient of beer. Today, *nshima* consists mostly of cassava, although many people still regard a mixture with grains as the real thing.[9] What induced people to change their diet so radically in favor of a crop as controversial as cassava? I shall look at the history of this change and ask about the underlying reasons.

A CHRONOLOGY OF INNOVATION

Indian cultivators in tropical South America were the first to domesticate cassava, and Portuguese conquerors there very quickly adopted it as their staple. The transatlantic slave trade, which began around 1500, established a strong link between Brazil and the West African coast, and cassava must have been introduced to Africa through this channel. Written sources first mention cassava cultivation in the Portuguese bridgeheads on the Angolan coast in 1608 (Loango) and in the 1620s (around Luanda).[10] Other crops imported from America, such as maize or groundnuts, were adopted much earlier; maize, for example, was grown in Angola as early as the mid-sixteenth century.[11] Nevertheless, there must have been considerable demand for cassava on the Angolan coast, as we know from the account of the British pirate Sir Andrew Hawkins, who seized a Portuguese vessel coming from Brazil in 1593. He described the cargo as "meale of cassavi which the Portingals call *Farina de Paw*. It serveth for marchandize in Angola, for the Portingals foode in the ship, and to nourish the negroes which they shall carry to the River of Plate."[12]

One plausible explanation for the relatively late introduction of cassava cultivation in Angola may be that the particular processing techniques cassava requires made a long period of experimentation and reorganization of the labor process necessary. Cassava contains poisonous hydrocyanic acid (HCN) in varying degrees, and its many varieties are accordingly subdivided into sweet and bitter ones. The HCN contained in the bitter varieties is most efficiently removed through a fermentation process before consumption. The practice of soaking the tubers in order to produce

fermentation was apparently the most striking innovation for African cultivators, since the Bantu root *bòòb*, "to be soaked" or "to become soft,"
became the word stem for cassava in most central African languages.[13]
Once the obstacles of processing had been overcome, cassava became in
the course of the seventeenth century *the* dominant cash crop along the
Angolan coast, serving as food for Portuguese settlers, foreign ships, and
above all slaves.[14]

Surprisingly enough, the remote interior of central Africa adopted cassava
much more rapidly than did the coast. The analysis of oral traditions and
linguistic evidence has led to the assumption that cassava cultivation in the
emerging Luunda (*Ruund*) empire, in what is now southwestern Zaire,
began before the mid-sixteenth century.[15] This means a jump of more than
1,500 km at a time when cassava was just being introduced on the coast
and communication was extremely difficult. Ruund's earliest contacts with
the Atlantic world, unlike later, more direct overland routes, apparently
went via the Lulua, Kasai, and Zaire rivers to the Kongo kingdom; i.e.,
they took a huge detour through the northern forests.[16] Cassava surpluses
brought in as tribute from all parts of the empire soon became the food
basis of the capital of Ruund with its large non-agricultural population. In
addition, the rulers ran something like a state farm, which was worked by
their slaves and "poor women."[17]

The Ruund empire, in turn, most probably passed on cassava cultivation
to the peoples of the Upper Zambezi, who likewise, it seems, eagerly
adopted this new crop. Linguistic analysis has shown a close link between
cassava terminology in the languages of the Upper Zambezi and the
Ruund peoples.[18] Oral traditions recorded among Angolan Luvale speak
of cassava having been brought to them by *Namuto* and *Samuto*, mythical
forebears whose origin is said to have been around the Lulua River, i.e., in
the Ruund area. And Zambian Luvale historians hold that their chiefs'
clan, *nama kungu*, which immigrated from Ruund, taught a more intensive
form of agriculture, along with other food production technologies, to the
resident acephalous population. The latter is described as having been
"very backward": "They hardly knew how to cultivate, preferring to eat
water lily plants and other such foods" (clearly a reference to a higher
importance of gathering in the pre-*nama kungu* food economy).[19] Interestingly, the decisive innovation reported here is mound cultivation (which is
characteristic for cassava), as opposed to the earlier form of cultivation on
ridges used for millets.[20] From the beginning cassava meant not merely a
new crop, but a whole new production system.

The introduction of cassava, however, should not be seen as something
that happened all at once. Rather we can assume it consisted of a long

process of importation and experimentation with ever new varieties, while others were dropped again; keen cassava growers make considerable efforts of this kind up to the present day. In the Angolan parts of the Upper Zambezi, 20 to 35 past and present varieties are known to Chokwe and Luvale peasants, and at least 18 different varieties, both bitter and sweet, are currently grown in Kabompo, on the Zambian side. Again, according to Angolan Chokwe cassava cultivators, the oldest-known varieties came from Ruund.[21]

The fact that immigrant political rulers apparently played a role in introducing the first varieties of cassava to the Upper Zambezi also provides some clues as to the origins and date of this event. Not only Luvale, but also Chokwe, Southern Lunda, and Luchazi claim that their chiefs' dynasties originate from Ruund, the major radiating center for political centralization and ethnic realignment in the central African savannah. But it seems unlikely that the chiefs actually carried the cassava technology with them when they arrived from Ruund. Their migration took place over a long period, with intermittent settlement. At least in the case of the Luvale and Chokwe, the original emigration from Ruund dates long before cassava could possibly have reached the area,[22] while the future Southern Lunda titles emigrated only much later, when cassava was already well established in the Ruund nuclear state. Those chiefs who immigrated early may have had a particular role as intermediaries, with more frequent contacts with their ancient homes, but these links were of a rather informal nature and hardly meant dependency. It can be assumed that these chiefs, as well as the other populations of the Upper Zambezi, adopted cassava growing through voluntary and decentralized types of contacts (e.g., gift exchanges, trade), rather than through political or economic pressure from Ruund.

Drawing together this evidence, the spread of cassava into the Upper Zambezi dates roughly between 1650, when the crop had certainly arrived in Ruund, and 1700, when the last of the new chiefs, the holders of the southern Lunda title of *Ishinde*, left the mature Ruund state to settle near the east bank of the Zambezi.

There seems to be little doubt that the introduction of cassava, along with other crops such as maize and groundnuts, was "a by-product of the earliest phases of long-distance exchanges" between coastal traders and inhabitants of the central African interior.[23] But pre-colonial world-market integration through the "Atlantic Zone" (J. Miller) was only just beginning at this time, at a very slow pace, and through a series of intermediaries. It thus seems unlikely that direct or indirect demand from outside markets spurred these innovations; reports from around 1800 by the first Portuguese-speaking traders to reach the Upper Zambezi already emphasize the abundance of cassava, besides bulrush millet and probably sorghum.[24] A dynamic within these societies must account for the introduction of cassava in the remote interior.

A RELIABLE FOOD

It has been argued, against neo-Malthusian pessimism, that "indigenous" agricultural change is a widespread feature in African history and that it reflects mainly an effort to adapt to climatic and soil conditions or to scarce natural resources (such as land, in cases of population growth), in situations where existing methods could no longer ensure a sufficient and reliable food supply.[25]

In fact, what first made cassava so attractive to Upper Zambezi cultivators, at least as a supplementary staple, was probably that it scores considerably better than millet with regard to yield, and particularly with regard to yield security, in their natural environment (see Table 1). Central African millet cultivators experience food scarcity and famine more or less regularly. Millets are relatively nutritious and popular in Africa, but their yield relative to area is low,[26] and the need to store seed and pre- and post-harvest losses reduce it even further.[27] Every year before the harvest, toward the end of the rainy season, some harsh "hunger months" have to be lived through.[28] Besides these seasonal variations, there has always been the risk of intermittent periods of drought. Minor precipitation shortfalls occur about every ten years, while major and catastrophic droughts lasting several years happen on average almost once in a lifetime, according to historical analysis.[29] Millet yields are highly susceptible to drought, while cassava is particularly drought-resistant.[30] Cassava can be harvested and replanted—this is often done plant by plant—at any time of the year without significant impact on yield; this also avoids peak demands on labor and hence risk. In addition, during the first year when cassava plants are still young, grain crops such as bulrush millet or maize can be planted in between them. Maize, which seems to have been introduced from Angola along with cassava, was originally grown only in small quantities and eaten green as a snack (Luvale *visakwola*, "vegetables"), another means of alleviating the scarcity of food toward the end of the rains.

In addition, most of the area is covered by a deep layer of loose and relatively acidic Kalahari sands, with which the fairly undemanding cassava plant copes much better than do grain crops. Grains are particularly problematic on the dry, thickly wooded uplands that fringe the depressions of major rivers and that had been almost unpopulated prior to the seventeenth

Table 1 Economic advantages and disadvantages of cassava as a staple crop compared with grains

Conditions	Advantages	Disadvantages
Soil	Requires fewer soil nutrients overall	Requires more potash More susceptible to high water table
Climate	Drought-resistant; therefore, carries less risk of crop failure	Prolonged maturation period at lower temperatures; in the Upper Zambezi about 2–3 years, depending on variety
Land and labor	Produces higher yield (relative to caloric energy per area) Requires less frequent shifting of fields (bush-clearing) Allows mixed culture in the first year(s) Permits greater flexibility in timing of field operations, no labor peaks Does not require bird scaring (as does millet) Does not require building of stores	Requires more effort in field preparation (mound building, green manure) Requires more labor for processing, particularly with bitter varieties (soaking, drying)
Storage	In-ground storage; therefore, fewer pre- and post-harvest losses	
Consumption	Requires no seed deductions Cassava leaves may also be used Allows mixed culture with complementary food crops	Lower nutritional value; therefore, more need for supplementary foods rich in proteins and vitamins.

and eighteenth century. Here the new crop proved to be particularly helpful. In the even more sandy, but seasonally flooded, open savannahs along the west bank of the Zambezi, a higher percentage of millet has been maintained up to the present day because a high water table is one of the few definite threats to cassava roots.[31]

Although cassava made the staple food supply much more reliable, a cassava-based diet posed new problems: it has a very low content of essential nutrients, especially proteins, compared to millet.[32] The peasants are well aware of this; they say that cassava has to be eaten in bigger quantities and that the feeling of satisfaction after eating lasts less long. They do not regard cassava as a complete meal in itself. For them, eating cassava *nshima* makes sense only if it is accompanied by its natural counterpart, a "relish" (Luvale *ifwo*) rich in these missing nutrients.[33] They are usually found in legumes such as beans and groundnuts, which can be easily interplanted with young cassava, and in leaves, often from the cassava plant itself. The most popular sources of protein, however, are game, fish, snared small animals, insects, or, rarely, livestock. Consequently, a diet based on cassava is tied to complementary hunting, fishing, and gathering for local consumption. The Upper Zambezi with its highly diversified mosaic of different ecosystems provides excellent conditions for all these activities. Significantly, the immigrant chiefs who brought cassava are also reported to have introduced important innovations that affected the productivity of ironwork (manufacture of weapons) and of flood plain fisheries.[34]

These non-agricultural ways of food production played a considerable role beyond that of meeting the residence groups' own consumption needs. The settlement structure consists of scattered, fairly independent "villages" of small lineage segments. Therefore, the increase of productivity in both agriculture (cassava) and fishing and hunting promoted specialization and a thriving regional trade between producers of crop surpluses in the eastern woodlands and hunters and, above all, fishermen in the western plains.[35] The two sides became so dependent on each other for their food supply that the east bank was nicknamed *nshima* (porridge) and the west bank *ifwo* (relish).

A WOMEN'S STRONGHOLD

Agricultural innovation, like any major technological development, involves much more than changes in the relationship between producer and nature. Even in societies organized along kinship lines, "the" producers can by no means be regarded as a homogenous mass: there are continued efforts to establish or challenge the asymmetrical power relations inherent in the kinship system. In segmentary lineage societies, the divisions of labor between men and women, elders and youths, are the most important social divides. In the Upper Zambezi, agriculture has always been a domain of women and was separated from the economic sphere of men perhaps even more than elsewhere in Africa.[36] Male-dominated forms of appropriating the wilderness (hunting, fishing, beekeeping, woodwork) played such an important role in this still very open environment that men, particularly the younger ones, were often away from their homes for considerable periods. Women have always done the bulk of cultivation work; the amount of agricultural work done by husbands or matrilineally related men varies individually, but the only tasks for which women can legitimately claim male assistance are the regular bush clearing to open virgin farm land and the provision of tools and grain stores.[37]

Seen in this context, the introduction of cassava cultivation, on the one hand, seems to suit the interests of men very well, because it reduces their labor input and makes their prolonged absence from home for the pursuit of their own activities even easier. Cassava makes little demand on soil nutrients and therefore requires less frequent shifting of fields to new land; it needs no grain stores and has a noticeably higher output per area than grain crops (see Table 1 and note 26). On the other hand, cassava requires more labor in what are considered in the area to be typical female tasks: careful preparing of seedbeds (mounds); incorporating organic matter in order to preserve soil fertility; harvesting (which is partly facilitated by mounding); and, above all, processing. The introduction of cassava cultivation meant, first of all, an increased workload for women.

Nevertheless, results of a recent research project suggest that women themselves may have had an active interest in cassava cultivation. Conventionally, they have to supply most of the family's food crops, just as men are responsible for the supply of animal protein, wooden tools, and buildings. Men's fields, if there are any, are used rather to feed their own visitors and friends than for family subsistence. But women can dispose independently of any surpluses produced from their own fields, even if the fields were provided by their husbands. If fields are owned (i.e., cultivated) jointly with their husbands, wives still have a right to half of the proceeds not needed for food. Even in the case of divorce or the husband's death, which usually means that the wife and children return to her maternal uncle's or brother's village, she can still claim half of the produce from her fields. Only the other half remains with her husband or his family, on the basis of land rights established through the initial act of bush clearing.[38] This claim provides a basis for women's economic independence, which is all the more important for them because of the high instability of marriage.[39]

Cassava cultivation, although requiring more effort from women, made them less dependent on always unreliable male support. It even increased to some extent their power vis-à-vis men, who became even more dependent

on their wives' or sisters' willingness to process food for them and for
their guests. In addition, it increased the amount of staple food women had
at their own disposal. Cassava surpluses strengthened the position of
women in the circulation of food and labor between village neighbors. Up
to the present day, a certain type of basket (nick-named *wayileyi*) filled
with cassava is regarded as equivalent to a certain amount of piecework on
cassava fields, or to fixed amounts of meat or dried fish, the typical male
products.[40] Today, women vigorously defend these standard rates against
rising prices for meat and fish on outside markets: "Men always destroy
the old prices," some women complain.[41] The relationship between men
and women very clearly expresses an idea, however exaggerated, of com-
plementarity as well as of competition between "male" (animal) and
"female" (vegetable) foods. Cassava became so much a part of female
identity that, for example, the root is now used in girls' initiation rituals.[42]
Economically, cassava growing made it easier for women, even for single
women, to secure a balanced diet and labor assistance. It enhanced their
economic independence even more when the crop began to acquire an
extra-village exchange value.

A BASIS OF AUTHORITY

But the opportunities of using cassava for the enhancement of economic
and social position have to be built up in a long process that reflects ecological conditions and the biological properties of the crop. The physical
conditions of the Upper Zambezi—its sandy soils; its altitude and distance
from the equator, which result in relatively long and cool winters—have
the effect of slowing down the plant's growth. In most local cassava varieties, the roots reach their full size only after 24–28 months,[43] and they
may stay in the ground for as long a period again, because they are harvested only for immediate consumption. A full cassava cycle, from field
preparation to the end of the harvest, may last up to four years. During this
period, new portions of cassava are planted annually (see Figure 4). Upper
Zambezi cultivators regard four fields in all stages of growth as a minimum requirement for economic self-sufficiency.[44] This means that cassava
cultivation requires considerably more initial investment in both time and
effort than grains, before a new producer becomes independent of others
for supplies of cassava and planting material (cuttings).

Not surprisingly, the producers who own the most numerous and size-
able cassava fields with standing crops are old people, often polygamist
men or single elderly women, who have not migrated for some time.

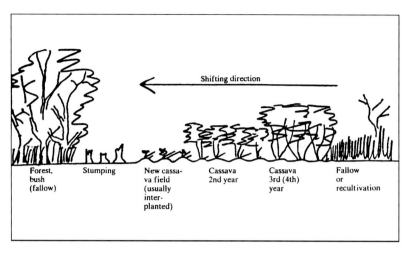

Figure 4 The cassava cultivation system in northwestern Zambia ("Luvale System"). From S. Schonherr, Lima Small Scale Farmer Crop Development (unpublished IRDP document, Kabompo/Eschborn, 1979), p. 12.

The introduction of cassava cultivation served the interests of such resident elders particularly because it enabled them to receive more visitors and much increased and prolonged their control over young people and over recent immigrants. A steady increase in the number of subordinate family members is a primary concern for elders in any kinship-based society, but it is one that is especially difficult to realize in this area with its extremely high spatial mobility, scattered population, and strong segmentation of lineages. Cassava cultivation became a means for seniors to attract more dependents (because it provided them with disposable food surpluses), and at the same time it prolonged the latter's dependency. In return for meal and cuttings, recently married spouses and newly arrived immigrants usually either have to give meat or fish or have to work the donor's cassava fields. This dependence affects a considerable number of people in the area, since migration has always been an important means of coping with social, economic, or political tensions. In 1986, for example, we observed large numbers of refugees from the Angolan civil war who worked the fields of Zambian peasants (many of them women) at a rate of one day's work for two days' food, in the form of cassava meal.[45] This sort of exploitation (on the basis of piecework relations, rather than unpaid family labor), combined with the durability of the cassava root, make an individual accumulation of food crops possible. And power over food, as so often, is converted into power over people, something that the local conditions have always made it difficult to achieve.

This political aspect of cassava cultivation seems to have been particularly important for the chiefs who invaded the area from the sixteenth century onward. Cassava production helped them to gather more dependents around them—relatives, wives, warriors, refugees, and visitors, but also large retinues of pawns and slaves. This may explain why oral traditions describe chiefs as pioneers and "teachers" in cassava cultivation. The new crop became a means for them to establish political rule among "people who largely retained their general characteristics of an acephalous society."[46]

The spread of the new chiefs' lineage groups over the Upper Zambezi, which had been remarkably peaceful in the earlier phases, assumed much more violent forms after around 1720, when the growing world-market demand for slaves spurred on their struggle for political power.[47] Violent strife and raiding between the dispersed residential groups had probably always been a feature of social relations, but now it spread and intensified with the force of an epidemic. One demographic consequence was the rapid clustering of followers around the palisaded strongholds of powerful chiefs who offered protection to the weak. Land was and generally still is abundant on the Upper Zambezi, where the average population density in 1980 was less than 3 persons per square kilometer. However, people are not evenly dispersed over the region but tend to flock to certain areas, today mainly to mission stations and administrative outposts with social and infrastructural facilities and to certain agricultural areas with good access to markets. The clusters around chiefs' headquarters may have been the earliest places where less frequent shifting of fields, a more permanent land-use pattern, and a higher productivity of caloric food output relative to area became imperative and where cassava cultivation—which fulfills all these requirements—spread most rapidly.

A SAFEGUARD FOR AUTONOMY

From the very beginning, cassava was probably also useful as a means for invading contenders for political authority to preserve their autonomy from more powerful neighboring states. They must have had a particular interest in becoming self-sufficient enough not to be driven by periodic famine to the more fertile river basins of the Kasai, Kwilo, Kwanza, or Zambezi (Bulozi floodplain), where they would have to submit themselves to those still in possession of food. For ordinary villagers a similar danger of losing their freedom as "famine refugees" must have made a highly productive staple crop such as cassava all the more valuable.[48]

When violence between and within ethno-political groups spread as a result of the slave trade, grain stores and even the standing crop in the fields were among the prominent targets. During raids, the attackers systematically plundered or destroyed stores and crops in order to starve the owners into slavery.[49] Food stealing became another threat to independence, particularly in areas where many travelers passed by, that is, near the main routes of pre-colonial long-distance trade.[50] Cassava appears to have provided salvation from the effects of these kinds of violence, too. Since the crop remains unharvested in the ground until it is actually needed, destruction or theft is much more difficult than with grains. In addition, Upper Zambezi peasants, contrary to their Angolan neighbors to the west, preferred the bitter varieties containing hydrocyanic acid. Precisely the fact that these require more treatment (soaking, drying) before they can be consumed than the better tasting sweet varieties seems to have been one reason for the preference: it affords a protection against both human and animal predators. Even today they usually mix bitter and sweet varieties at random on the same field, partly as a deterrent for thieves and elephants.[51]

Other more qualitative food problems resulted, however, from these tactics. The smell and taste of fermentation in soaked cassava is unpleasant, not only to the taste of other peoples in Zambia, but also for Upper Zambezians themselves. One observer even found that "the older generation indeed hold that the odour of damp cassava flour introduced into a house will upset the efficacy of protective charms." He described the invention of specific drying techniques as one way to cope with this problem. High, solid racks for sun drying have replaced sophisticated and once ubiquitous grain stores in Upper Zambezi villages. For the rainy season, a system of drying cassava near the fire *(kusota)* was developed, which is unknown in other parts of Zambia.[52]

It seems, in general, that during the nineteenth century worsening social relations increased the danger of food shortages and famine. As a result, cassava gradually became more dominant as a staple food, particularly on the wooded uplands: "All the Balonda cultivate the manioc or cassava excessively" and "manioc is the chief article of cultivation" Livingstone noted in his diary in 1854, when he first visited the Lunda areas east of the Zambezi; he observed "houses surrounded by gardens of manioc, which they seem to regard as their staff of life."[53] Apparently, the peasants were prepared to put aside considerations of taste, encouraged, perhaps, by the example of their Portuguese-speaking trading partners who also subsisted on manioc meal.

A WAY TO THE MARKET

Another, increasingly important reason for the expansion of cassava cultivation was a broadening in the opportunities to make use of food surpluses.
An intense regional trade, to a large extent in foodstuffs, had been carried
on since before the nineteenth century. This pattern of regional exchange,
typical of central Africa, appeared on the Upper Zambezi in a particularly
decentralized form, involving individual petty producers and traders. In
neighboring, more centralized societies such as Ruund or Bulozi, in contrast, the circulation of foodstuffs functioned much more in the way of
tribute collection and redistribution through the hands of the rulers.[54] This
decentralization helps to explain why Upper Zambezi peoples subsequently
took such an active part in long-distance trade within the "Atlantic Zone"
of the pre-colonial world market. Cassava, again, became an important
medium in this market integration. Large numbers of caravan travelers—
traders, slaves, and porters—crossed the area in various directions, while
others stayed there for months to buy slaves, ivory, beeswax, and wild rubber for export.[55] They were all continually searching for food provisions,
mainly cassava flour. Food was bought at villages en route, at the trading
camps that went up all over the area, and even in remoter villages, when
hungry travelers roamed the bush in search of it.

While many producers seem to have been very actively interested in
finding new customers for their surplus,[56] foreign travelers often had to
use the existing system of regional food trade to obtain cassava and other
commodities. Chokwe cultivators, for example, would sell cassava flour to
the traveler only in exchange for dried fish, which he first had to procure
somewhere else along the route.[57] A Luvale trader who wanted to buy
wild rubber collected by remote Lunda forest dwellers, in order to sell it in
bulk to Angolan middlemen, had to offer them fish. The fish he had to buy
beforehand from fishermen on the other side of the Zambezi, in exchange
for cassava. Large cassava fields were, thus, the "initial capital" on which
this trader's business was founded.[58]

Again, social differences are significant. Men seem to have been
involved in trading crops to some extent, but they either traded on account
of their wives or at least depended on them to process the meal. Their main
business was the production and sale of "legitimate" export articles—ivory,
beeswax, and wild rubber. Cassava, predominantly a female product,
offered women for the first time, therefore, the opportunity to gain direct
access to imported goods, mainly cloth, certain beads, salt, and copper
ornaments, which had quickly become "currencies" in all manner of social
transactions. The fact that not only chiefs, elders, and some notables (as in

some neighboring societies), but also ordinary women and men were able to enter external markets, made cassava cultivation all the more attractive and accelerated "commercialization" and "monetarization" within the area.

The imposition of colonial rule shortly after 1900 meant then a slump in market integration and commodity production, not its beginning. The colonial boundary trisected the historical unity of the area between Northern Rhodesia (Zambia), Angola, and the Congo Free State (Zaire). The area that is now Zambezi and Kabompo Districts was cut off from the established trade routes to the west; in addition, demand for the leading export commodities collapsed. The Poll Tax forced many young men to work for certain periods of time as migrant laborers in distant mines and towns in order to earn coined money. Customary male absenteeism from agriculture, already favored by pre-colonial long-distance trade which had caused men to be away for prolonged periods as slave-raiders, ivory hunters, beeswax and rubber collectors, caravan porters, and traders, increased even further at this point. Cassava enabled women to maintain a sufficient base for local subsistence even without male labor. In other words, it looked as if the Upper Zambezi was doomed to become just one of the hopeless labor reserves of southern Africa.

Colonial intervention was certainly an important aspect of the expansion of cassava cultivation during the nineteenth and twentieth centuries.[59] But in the Upper Zambezi colonial intervention did not destroy peasant commodity production or, rather, reduce it more or less to a level of "subsistence production," as much as it did elsewhere in southern Africa. After a period of depression, the peasants found new marketing opportunities for their products, which must have provided more than a merely supplementary income, since throughout the colonial period the incidence of labor migration from what is now Zambezi and Kabompo was among the lowest in Northern Rhodesia.[60] During the later colonial era, cassava became more and more the dominant local market product. This dominance appears to have been the driving force behind a further dramatic expansion of cassava as the staple crop. Only then was the process which had begun in the nineteenth century of substituting cassava for millet (as opposed to the earlier supplementing of one by the other) completed.

To quote a contemporary observer, the land-use system in the Northern Rhodesian (now Zambian) portion of the Upper Zambezi underwent "an almost unique change [which came] about largely through the initiative of the people concerned, and certainly without any activity of the Agricultural Department, ... due to the great decrease in the cultivation of bulrush millet."[61] When in 1932–34 the first systematic land-use survey was undertaken, bulrush millet still played an important role alongside cassava cultivation. What the surveyors then called the "Northern Kalahari Woodland System" was based on an initial planting of bulrush millet on freshly cleared virgin land, followed by one or more cycles of cassava in the subsequent years, and a long fallow after a maximum of six to seven years. The ratio of harvested area of bulrush millet (including intercultures) to cassava ranged between 2 : 1 and 2 : 3.[62]

In the 1950s, when the next surveys were carried out, the regular fallow periods and clearing of new fields ("shifting cultivation") necessary for millet cultivation had been almost completely abandoned in favor of a semi-permanent cultivation of cassava. Fields were found to have been planted continuously with cassava for up to 29 years with no sign of decreasing fertility, an astounding figure for "traditional" tropical agriculture. Cassava had become the main crop on almost the entire cultivated area. Beans, groundnuts, maize, and other crops, though rarely bulrush millet, were interplanted in the first one or two years. The total cultivated area per household (4–5 people) was on average 2.4 hectares.[63]

Two kinds of markets for cassava were stimulating this change during the colonial period: demand from a growing and at least temporarily non-producing local population, and demand from neighboring regions that normally relied on grains but were hit by growing food shortages. The first market developed mainly through the food rations that the administration and missions gave to their local employees and pieceworkers, through labor agencies that had to feed newly recruited migrants on their journeys, and through the first mission-run boarding schools and hospitals. These institutions acquired cassava and other foodstuffs through "meal contracts" awarded to local white traders. The traders bought up the cassava flour of a very large number of petty producers at their shops and at seasonal buying stations scattered over the Balovale and Kabompo districts, which then had an adult population of about 45,000. Toward the end of the colonial period, local market demand for cassava flour was estimated to be around 470 metric tons per annum within Balovale, the bigger district, alone.[64]

An informal kind of local demand came directly from male government employees and returned migrants: outside the area, they had developed a taste for a strong homemade gin called *kachasu* or *lituku*. At home, hitherto, young men had not easily found access to strong alcoholic beverages, such as the customary honey beer. Village women quickly grasped the opportunity to distill *lituku* and to sell their cassava (and some maize) in this processed form, diverting a sometimes considerable share of men's income into their pockets. Rather symbolically, they employed gun barrels, for which the men had little use after the imposition of *Pax Britannica*, as their main utensil for distilling.

As to the external market, from the early 1920s white traders in Balovale (today Zambezi) began to supply "meal contracts" in neighboring Barotseland (today Western Province) that were much bigger than the local contracts. Officials there were increasingly worried about a steady decline in grain production, probably a consequence of the liberation from tribute relations of Lozi subject peoples who lived on the surrounding uplands and had to supply the floodplain with grains.[65] Unusually high floods, locust invasions, and droughts finally triggered serious famines during the 1930s. In this period, the Upper Zambezi began to be called the "Granary of Barotseland," supplying about half of its enormous demand for food—mainly with cassava meal. At the same time, seasonal famines increasingly occurred in the sorghum-growing Kaonde area to the southeast. "Official" exports of cassava from the Upper Zambezi to both these areas rose from 63.5 metric tons in 1922–23 to well over 1,000 tons annually during the copper boom in the late 1940s and early 1950s.[66]

But peasants and petty traders from Balovale and Kabompo rapidly found their own ways into the new outside markets. They undertook tedious journeys by dugout canoe or bicycle to channel "informally" about one half again of the official shipments of cassava to their suffering neighbors. They exchanged it either for fish or for slaughter cattle which were taken home to Balovale. Today, with a much reduced demand from Western Province, one bag of cassava still buys one bundle of fish, and four to five bags one cow, which at Zambezi prices means a profit margin of 200 to 300 percent.[67] And Kaonde customers sometimes even paid by piecework on their suppliers' cassava fields.[68] It is obvious that this trade was conducted as a very efficient extended version of the earlier forms of regional and local circulation.

AN ALTERNATIVE TO "MODERNIZATION"

The new state embodied in the colonial administration was, however, much less happy than were the peasants and petty traders with this brisk trade in food-stuffs, which resulted in vastly extended cassava cultivation in Balovale East and Kabompo. It is true that the administration itself partly depended on the peasants' cassava sales, which provided an additional source of income that enabled villagers to pay taxes and formed the food basis for the growing number of local government employees. But its dependence was reluctant, and its officers increasingly grumbled about cassava as "an undesirable crop," a sign of backwardness.[69] In their eyes there seemed to be few long-term prospects for developing cassava as a cash crop. This may have been partly because cassava offers less scope for "modernization" (new varieties, fertilizer, mechanization) than do grain crops.[70] A common argument, at any rate, was the remoteness of the area, which made transport costs for exporting bulky, low-value goods such as cassava to the urban markets of the "Line of Rail" prohibitive. These markets were much nearer to the "white" commercial farming areas that were originally supposed to supply the entire country's market demand for food. In reality, though, transport costs from the "Line of Rail" made food *imports* equally prohibitive, which explains the market niche for peasant producers within this rural periphery.

The other main argument used increasingly to discredit cassava as a backward subsistence crop was its relatively low dietary value.[71] Excessive sales, it was feared, threatened rural nutrition: "people used to get short of food, they used to take down [to Bulozi] so much cassava... [that they even took] up the cassava which should have stayed one more year in the ground," one former colonial District Commissioner told me.[72] Beginning in the late 1920s, but particularly after 1945, continuous efforts were made to persuade "native growers" to cultivate more maize, rice, and groundnuts.[73] Cassava exports to Bulozi (Barotseland) were restricted and completely banned in years with poor grain harvests.[74] There were repeated attempts to keep cassava prices at a low level. The Forestry Department enforced a number of conservation measures, partly against allegedly excessive bush clearing and soil degradation resulting from the expansion of cassava.[75]

Curiously enough, the colonial administration in other, millet-growing parts of the country not only encouraged, but sometimes even enforced cassava cultivation as a hedge against famine. In Northern Province, with its different social structure, these attempts met with peasant resistance and contributed to very bad feelings against cassava among the population, according to one report "mainly because the women object to the extra work entailed in reducing the root to the palatable form of porridge."[76]

Peasant producers in Zambezi and Kabompo, however, resisted government agricultural policy against cassava. For a long time, they went on expanding their cassava production fairly successfully, unimpressed by the outspoken policy of curbing "overproduction of cassava" and "encouraging other, more economic crops."[77] What made the peasants continue their cassava production for regional markets was certainly not conservatism, but precisely that "highly developed economic instinct" that, contradictorily enough, colonial administrators in the area found equally remarkable. High transport costs and also white traders' profits locally much reduced the higher prices other crops fetched on copperbelt markets. Marketing problems were also created by the Grain Marketing Board, in the interest of white farmers in the "Line of Rail" who feared African competition.[78] Another apparent reason for the peasants of Balovale and Kabompo to keep to their own staple, cassava, was that it protected them from dependence on new inputs such as seed and fertilizer and from control by extension agents.[79]

The peasants did, in fact, also increase the production of other crops, but they were mainly crops that could be easily integrated into their autonomous cassava-based agriculture. Groundnuts, in particular, can be easily inter-planted with first-year cassava, have a positive effect on soil fertility (fixing nitrogen, rather than requiring fertilization), reproduce their own seed, and are grown mainly by women. These reasons probably explain why during the late colonial period groundnuts (and not maize) became the second most important peasant surplus crop (next to cassava) in Balovale and Kabompo and the only regular agricultural export to the "Line of Rail."

In 1962, there was still four times more cassava than maize marketed in Balovale. But only six years later, after political Independence, cassava had completely disappeared from official marketing records, while the output of maize had increased by 50 percent.[80] This shift meant that the large majority of peasant producers, many of them women, had suddenly lost their main avenue to the market. Peasants subsequently reduced their average cultivated area from about 2.4 hectares (in 1957) to only 1.2 hectares per household (in 1979), but cassava still dominated 83 to 100 percent of the area, according to locality.[81] The reasons for this sudden slump are to be sought less in the very generous support the post-Independence government gave (through loans, machinery, and so forth) to a few cooperatives and "progressive farmers," than in certain long-term historical changes.

One of these changes was the spread of maize consumption among urban consumers, including government employees in remote district centers. The origins of this urban image of maize consumption seem to be linked to the pattern of food rationed out to mine workers, the "labor aristocracy," throughout southern Africa, as well as to the Northern-Province background of many of today's educated elite in Zambia. In the political arena, urban dwellers and their organizations, namely, the trade unions, also pressed successfully for, and subsequently defended, the present high level of subsidies for maize, against which cassava cannot compete. Recent government attempts to cut subsidies on maize provoked serious riots in the "Line of Rail" towns in December 1986 and June 1990. Another development detrimental to the sale of cassava was the increase of maize supplies within Western Province (Barotseland). Much of the production occurred in the Kaoma area, with the help of considerable numbers of Luvale and

Lunda immigrants from the Upper Zambezi; the balance was brought in on a new road from the commercial farming areas on the "Line of Rail." This increase enabled the inhabitants of Bulozi to return to a grain-based diet.[82]

A third important reason for the expulsion of petty cassava producers from the market was the creation of a government monopoly on food marketing. The parastatal marketing organization (NAMBoard) ran fewer and less effective buying stations and bought only in large quantities by the full bag. Cassava was not accepted at all for marketing until 1982. Consequently, the once thriving cassava trade was reduced to relatively insignificant quantities in "informal" channels, mainly supplying the lower ranks of local government workers.

During the last few years, however, a foreign-funded development project that emphasizes the "small-scale producer" has effectively introduced a new standardized system of grain cultivation to peasant agriculture in Kabompo and Zambezi, with maize in the east and rice in the west. At the same time, these crops are gradually gaining importance as staples even within the rural areas. For the first time in 300 years, there is now a trend reversal against cassava in the Upper Zambezi. To ask about the reasons of this new turning point would bring us onto different ground. But although a majority of the peasants now respond "enthusiastically" to maize, cassava still remains by far their dominant crop. In this field, they hardly accept even the minor modifications offered by the development project. For example, peasant participants have shown little inclination to interplant their cassava with "improved" maize varieties instead of growing it purestand (a recommendation that the project viewed as an adaptation to local practices), and they have not been interested in fertilizer or extension advice for their cassava fields.[83] It seems as if the peasants under the pressure of a changed market situation have accepted some outside interference in their land-use system, but they continue to regard cassava as the basis of their autonomy, which they are willing to defend even against a "development" type of intervention.

CONCLUSION

Although cassava is not indigenous to any part of Africa, its introduction to the Upper Zambezi was clearly the initiative of the indigenous population. Bearing in mind the fundamental implications for land-use systems, labor processes, and patterns of consumption this innovation had, it would indeed be possible to speak of an "indigenous agricultural [and dietary] revolution," following P. Richards.[84] The history of cassava in the Upper Zambezi shows, however, that this was not a revolution in the sense of a rapid and single event. It happened in several stages over a period of three centuries: the rapid introduction of cassava as a supplement to grain crops (millets); its slow expansion; and its acceleration only much later, when it became the substitute for grains. In more recent times, under different conditions, peasants have resorted to a strategy of non-innovation and have maintained or even defended cassava against attempts to reintroduce grain cultivation (mainly maize). The land-use patterns and diet of African peasants should be seen as a field of continuous experimentation and adaptation, quite contrary to still widespread prejudices concerning a "stagnant" rural economy caught in "traditional behavior." The case of cassava shows particularly well how little influence agricultural research institutions often have on these processes; on the contrary, they could learn a lot from peasant experience.

I asked at the beginning why peasants in the Upper Zambezi put so much effort into the adoption of a new staple crop that many of their neighbors, and probably initially they, too, regarded as "poor food." The reasons must be sought in several different but interacting dimensions. Cassava offered, first of all, clear advantages with regard to the economics of production, for the sake of which the peasants were apparently prepared to undergo major changes in their diet. Poor soils, climatic insecurities, and uneven seasonal distribution of labor requirements meant, and still mean, increased risks of crop failure under grain cultivation, and this probably accounted for the rapid introduction of cassava as soon as it became available in the seventeenth century. Cassava-based mixed cropping systems, in combination with other activities, seem to follow an "eco-logic" of adaptation to difficult or scarce natural conditions. At the same time, they appear to serve the well-known peasant "subsistence logic" of securing the food base, which is by no means necessarily a conservative factor.[85]

These explanations, however, seem insufficient. The expansion of cassava cultivation from the nineteenth century onward increasingly contradicted the model applied so far of optimal interaction between the individual producer and nature. With increasing cassava production, the *total* amount of labor required for nutrition probably increased as well, if processing and the need for supplementary foodstuffs for a balanced diet are taken into account. Rather than being a "lazy man's crop," cassava meant a shift of labor toward other activities, in addition to increasing the work load of women. In recent years, plant pests such as the mealie bug or mosaic disease have spread very rapidly in the endless peasant cassava fields of the Upper Zambezi. At the same time, game and fish resources are becoming increasingly scarce. A state of "ecological equilibrium" may have long since been disturbed. Maize cultivation, however, which is expanding now instead, appears to be ecologically harmful as well and nutritionally not much of an improvement—this lesson may be learned from other countries.

Such inconsistencies suggest that other factors are also at work. The history of cassava cultivation has shown that an understanding of the dynamics of agricultural and dietary change may be reached only by taking the wider historical context with its various social forces into consideration. In the case of the Upper Zambezi the decisive historical context has undoubtedly been the expansion of the world market. Here, cassava cultivation acted as a catalyst for increasing market integration in several ways.

To start with, it appears that cassava—perhaps similarly to potatoes in parts of Europe—became a means of cushioning the effects of capitalist penetration. One could argue that a sufficient supply of calories resulting from increased female work in cassava cultivation subsidized the extraction of (male) surplus labor through pre-colonial long-distance trade and the colonial system of circulating labor migration, though in the long run it was at the expense of a balanced diet.

But cassava has always played a double role. It has been not only a use-value but from the very beginning also an exchange value, and the priorities between these two have changed constantly over the past centuries: introduced in Angola originally as a cash crop, then adopted in the Upper Zambezi as a reliable food for the producers themselves, it became the main item of regional commodity production up to Independence. Subsequently, it was again degraded to a "subsistence crop"; but this may not be the last word in view of the Zambian government's recent attempts, under the pressure of economic crisis and international creditors, to re-establish an urban market for cassava. On closer examination it seems, therefore, that the expansion of cassava cultivation followed much less a rationale of peripheral-capitalist subsistence production than a logic of "petty commodity production."[86] Drawing on a dense network of regional food trade—basically an exchange of "calories for protein"— cassava became a major means of access to money and basic industrial commodities for local producers, many of them women, outside export production and labor migration.

Both commodity production and local "subsistence" always involve processes of circulation of, and questions of control over, land, labor, foodstuffs, and other essential goods. On this level, we find yet another explanation for the adoption of cassava: it was a useful instrument in the existing network of social interactions and power struggles. Although the new crop meant more work for them, it was attractive to women because it gave them greater independence from male contributions in production and more bargaining power in the village division of labor as well as vis-à-vis the market. This does not mean, however, that cassava led to more social equality: it only altered the power hierarchy. Cassava cultivation enabled resident elders, both men and women, to accumulate control over younger people and particularly immigrants; and it enhanced the political influence of chiefs. Cassava cultivators in general found it easier to resist government intervention in their productive base and, indirectly, capitalist pressure for proletarianization, that is, dependence on wage labor outside the area instead of local commodity production. Peasants in the Zambezi and Kabompo districts of Zambia were prepared to be looked upon as "just cassava eaters" by officials and "progressive farmers" as long as this gave them greater economic independence.

NOTES

The data on which this article is based mostly originate from a series of field research stays in Zambezi and Kabompo between 1979 and 1986 and include a variety of surveys and individual interviews, published oral traditions and early travelers' reports, colonial administrative records, and interviews with ex-colonial officers. I learned a lot about the strategies and views of village women concerning cassava from the excellent fieldwork done by Josefine Beck and Sabine Dorlöchter in 1986. I am also grateful for discussions of the views contained in this article, particularly with members of the Bologna Workshop and with Kate Crehan, now of New York.

1. Oral testimony by S. N., farmer and ward chairman in Kabompo, 18 June 1983.
2. Oral testimony by J. S., Zambezi, 21 Oct. 1986, kindly passed on by K. Crehan.
3. S. K. Hahn and J. Keyser, "Cassava: A Basic Food of Africa," *Outlook on Agriculture* 14, 2 (1985): 95; J. H. Cock, *Cassava: New Potential for a Neglected Crop* (Boulder and London: Westview, 1985), pp. 1–11.
4. For Northern Rhodesia/Zambia see, for example, D. G. Cowsey, J. R. Shaw, and A. Lesslie, Report to the Development Bank of Zambia on a Study to Determine the Feasibility of an Extension of Cassava Production on a Commercial Scale in Zambia (unpublished, Lusaka: Development Bank of Zambia, n.d. [ca. 1977]), p. 16. Serious agronomic research on cassava in Africa began only in the 1960s, and, subsequently, the focus of discussion shifted from the crop as such to the question of sweet vs. bitter varieties (Dr. Peter Ay, personal communication).
5. See K. Crehan and A. von Oppen, "Understandings of 'Development': An Arena of Struggle. The Story of a Development Project in Zambia," *Sociologia Ruralis* (1988), p. 126; and J. Redinha, "Subsídio para a história e cultura de mandioca entre os povos do nordeste de Angola," *Boletín do Instituto de Investigaçâo Científica de Angola* (1968), p. 98. A typical slogan displayed at the entrance of Zambezi's "Farm Training Center" is "Laziness is an enemy of Zambia."
6. In the late 1970s, only 47 percent of rural households in Zambia grew any cassava, compared to 84 percent for maize (see A. Marter, *Cassava or Maize?* [Lusaka: Rural Development Studies Bureau, 1978], p. 5).
7. In the five central African countries surrounding the Zaire basin (Angola, Zaire, Central African Republic, Gabon, Congo) compared to southern Africa (including Zambia,

excluding the Republic of South Africa), the percentages of staple crops in total food production 1981–83 (measured in cereal equivalents) were as follows:

	Millets	Maize	Cassava
Central Africa	1.1%	10.6%	75.1%
Southern Africa	5.3%	48.2%	18.9%

(The table is calculated from figures given in C. Hiebsch and S. K. O'Hair, "Major Domesticated Food Crops," in *Food in Subsaharan Africa*, ed. A. Hansen and D. McMillan [Boulder: Westview, 1986], p. 179.)

8. J. Hoover, "The Seduction of Ruwej" (Ph.D. diss., Yale University, 1978), p. 331; W. O. Jones, *Manioc in Africa* (Stanford: Stanford University Press, 1959), p. 66.

9. C. M. N. White, *A Preliminary Survey of Luvale Rural Economy* (Lusaka: Rhodes-Livingstone Institute, 1959), p. 17. The former importance of millet is reflected, for example, in the Luvale term for the annual custom of eating the first fruits: *kutoma masangu* , literally, "to eat bulrush millet" (ibid.).

10. See C. de Ficalho, *Plantas Uteis da Africa Portuguesa* (Lisbon: Agéncia Gêral das Colónias, 1947), p. 252f.; J. Vansina, "Finding Food: A Plea," *African Economic History* (1979): 12; J. Redinha, "Subsídio," p. 96.

11. M. Miracle, *Maize in Tropical Africa* (Madison: University of Wisconsin Press, 1966), pp. 93–95.

12. Quoted in W. O. Jones. *Manioc*, p. 62.

13. J. Hoover, "Seduction," p. 579.

14. W. O. Jones, *Manioc*, p. 63.

15. J. Redinha. "Subsídio," p. 106: J. Hoover, "Seduction." p. 332 n. 14.

16. J. Redinha, "Subsídio," p. 105.

17. J. -L. Vellut, "Notes sur les Lunda et la frontière luso-africaine, 1700–1900," *Etudes d'histoire africaine* 3 (1972): 74, 78.

18. J. Hoover. "Seduction," p. 579.

19. J. Redinha. "Subsídio," p. 102; M. K. Sangambo, *The History of the Luvale People and Their Chieftainship* (Mize, n.d. [2d ed. ca. 1985; 1st ed. 1979]).

20. R. J. Papstein, "The Upper Zambezi: A History of the Luvale People, 1000–1900" (Ph.D. diss., UCLA, 1978), p. 219.

21. J. Redinha, "Subsídio," pp. 99–103; A. von Oppen. E. Shula, U. Alff et al., LIMA Target Group Survey, Final Report, (unpublished IRDP project document, Kabompo, 1983), p. 108.

22. R. J. Papstein ("Upper Zambezi," pp. 118, 123) assumes a late fifteenth-century date of departure for the Imbangala, Chokwe, and Luvale senior political titles.

23. T. Q. Reefe, "The Societies of the Eastern Savannah," in *History of Central Africa*, ed. D. Birmingham and P. M. Martin (London: Longman, 1983), 1:190.

24. A. da Silva Teixeira, "Relaçâo da viage q fis desta cidade de Benguela para as do Louar, no anno de 1794"; and Anon., "Derrota de Benguella para o Sertâo [1803]"; both in *Apontamentos sôbre a colonizaçâo dos planaltos e litoral do sud de Angola*, ed. A. de Albuquerque Felner (Lisbon: Agencia Gêral das Colónias, 1940), 1:237, 2:24–25.

25. See E. Boserup, *The Conditions of Agricultural Growth* (London: Allen and Unwin, 1965); P. Richards, On the South Side of the Garden of Eden: Creativity and Invention in Sub-Saharan Agriculture, unpublished seminar paper, University College, London, n.d. (ca. 1986).

26. Bulrush millet (and sorghum) yields are about 600–700 kg per hectare under "traditional" African smallholder conditions, compared to an average of about 9,000 kg/ha for cassava

(with a period of approximately three years from planting to complete harvest, i.e., 3,000 kg/ha per year) under western Zambian conditions (Minster Agriculture Ltd., *Farm Survey Kabompo District. Final Report* [Thame/Eschborn: German Agency for Technical Cooperation, 1982], Appendix 7–2; A. Marter, *Cassava or Maize?*, p. 32).

27. Birds, rodents, and insects cause regular pre- and post-harvest losses for millets, while large game (elephants) are the only serious threat to the cassava root.

28. A classic in the analysis of this problem is A. Richard, *Land, Labour and Diet in Northern Rhodesia* (Oxford: Oxford University Press, 1939), on the Bemba in Northern Province.

29. See J. C. Miller, "The Significance of Drought, Disease and Famine in the Agriculturally Marginal Zones of West-Central Africa," *Journal of African History* 23 (1982): 21ff.

30. See Cock, *Cassava*, p. 18. Climatic variations do affect the above-ground parts of the plant, but there is no direct relationship to the growth of the tubers (M. J. T. Norman et al., *The Ecology of Tropical Food Crops* [Cambridge: Cambridge University Press, 1984], pp. 230–234).

31. See note 62, below.

32. Bulrush millet, for example, contains about 13% crude protein, maize about 9.5%, compared to only about 2.8% for cassava meal (when reduced to the same water content as grains) (C. Hiebsch and S. O'Hair, "Food crops," pp. 182–183)

33. Personal observations.

34. M. K. Sangambo, *History*.

35. M. K. Sangambo, *History*, p. 70; R. J. Papstein, "Upper Zambezi," p. 230. Dried fish, for example, is still the most important export article from the area.

36. See V. Turner, *Schism and Continuity in Ndembu Village Life* (Manchester: Manchester University Press, 1957), pp. 21ff.; C. M. N. White, "The Role of Hunting and Fishing in Luvale Society," *African Studies* (1956), p. 85ff.

37. See J. Beck and S. Dorlöchter, " 'Wahileyi': Women's Agricultural Activities as a Basis for Subsistence and for Their Economic Independence," in *Is Small Beautiful? Five Case Studies on Rural Economic Activities and the Impact of Development Projects in the Zambezi and Kabompo Districts* (*NW Zambia*), ed. K. Crehan and A. von Oppen (Berlin: Institut für Soziologie, Freie Universität, 1987), pp. B50f., B56f.

38. J. Beck and S. Dorlöchter, "'Wahileyi'," pp. 53ff., 81f. See also C. M. N. White, *Preliminary Survey*, p. 21f.; A. Spring and A. Hansen, "The Underside of Development: Agricultural Development and Women in Zambia," *Agriculture and Human Values* 2, 1 (1985): 63.

39. C. M. N. White, *Luvale Social and Political Organization* (Lusaka: Rhodes Livingstone Institute, 1960), p. 40f.; A. Spring, "Women's Rituals and Natality among the Luvale of Zambia" (Ph.D. diss., Cornell University, 1976), p. 187f.

40. The Luvale term *wayileyi* (Lunda-Ndembu *wahileyi*) "translates literally as 'where were you' and is an abbreviated form of the derogatory unspoken question that accompanies this basket. 'Where were you when your friends were out working?' Self-sufficiency in the basic staple is valued, and everyone should assure their staple food supply. If a person must purchase food, local people attribute this to being too lazy to work hard at cultivating their own fields" (A. Hansen, "When the Running Stops: The Social and Economic Incorporation of Angolan Refugees into Zambian Border Villages" [Ph. D. diss., Cornell University, 1977], p. 215ff.).

41. J. Beck and S. Dorlöchter, "Frauen als 'Opfer der Entwicklung'? Strategien und Handlungsspielräume afrikanischer Kleinbäuerinnen zur Sicherung ökonomischer Unabhängigkeit" (Diplom thesis, Freie Universität Berlin, 1988), p. 168.

42. For a description see C. M. N. White, *Tradition and Change in Luvale Marriage* (Lusaka: Rhodes-Livingstone Institute, 1962), p. 10.

43. D. G. Cowsey, J. R. Shaw, and A. Lesslie, *Extension of Cassava*, p. 46. In tropical lowlands the maturation period is only 12–15 months (ibid.).

44. J. Beck and S. Dorlöchter, " 'Wahileyi'," p. B33.

45. Instead of being a burden, as was alleged by Zambian administrators (see, for example, *Times* of *Zambia*, 22 Aug. 1986), the resident population turned the refugees into an

asset for local food production. For a more detailed analysis of this phenomenon see A. Hansen, "When the Running Stops," p. 215ff.

46. C. M. N. White, *Social and Political Organization*, p. 44.
47. See R. J. Papstein, "Upper Zambezi," p. 179f.
48. According to J. C. Miller, "Significance," p. 28f., major droughts in west-central Africa were one typical event that produced hostages or "slaves."
49. R. J. Papstein, "The Upper Zambezi," p. 171.
50. See, for example, C. Harding, *In Remotest Barotseland* (London: Hurst and Blecket, 1904), p. 91.
51. See Ficalho, *Plantas Uteis*, p. 250; J. Redinha, "Subsídio," pp. 101, 102; A. von Oppen, E. Shula, and U. Alff, *LIMA Survey*, p. 108.
52. C. M. N. White, *Preliminary Survey*, p. 18.
53. I. Schapera, ed., *Livingstone's African Journals, 1853–1856*, (London: Chatto and Windhus, 1963), 1: 36, 46, 65.
54. In the Ruund empire, much tribute *(mulombo)* had to be paid in the form of cassava flour to feed officials and inhabitants of the capital (see note 17, above). In Bulozi, food crops from the "King's Gardens," which were worked by subject peoples in areas surrounding the floodplain, made up most of the tribute that flowed into the capital for the same purpose (E. Hermitte, "An Economic History of Barotseland, 1800–1940" [Ph.D. diss., Northwestern University, 1974], p. 141).
55. Slave caravans usually comprised several hundred, sometimes thousands of people; caravans carrying "legitimate goods" were smaller, perhaps 50 to 60 people on average, but more frequent. It has been estimated for the 1880s that some 50,000 Ovimbundu, the main group of Angolan middlemen, were involved in trading in the interior, which means they either crossed the Upper Zambezi at least once a year or stayed there for up to six months. See J.-L. Vellut, "Lunda," pp. 91, 139; L. M. Heywood, "Production, Trade and Power. The Political Economy of Central Angola, 1850–1930" (Ph.D. diss., Columbia University. 1984), pp. 153, 173; and various travelers' reports.
56. I. Schapera, ed., *Livingstone's African Journals*, passim, gives many instances of this.
57. V. L. Cameron, *Across Africa* (London, 1877) 2:169.
58. Oral testimony by Y. S., Dipalata Area, Zambezi, 21 Oct. 1986.
59. See A. von Oppen, "Abwanderung, Arbeitskraftentzug und Lebensbedingungen in einer peripheren Region Zambias," *Zeitschrift für Wirtschaftsgeographie* 29 (1985): 92f.
60. C. M. N. White, *Preliminary Survey*, p. 48.
61. Ibid., p. 24. Similarly, a great increase in the percentage of cassava was observed in the 1950s in Mwinilunga (Lunda Ndembu), where in 1940 a lot of fingermillet had still been grown (C. M. N. White, "Factors in Luvale Social and Political Organization," *African Studies* 14, 3 [1955], p. 112).
62. This system was observed in its purest form among the Luvale west of the Zambezi; the importance of millet declined and cassava (interplanted with grains) was increasingly planted in even the first year of cultivation the farther one got toward the eastern uplands inhabited by Luchazi, Mbunda, and Southern Lunda, successively. This led the surveyors to fall back on a current ethnicist and evolutionist terminology, and to classify the "Luvale system" with its higher percentage of millet and frequent shifting of fields as more "backward" than the land-use pattern of neighboring groups. But it was the same authors who realized for the first time that "the practice adopted depends as much on the soil obtained for cultivation as on custom" (C. G. Trapnell and J. N. Clothier, *The Soils, Vegetation and Agricultural Systems of North-Western Rhodesia* [Lusaka: Government Printer, 1937], pp. 31–32).
63. C. M. N. White, *Preliminary Survey*, pp. 24–28.
64. *Marketing Report Balovale* 1963, National Archives of Zambia (NAZ), file MA 169/3.
65. E.g., *Annual Report Barotse District* 1928 (NAZ, file ZA 7/1); see also E. Hermitte, Economic History, pp. 299–301.

66. *Annual Reports Barotse/Western Province* 1935, 1939, 1948 (NAZ, file SEC 2/71). The maximum was reached in 1953, when 1247 t of cassava meal, plus over 700 t of other crops (groundnuts millet, maize, rice, and beans) were exported from Balovale/Kabompo (*Annual Reports Balovale and Kabompo*, NAZ, file SEC 2/136).
67. Oral testimony by D. C., Dipalata Area, Zambezi, 16 Oct. 1986.
68. C. M. N. White, *Preliminary Survey*, p. 41.
69. *Annual Report Balovale* 1953 (NAZ, file SEC 2/136). This modernist view is expressed in even plainer terms in the *Northern Rhodesia Annual Report on African Affairs for 1960* (Lusaka: Government Printer, 1961), which alleged that "the [Northwestern] Province generally adheres rigidly to the traditional forms of cultivation and a restricted subsistence economy" (p. 9)—against better knowledge.
70. In addition, annual crops such as grains fit much better into the one-year budget plans of research and other institutions (communication by Dr. P. Ay).
71. See, for example, *Annual Report Balovale* 1951 (NAZ, file SEC 2/135); also C. G. Trapnell and J. N. Clothier. *The Soils*, §191; C. M. N. White, *Preliminary Survey*, p. 19.
72. Interview with Mr. O. -E., ex-administrator, 2 Nov. 1987.
73. See, for example, C. G. Trapnell and J. N. Clothier, *The Soils*, §191.
74. See, for example, *Annual Report Barotse District, Balovale Subdistrict* 1928 (NAZ, file KDE 8/1); *Kaonde Lunda Province 5-Year Development Plan* 1943, Schedule 8 (NAZ, file SEC 2/279). The legal basis of these market restrictions was mainly the "Native Foodstuffs (Control of Acquisition) Ordinance" of 1940.
75. See, for example, *Northern Rhodesia Annual Report on African Affairs for 1953* (Lusaka: Government Printer, 1954), p. 22.
76. *Northern Rhodesia Annual Report on Native Affairs for 1930* (Lusaka: Government Printer, 1931), pp. 12–13. See also D. G. Cowsey, J. R. Shaw, and A. Lesslie, *Extension of Cassava*, p. 16f.
77. *Annual Reports on African Affairs*, Balovale 1954 and 1952 (NAZ, SEC 2/135); also *Annual Reports* 1948, 1949 (NAZ, SEC 2/155–156).
78. See, for example, *Northern Rhodesia Annual Report* 1953, p. 22: *Northern Rhodesia Annual Report on African Affairs for 1959* (Lusaka, Government Printer, 1960), p. 32; *Annual Report Balovale* 1949.
79. Various oral testimonies.
80. *Marketing Report Balovale* 1963 (NAZ, file MA 169/3); *Data Book North-Western Province* (Lusaka: Office of National Development and Planning, 1968).
81. A. von Oppen, Wanderarbeit, Unterentwicklung und Lebensbedingungen in einer peripheren Region Zambias: Der Kabompo-Distrikt (Diplom thesis, Freie Universität Berlin, 1981), p. 159.
82. Interview with J. H., former colonial official, 9 Dec. 1986.
83. A. von Oppen, E. Shula, and U. Alff, *LIMA Survey*, p. 117; K. Crehan and A. von Oppen, "Understandings of 'Development'," p. 138.
84. P Richards, *Indigenous Agricultural Revolution* (London: Allen and Unwin, 1985).
85. See also, for example, J. C. Scott. *The Moral Economy of the Peasant* (New Haven and London: Yale University Press, 1976).
86. See H. Bernstein, "Capitalism and Petty Commodity Production," in *Rethinking Petty Commodity Production*, ed. A. M. Scott, special issue of *Social Analysis* 20 (1986): 20.

3. THE COOK, HIS WIFE, THE MADAM, AND THEIR DINNER: COOKING, GENDER AND CLASS IN ZAMBIA

Karen Tranberg Hansen

Northwestern University, Anthropology Department,
Evanston, IL 60208-1310, USA

This article concerns the effects of the colonial encounter and recent changes in food availability on cooking practices in urban Zambia. Highlighting issues of gender and household dynamics, the article draws on my research into urban domestic service in colonial and postcolonial Zambia (Hansen 1989).[1] The skills, including European cuisine, taught to male African servants in white colonial households were imparted with the assumption that this new knowledge would be transferred to African homes and thus contribute to introduce western-derived patterns of behavior and consumption.

As I demonstrate on the pages that follow, the significance of cooking in this encounter had less to do with ingredients and skills than with matters internal to African households. In the post-colonial era, where the majority of employers of servants are black Zambians, the standard Zambian meal of starch and relish holds top rank in daily eating habits with western foods having mainly snack, or special occasion functions. Thus both in colonial and postcolonial servant employing households in Zambia, cooking practices constitute a gender, race, and class divided battlefront on which African gender and household dynamics confronted new dishes and foodstuffs that required different methods of preparation and serving. The continued valorization of the standard Zambian meal throughout these processes testify to the complexity of dietary transformations, and above all it demonstrates the centrality of household dynamics to our understanding of persistent food habits.

From the early colonial period in what then was Northern Rhodesia until today in the cities and towns of Zambia, domestic service has been a crucial wage occupation for a large proportion of men and, after independence in 1964, an increasing number of women. The work experiences of cooks between then and now have changed and the consequences are vexing. After a brief discussion of cuisine and cooking, I first explore the kitchen as a battlefront between tools, people, and ideas that produces not only meals but particular social relations that have to do with gender and class. Then I enter some colonial servant employing households, examining the servants' acquisition of skills. I next describe the extent of transfer of cooking skills to African households, raising questions about the transformative capacity of this aspect of the colonial encounter and about gender. And lastly I turn to the work of postcolonial servants, exploring reasons for the levelling out of cooking practices from a cuisine of luxury to cooking of necessity.

COOKING AND THE COLONIAL ENCOUNTER

For an analysis of cooking, Jack Goody takes us to the door of the household in his study of the difference between the cuisines of West Africa and those of Europe and Asia. Criticizing Claude Levi-Strauss's binary abstraction of culinary systems into so many recipes (1970, 1973, 1978) and Mary Douglas's cultural grammar of meals (1971; Douglas and Nicod 1974), Goody proposes a comparative explanation in terms of local economic production and social differentiation (1982: 17–39). Cooking, he argues, needs to be analyzed in the context of the total process of production, preparation, and consumption of food. He suggests that we find a "high" cuisine where people have differentiated access to resources. The extreme form of this differentiation is the allocation of special foods to specific roles, offices, or classes and a gulf between them not only of quantity, but of quality, of complexity, and of ingredients (1982: 99). He also notes that the "high" and the "low" cuisines are divided sexually, and that hierarchy, specialization and elaborate cooking are associated with men as cooks. Only in societies such as in Africa did women cook at the courts of kings, yet Goody qualifies, not as household servants but as wives. What is also different in Africa, he says, is the virtual absence of alternatives or differentiated recipes either for feast or for class.

Having explained why most precolonial African societies lack a differentiated cuisine, Goody discusses the impact of industrial cooking on food and consumption style, and the creation of a new mix of diets everywhere. He observes a "tendency towards the homogenisation of taste that accompanies the industrial processes of the world system," closing consumption gaps in the more advanced countries and opening them in the more peripheral (1982: 189). When people add on elements of western consumption, modifying their local forms of cooking without giving it up, Goody speaks of culinary diglossia (1982: 184). He is careful to note that "the direction of these changes is not determined by the world system alone. The nature of the indigenous societies is of prime importance; so too is the nature of the particular colonial encounter" (1982: 183).

Goody's acknowledgement that styles of cooking are shaped also by the particularities of the encounter between colonial culture and indigenous practices opens many interpretative possibilities. In his study of the rise of sugar consumption in the West, Sidney Mintz recognizes the complicated and many-sided forces involved in changing consumption patterns. He argues: "patterns will not yield unless the conditions under which consumption occurs are changed—not just what is worn, but where and when, and with whom; not just what is eaten, but where and when, and with whom" (1986: 194). The state and the market are not the only forces that provoke shifts in consumption styles. An account of such changes needs to take us *inside* the household and reckon with the ideological in a wide sense of that term. As my discussion of cooking in domestic service will illustrate, this aspect certainly ties in with the socio-economic pattern, but does not reflect it in any straightforward way.

When British colonial officials in Northern Rhodesia attributed a "distinct educational value" to domestic service, they were thinking of their African men servants whom they believed they might "make over" and civilize, instilling new skills, notions of individual responsibility and morality, and values of work, time, order and cleanliness which they would apply to improve their own household organization (Hansen 1989: 27).

But the meanings of these new skills were not self-evident to Africans. They were refracted through notions of class condescension and racism that were central to the molding of colonial domestic service conventions in Northern Rhodesia. The difference between European and African diets constituted an important social and cultural barrier that was not erased by the African cook's work in colonial households. Thus cooking has ambiguous meanings caused by the different experiences people have of it, or, in Pierre Bourdieu's words, caused by the dispositions, "they derive from their position in economic space" (1984: 101). Cooking meant different things, depending on one's place in a race divided and class structured society, and, as I discuss shortly, on gender. While that oppressive opportunity structure scarcely allowed the transformation of Africans in the image of Europeans, it did not preclude them from reworking colonial notions of domesticity and civilization on their own terms. In short, domestic work, the colonial kitchen, styles of cooking, are influenced by more than household management with tools and resources, the distribution of power in the economic sphere, and lifestyles and tastes (Davidoff 1976, Douglas 1971). It is also affected by the meanings people attribute to cooking, by their ideas about who does it and where, and thus it is about the construction and possible transformation of particular social relationships.

CUISINE, RACE, AND CLASS

Colonial whites considered Africans to be members of societies so totally different from their own in social, cultural, and moral outlook that they had to be "broken in," worked, and handled, in short to become domesticated.[2] In private household service white women faced the task of turning African men whom they considered as "raw natives" into domestic workers, skilled at "keeping house like in London" under circumstances where many amenities were lacking. Most colonial households employed a fair number of servants. So there were separate cook, house, laundry, scullery, wood, water, garden boys, and so forth. From the point of view of the employer, these men servants formed a hierarchy of domains between kitchen, home, and grounds in a strict division of labor with the kitchen at the top.

Domestic work was hard work. It was labor intensive and largely done without the use of labor saving appliances even when vacuum cleaners, floor polishers, washing machines, and a variety of kitchen gadgets became more readily available. The colonial servant's job was specialized. He was cook, tableboy, houseboy, or worked on the grounds, and he could look forward to advancement through the ranks.

Because employers considered them to be simple, they also thought that their servants were impressionable. Just what skills did such men acquire during their life-long work in domestic service? They did not enter domestic service with ready-made skills, but were trained. As cooks, men were taught and expected to prepare a differentiated cuisine. Using a variety of locally available and imported foodstuffs, African cooks were crucial to their employers' efforts at reproducing a familiar lifestyle. Some cooks could read recipes, others committed them to memory. They were taught and coached by their madams, who expected them to be able to prepare coffee and tea, and breakfasts; to make bread, cake, and pastry; soup stock and sauces; to master the arts of boiling, frying, and roasting of meat, poultry, and fish; and to prepare a variety of desserts (Bradley 1939, 1948, 1950: 19–20). It is not surprising that cooks who had worked for many different white employers were proud of their specialized skills.

Aside from acquiring knowledge of cuisine, such men servants learned to observe etiquette and manners. The serving of tea is one example of etiquette servants learned as workers in a labor process that was hierarchically structured in social and spatial terms. When on duty, servants wore uniforms, but rarely shoes; they were not supposed to talk unless they were spoken to; they were usually called by their first name and referred to as "boys;" they were not to use the facilities of the main house. There was subordination and discipline everywhere. Although many servants lived in small shacks at the end of their employers' gardens, this space was not theirs for they were considered always available. Their lives when off work were not really private, for the employers decided whether spouses and dependants could live in, when and which visitors could call, and what sort of leisure time activity might be undertaken.

Some employers and some Africans believed that the servants' privileged knowledge of the European way of life led to their easy way with African women. Chief among the activities white householders related about their men servants were drinking, gambling, and sex. Employers often attributed their servants' tardiness on Mondays to weekend brawls, drinking, and cavorting with women in the compounds. The stereotype of the servant as womanizer struck a cord in a snappy song by popular musician Alick Nkatha in the 1950s. The song depicts the servant pursuing a beautiful woman with promises of morning coffee, toast and butter, and "so many dresses you'll be changing clothes all day" (Fraenkel 1959: 51–2). Whether or not this stereotype reflected reality, many employers preferred to hire married men as their servants, with the assumption that a married man takes his job seriously since he has wife and dependents to provide for.

My discussions with colonial menservants, their wives, and their employers converge on one issue: the disassociation of African men's paid domestic work from any female gender connotation. Domestic service was a "job of work" which men learned from their employers. It was wage labor. And men did wage labor; women stayed home. In short, the work of African servants was skilled work, men's work.

COOKING, GENDER, AND URBAN AFRICAN HOUSEHOLDS

Did men servants apply these skills in their own context of living? An answer to this question is ambiguous, for it depends not only on cultural practices based on gender, and age that informed interpersonal interaction in African households, but also on the restrictions colonial rules and regulations placed on the transfer of western derived notions of domesticity to

African homes. Gender relations in African households required women to feed the family. The standard meal Zambian women cooked consisted of a starchy staple and a relish of vegetables, meat or fish eaten with it, the difference between rich and poor being largely one of quantity eaten rather than of quality of ingredients and elaboration of preparation. Strong connotations of taste surrounded this standard Zambian meal. Thus, starch and relish must be served together for a meal to taste good and be properly satisfying.

To be sure, there were variations over this meal pattern. For starches, there were sorghum, millet, cassava and maize. The cultivation and consumption of maize increased during the colonial period when maizemeal became the staple for the rapidly growing urban populations. Rice production has been introduced more recently. In addition, different regions had their own specialities; some groups ate rodents, others fish. The relish might contain more or less meat, chicken, fish (dried or fresh, roasted or fried), and insects. It included many different vegetables (e.g., greens, beans, groundnuts, mushrooms).

There were several ways of preparing the relish. The most common procedure makes use of cooking oil, onions and tomatoes. Then there is the use of grated groundnuts. Another method adds baking soda to ocra, at times including onions and tomatoes. And salt, if available, adds taste to the Zambian meal which does not commonly include the red hot pepper that so spices the standard meal in much of West Africa. Oil seeds, onions and tomatoes are not indigenous crops in Zambia. In so far as Zambians today consider them to be basic ingredients of a proper meal, they represent a recreated tradition that is a product of fairly recent history. But in the final analysis, these practices do not produce differentiation in Goody's sense, but constitute variations of exclusion or inclusion on the shared basics in the starch/relish theme.

From my own study, I know of no one single instance of African men servants exercising their skills in preparing, say, Irish stews or roasts in their own households. There, cooking was a woman's task, and the work of a servant, a skilled cook, was a "job of work" that ceased on the threshold of his own household. Aside from cooking being defined as women's work in the African household context, prohibitive food expenses and unaffordable kitchen technology contributed to the continuity of African meal patterns in spite of the new skills and knowledge of cuisine that African men acquired in colonial household employment. European cuisine would under all circumstances have been too expensive for most servant households. The rapidly growing consumption of tea, refined sugar, white bread, cooking oil, and jams, reported in urban surveys from the late 1930s onward, was added onto African diets but did not transform the standard meal pattern of starch and relish (Bettison 1959, Thomson 1954, Wilson 1942: 211–31, Woodruff 1955: 70). Even if African men had wanted to apply their acquired skills in cooking within their own kitchens, their wages were too low to allow the purchase of the requisite ingredients. This wage differential determined by the color bar was built into the organization of commerce and retail on the assumption that African diets, and consumption patterns in general, were different from Europeans'. Separate butcheries and special sections for African customers in European shops sold lesser quality meat, known as "boys' meat."

Even if wages had allowed the purchase of prime cuts, the kitchen technology in most urban African households would have complicated their preparation. Even if the employers' house had electricity and piped water, servants' quarters rarely included such amenities. Cooking was done by charcoal fuel, often out of doors, and most households possessed but one charcoal brazier. If undertaken inside, cooking produced smoke and grime. This time consuming process was best suited for the preparation of an inclusive relish, rather than for many individual dishes.

Wages, finally, were too low to enable servants to create the kind of home envisioned in the European derived domesticity ideal: organized around values of order, privacy and domestic bliss. Servants' quarters were typically one- or two-roomed affairs, at times shared by several servant households. Such housing (not houses) affronted African notions of propriety between the sexes and the generations, forcing a man to sleep in the same room as his wife and children, and causing embarrasment about where to bathe and dress.

AFRICAN WOMEN, DOMESTIC SKILLS AND CLASS

If men servants were to set an example with their new skills, they would first have had to reorganize their own homes and, in particular, redefine their women's cooking practices. While colonial authorities attributed civilizing functions to domestic service in white households, that is to say, to African men's work, they blamed African women for the slow development of "proper homes." But better housing, better wages, and training for African women were slow in the offing. And had it not been for the white employers' need for creature comforts, they cared little about how their household workers lived. This is demonstrated in a discussion during the 1940s about how many servants white employers in civil service were entitled to and how to house them. There was no agreement about whether servants should live in and be allowed to have wives and dependants with them. In the view of most whites, African women meant trouble. Having African wives and children on the premises would cause noise and uncleanliness, yet without some permanent female company, servants would probably solicit women's services when off work, and this would adversely affect their constancy in work (Hansen 1989: 172–3).

In the colonial white view, urban African women sat around and were lazy; or they solicited men while their partners were at work. They were slow to take to the domestic science and homecraft classes that philanthropic groups, mainly churches, began to organize from the mid 1930s (Hope 1944, Powdermaker 1962: 109, Taylor and Lehmann 1961). The debate about recruiting African women into domestic service during the post World War II years when the mining economy boomed and men's labor was needed elsewhere, attributed women's poor potential as servants to their alleged loose morals. Although this debate overtly concerned skills, it conflated gender and sexuality (Hansen 1989: 120–38). Speaking in the language of skills, i.e. cooking, colonial employers agreed with their African men workers that African women could not cook, that is to say that they had not mastered the skills of a differentiated cuisine.

The few African women who did work in colonial households were hired as nannies. They did not relieve white women of the chief tasks of child care, but watched the children, pushed the pram, and washed the nappies, something which "nurse boys" also did, and in larger numbers than women. They may have worked as Betty Kaunda did in the early 1940s, long before she became the ex-president's wife, looking after the district officer's baby for a couple of hours after school. She worked in this capacity in a succession of colonial households until she left home for boarding school (Mpashi 1969: 15–7).

Most of the African women who acquired western-derived domestic skills did not do so in white households. The chief outlet for the ideological aspect of domestic science was the homecraft courses organized by church and mission groups and the newly established (1952) welfare department (Mann 1959, NAZ/NR 5/512 1949–59). Such courses were not organized for the purpose of enabling African women to replace the skilled male cooks in paid domestic service or to engage in other forms of wage labor. They aimed at instilling notions about proper homes and to upgrade the home life of the emerging African elite by making women into suitable wives, skilled in nutrition, baby care, simple cooking, house cleaning, and handicrafts. The cultural arrogance, paternalism, and gender assumptions that informed such teaching are exemplified in cookbooks for Africans (e.g., Kaye 1939, Cartwright and Robertson 1957), in recipes for European-type dishes like scotch eggs and chocolate cake (African Listener 1955: 7), and columns about how to dress well, with matching handbag, shoes, and hat (African Listener 1957a: 12, 1957b: 9) featured in magazines the colonial information service published for elite Africans.

It is difficult to assess the impact of domestic science education on the many African women who were exposed to it, yet it is certain that the results occasionally were at variance with the white teaching staff's intentions.[3] When Betty Kaunda's and Salome Kapwepwe's husbands had been appointed ministers on the eve of independence, they moved from tiny houses in the African township, Chilenje, into larger government houses. They certainly enjoyed having more space as their households, including extended family members, numbered eleven and eight respectively. To help them run their homes, they employed male domestic servants, Mrs. Kapwepwe three, and Mrs. Kaunda, who was looking for an expert cook, had two. Cooking in such elite households was thus not done by women, but by men cooks. These households had not switched entirely to European-type food, for as Mrs. Kapwepwe explained: "we usually receive many visitors from our home district in the Northern Province who are not used to the European-type food" (Nshila 1963: 40–1).

In short, those African households that opened up for a partial penetration of European notions of domesticity were mainly those that were better off, where men certainly did not make a living as domestic servants, and wives did not cook on a regular basis. Rather than creating better homes and wives, colonial domestic service practices reproduced distinctions between emerging Zambian classes and between women and men. For most of the colonial period in Northern Rhodesia, racial distinctions built into the material organization of daily life prevented African men servants from transferring the skills they acquired from domestic work for whites to their own households. Urban housing arrangements clashed with African notions of gender, age, and space, and normative assumptions about gender and about standard Zambian meals made men servants, then and now, resist the transfer of their cooking skills to their own households where the preparation of starch and relish based meals remained African women's work.

COOKING AND GENDER IN POSTCOLONIAL HOUSEHOLDS

Paid domestic service in postcolonial Zambia has changed in many respects, particularly among the employers who today predominantly are black Zambians.[4] The nature of the work undertaken in private households has changed as well. The colonial staff of specialized men servants has largely been replaced by one general servant. The exception to this is a tiny segment of the servant employing classes whose workers often are paid via company payroll. The general servant is a man who works inside the house and on the grounds. When asked to cook for his black Zambian employers, he complains of doing "women's work." This does not mean that domestic work has become a woman's job, for men servants outnumber women by far. Men still take servant jobs because they have few other choices. But they bitterly resent the subordination they experience in the work relationship to their black Zambian employers who demand that they do everything within the house and on the grounds, including the cooking of Zambian food, which is women's work.

The gradual levelling out of distinct task specializations into the work of the male general servant is a product of an ongoing recomposition among the employing classes: from white colonial employers mainly of British background to black Zambian employers, and within the steadily declining number of whites, a shift from largely British colonists to expatriates from many different parts of the world. Servants who worked for colonial employers will tell you that today even *wazungus* (whites, expatriates in general) eat *nshima* (maize porridge). This does not mean that expatriates regularly eat the urban Zambian food staple of maize porridge, but that women expatriate householders themselves do most of the cooking which is less elaborate than the cuisine served up by the colonial cook.

The last, but certainly not least noticeable change between the colonial period and the present is that larger numbers of women than ever before are employed in private households.[5] As I noted above, it was not the growing entry of women but the gendered meaning of cooking in Zambian households that long-time servants have in mind when they speak of domestic service becoming a "woman's job." For women are not taking over men's jobs but are hired chiefly as nannies. Because of their substandard wages and poor treatment, Zambian women consider domestic service as a job best to be avoided. When they do take a job as paid help in private households, it is as a last resort and mainly because of lack of household support.[6] They quit their nanny jobs as soon as they find something better, either a man to take care of them, or some economic means with which to start an informal sector activity. And only because they need child care do Zambian women employers tolerate their nannies, of whom they see several come and go throughout their childbearing years (Hansen 1990).

When they have had it with their nannies and/or when they can afford it, Zambian women hire men servants whom they in any case consider to be better domestic workers and, to be sure, better cooks. Yet cooking is a contested domain because of its implications about status/class and its sexual connotations. In my Lusaka survey, I came across Zambian civil servant households in which the male cook prepared "English" food (e.g. meat and boiled vegetables, served separately) for the household head, and the wife cooked Zambian food (*nshima* and relish) for herself and the children. In not-so-well-off households without cooks, I found the nanny making the children's food, while the wife took special care in the preparation and serving of her husband's Zambian meal. Many such husbands are still served separately and not simultaneously with the rest of the household.

In such households, a satisfactory meal today does not differ much from that Audrey Richards described for the rural Bemba in the 1930s. Such a meal "must be composed of two constituents: a thick porridge … and the relish … eaten with it" (1969: 46). Outside of the household, buns (and other bread products, if available), tea, soft drinks, and bottled beer, and a variety of prepared snacks (e.g. sausages, meat pies, samosas as well as *nshima* and relish) are consumed by urban wage workers on their lunch breaks. But neither during the colonial period nor at present has this consumption altered the basic procedures of Zambian cooking nor the composition of the standard Zambian meal: starch and relish.

When Zambian female householders claim that their women servants are poor cooks, they are not speaking of meals per se but of the sexual connotations of meal related behavior and the possibilities entailed in the woman servant's making and serving of meals to the male household head. As in several other parts of Africa (e.g. Clark 1989), the wife's preparation of food for her husband is a central obligation of marriage in Zambia. Receiving cooked food thus becomes symbolic of the legal and economic relationship between husband and wife. "Hence," according to Audrey Richards' observations from the 1930s, "it becomes a privilege and a matter of pride" for wives to attend to their husbands' food (1969: 129). The symbolic meanings and sexual connotations about preparing and receiving cooked food have not altogether disappeared from postcolonial urban Zambian households. The tensions they create between female householders and women servants give rise to many fears, among them allegations of women servants adding love potions to the relish.[7] Since the wife wishes to reduce the likelihood of compromising sexual encounters, she insists on being in charge of cooking her husband's meals herself.

SPECIAL OCCASIONS FOOD,
STANDARD MEALS, AND FOOD ACCESS

While much of what goes on in Zambian kitchens today calls forth notions of *déja vu*, the possibilities for cooking innovations remain potentially wide open, due to external influences. The food pages of a locally pub-lished women's magazine, *Woman's Exclusive*, do not differ much from those in the West. Its "cookery corner" features neither "traditional" foods, nor the colonial period's "English-type" cooking, but a blend of recipes from all over the world (1984a, b, 1989). Its readers, who in all likelihood have little practical involvement in the kitchen and employ both cooks and nannies, comprise among others the tiny jet-set who go on shopping trips abroad and run Lusaka's small boutiques. They are among the television viewing Zambian audience who watched Maggie Kaweche's cooking show "The Solution" in the mid-1980s. Ms. Kaweche, about whose mari-tal status rather than her cooking newspaper readers and television viewers wrote many enquiring letters, never wore an apron but sported the latest fashions and different hairstyles at each show while demonstrating how to prepare savory soups, pork chops, lemon meringue, and other delicacies on her electric stove, using beater, blender, and the newest in kitchen tech-nology. She did at times, when sponsored, include recipes using Zambian products such as sorghum and groundnuts.

While entertaining, the impact of Maggie Kaweche's cooking lessons was limited.[8] Viewers were watching Maggie, not her cooking, and the greater part of the urban population does not have electricity, nor does the rest of the country. The proportion of households with electricity increased from only 11.9 to 17.9 percent between 1969 and 1980. In the most urban-ized areas, that is the Copperbelt and Lusaka Provinces, electricity was available between 30 and 40 percent of the households in 1980. Nearly eight out of ten households in the urban areas depended on wood fuel and/or charcoal for cooking in 1980. This means that electricity served mostly lighting purposes and that only a small proportion of electrified households used this source of power for cooking (Republic of Zambia 1985: 45). Many households do not possess an electric stove and if they do, they may use it for special occasions rather than on a regular basis.

Special occasions include *kitchen parties*, the all-women's celebrations held before marriage when female relatives and friends get together, bring-ing presents "for the kitchen" and money, and in ribald performance style, tell the prospective bride about her duties and responsibilities in marriage. There is much banter, talking, singing, dancing, and drinking of beer. And food is served in an assemblage that throws light on the nature of festive cooking in Zambia and its appropriation of items from elsewhere. Among the foods on the plastic wrapped plate each guest received at a Lusaka kitchen party in a middle-income household in July 1989 were the following: a piece of chicken, a boiled egg, a samosa, a sausage, cabbage, beans and rice. I do not recall if there was a roll, for flour was a scarce item then, and bread was mainly available on the black market. The individual serving at the kitchen party provides a striking contrast to the usual meal served out of one pot and ritual occasions where food is served jointly. In more lavish, or scaled-down versions, such individually served meals are consumed at kitchen parties held at all class levels, except the poorest, in Zambia's towns.

Save among households of the powers that be, the few really wealthy citizens (who have differential access to consumer goods and perhaps even generators) and those in the direst of straits (who are reduced to eating *nshima* only), day-to-day cooking practices in postcolonial urban Zambia have much in common. The widely shared notion that a satisfactory and tasty meal must consist of starch and relish helps in part to account for this commonality of meal patterns. But so do restrictions which economic conditions are placing on the emergence of a differentiated cuisine. All households are affected by cuts in the supply of water and electricity. Those who have cookstoves, keep the brazier and a supply of charcoal ready. Thus, the consumption styles of servants and their black Zambian employers hardly differ, except in magnitude and diversity of relish and thus in protein content and source. This is largely due to the strained economy and many temporary bottlenecks in the distribution system that are forcing rich and poor, expatriates and Zambians, to shop in the same places. Recurrent scarcities of most basic consumer goods (e.g. maize-meal, charcoal, cooking oil, sugar, salt, flour, rice, soap, and detergent), spices and condiments notwithstanding, are in part to blame for the shift from the cuisine of luxury in colonial households to the cooking of necessity in most urban households today.

In so far as such shortages are a product of the efforts toward economic restructuration imposed on the government by international loan and aid providers, they tell a revealing tale of how IMF priorities are hitting Zambian kitchens (cf. Bolles 1983). A recent Lusaka survey indicates that economic stringencies are forcing poor households to cut down on protein sources, reduce the number of meals per day, or even eat *nshima* without relish, with dire consequences for the nutritional status of those who always ate least and last: women and children (Muntemba 1987: 24–6). Finally, food access depends not only on the relationship between local production and imports, externally imposed demands, and gender and age distinctions in consumption, but also on food aid, especially of maize, rice, and wheat, that give foreign governments and philanthropic groups a new role in shaping Zambian kitchens (cf. Khare 1986, Lindenbaum 1986).

CONCLUSION

Ideas about cooking and domestic work in Zambia are linked to the changing historical relationship between this part of southern Africa, and of Africa, to the West, to the process of decolonization, and to the internationalization of formerly distinct consumption styles. They are also becoming affected by IMF priorities and foreign food aid (Friedmann 1990, Raikes 1988). Yet this is not a story of straightforward cultural continuity or of wholesale Westernization. The adoption of styles of cooking and domestic arrangements in postcolonial Zambia has developed its own diglossia that is shaped by the slowdown of the economy and by practices pertaining to gender and household organization.

Such culinary diglossia, Goody suggests, gives rise to a relatively stable situation that is "part of an emergent system of socio-cultural stratification" (1982: 184). In postcolonial Zambia, food habits clearly have lost much of their past significance in setting boundaries between groups. Except for variety and quantity of relish, everyday meals share the same basic ingredients and are much alike across the urban Zambian class spectrum. Because of problems in the supply of power and commodities, the cookstove and the charcoal brazier coexist as do their distinct social usages. Today, the great mass of the Zambian urban population is setting food consumption styles regarding standard meals and in the process eliminating differences between cuisine and cooking in more ways than one: between classes, broadly speaking, and between local and external influences. But while food habits no longer serve as a powerful means for the marking of social boundaries, cooking, and the question of who cooks, continue to do so. When reduced to their simplest ingredients, the processes that are shaping food behavior in Zambian kitchens reveal themselves: men work as professional cooks, wives prepare meals for husbands, and nannies feed children.

ACKNOWLEDGEMENTS

This paper is based on research funded in 1982 by the McMillan Fund and the Office of International Programs at the University of Minnesota, from

1983 to 1985 by the U.S. National Science Foundation grant no. BNS 8303507, by a grant from the U.S. Social Science Research Council and the Africa Committee of the American Council of Learned Societies in 1988, and by faculty grants from Northwestern University in 1985, 1986, and 1989. This chapter represents a significantly revised version of a longer paper included in Hansen (1992).

NOTES

1. My study draws on extensive archival research in Great Britain, Zambia and Zimbabwe begun in 1982, and field research in Zambia 1983–84, 1985, 1988, and 1989, including the collection of life history data from retired employers of colonial servants in Great Britain and Zambia, elderly servants, and a sample survey in 187 servant employing households in middle- to upper-income residential areas in Lusaka, involving separate interviews with the chief domestic servant and the employer.
2. Because of the nature of my sources, most of my discussion of colonial European, or white, attitudes refers to the British. The fact that African, Asian ("Indian"), and Afrikaans-speaking households also employed servants does not mean that the master-servant relationship in British households was atypical or out of the ordinary. On the contrary, since the British were the dominant group in political terms, they set the norms and standards against which social interaction and practices were evaluated.
3. Neither the education nor the welfare departments had much success with their homecraft classes and clubs for women in the African townships. The white staff of the departments realized this, as indicated, for example in NAZ/NR 2/27 African Welfare, General Correspondence, 1944–54, and NAZ/NR 2/512 Native Education, Female, 1949–59.
4. In my sample survey of 187 servant employing households in Lusaka, 42 percent of the employers were Zambian, 33 percent whites, and 25 percent Asians.
5. These 187 households employed among them a total of 311 full-time servants, 232 of whom were men and 79 women. Focusing on the chief domestic worker in these households, we interviewed 131 men and 56 women. Most of these women were employed as nannies. I suggest that women comprise between one third and one fourth of this occupational group.
6. Thirty-five percent of the women servants in my sample survey were married and lived with their husbands (compared with 67 percent men), 13 percent had not married (compared with 20 percent men), and 52 percent (compared with 13 percent men) were either divorced, widowed, or living away from their spouses and supporting children without receiving financial assistance from a man on a regular basis.
7. Some Zambian women will go to great expense to buy love medicines to attract a man's love and ensure his financial attention. On this, see Keller (1978) and Jules-Rosette, especially her discussion about urban medicine (1981: 129 168).
8. According to Deborah Spitulnik, Radio 4, a new radio channel in Zambia, launched in 1989, aired a call-in cooking program "In the Kitchen" some time during 1989. The listeners who called in comprised three broad categories: 1) male servants providing detailed explanations of recipies they cooked for expatriate employers; 2) Zambian teenagers from urban elite households who seemed to be reading recipies from European cookbooks, e.g. for chocolate cake with icing, apparently making up a familiarity with fancy cooking they did not have (nor would the ingredients be readily available for purchase); and 3) persons cooking Zambian food like *nshima* and *kapenta* (dried fish) who had a hard time giving "recipies" for procedures of cooking which everyone is supposed to know. Like the television show "The Solution," the potential impact of the radio program was limited, in this

case to those literate in English who happened to be "at home" at 10 am. in the morning when the program went on the air, and who had access to a telephone (Deborah Spitulnik, personal communication, October 17, 1990).

REFERENCES

African Listener. 1955. "Recipes." 41: 7.
———. 1957a. "The Well-Dressed Woman. Part 1." 63: 12.
———. 1957b. "The Well-Dressed Woman. Part 2." 64: 9.
Bettison, David S. 1959. "Numerical Data on African Dwellers in Lusaka, Northern Rhodesia." *Rhodes-Livingstone Communication*, no. 16.
Bolles, A. Lynn. 1983. "Kitchens Hit by Priorities: Employed Working-Class Jamaican Women Confront the IMF." In J. Nash and M. P. Fernandez Kelly, eds., *Women, Men and the International Division of Labor*. Albany: State University of New York Press, pp. 138–159.
Bourdieu, Pierre. 1984. *Distinction: A Social Critique of the Judgement of Taste*. Cambridge, MA: Harvard University Press.
Bradley, Emily. 1939. *A Household Book for Africa*. London: Oxford University Press.
———. 1948. *A Household Book for Tropical Colonies*. London: Oxford University Press.
———. 1950. *Dearest Priscilla: Letters to the Wife of a Colonial Civil Servant*. London: Max Parrish.
Cartwright, D., and C. Robertson. 1957. *How to Cook for Your Family*. Published in association with the Northern Rhodesia and Nyasaland Publications Bureau. London: Longmans, Green and Co.
Clark, Gracia. 1989. "Money, Sex and Cooking: Manipulation of the Paid/Unpaid Boundary by Asante Market Women." In H. Rutz and B. Orlove, eds., The Social Economy of Consumption. *Society for Economic Anthropology Monographs*, no. 6. Washington, DC: University Press of America, pp. 323–348.
Davidoff, Leonore. 1976. "The Rationalization of Housework." In D. L. Barker and S. Allen, eds., *Dependence and Exploitation in Work and Marriage*. London: Longman, pp. 121–151.
Douglas, Mary. 1971. "Deciphering a Meal." In C. Geertz, ed., *Myth, Symbol, and Culture*. New York: W.W. Norton, pp. 61–82.
———. ed. 1984. "Standard Social Usages of Food." In M. Douglas, ed., *Food and the Social Order: Studies of Food and Festivities in Three American Communities*. New York: Russel Sage Foundation.
Douglas, Mary, and M. Nicod. 1974. "Taking the Biscuit: The Structure of British Meals." *New Society* 19(December): 744–747.
Fraenkel, Peter. 1959. *Wayaleshi*. London: Weidenfeld and Nicolson.
Friedmann, Harriet. 1990. "Family Wheat Farms and Third World Diets: A Paradoxical Relationship Between Unwaged and Waged Work." In J. L. Collins and M. Gimenez, eds., *Work Without Wages: Domestic Labor and Self-Employment Within Capitalism*. Albany: State University of New York Press, pp. 193–213.
Goody, Jack. 1982. *Cooking, Cuisine and Class: A Study in Comparative Sociology*. Cambridge: Cambridge University Press.
Hansen, Karen Tranberg. 1989. *Distant Companions: Servants and Their Employers in Zambia, 1900–1985*. Ithaca, NY: Cornell University Press.
———. 1990. "Body Politics: Sexuality, Gender, and Domestic Service in Zambia." *Journal of Women's History* 2(1): 745–765.
———. ed. 1992. *African Encounters with Domesticity*. New Brunnswick, NJ: Rutgers University Press.
Hay, Hope. 1944. "An African Women's Institute." *Oversea Education* 15(3): 104–107.

Jules-Rosette, Benetta. 1981. *Symbols of Change: Urban Transition in a Zambian Community*. Noorwood, NJ: Ablex Publishing Corporation.

Kaye, Elsie A. 1939. *A Cookery Book for Use in African Schools*. Approved by the African Literature Committee of Northern Rhodesia, available through the International Committee on Christian Education for Africans. London: the Sheldon Press.

Keller, Bonnie B. 1978. "Marriage and Medicine: Women's Search for Love and Luck." *African Social Research* 27: 565–585.

Khare, R. S. 1986. "Hospitality, Charity & Rationing: Three Channels of Food Distribution in India." In R. S. Khare and M. S. A. Rao, eds., *Food, Society, and Culture: Aspects in South Asian Food Systems*. Durham, NC: Carolina Academic Press, pp. 277–296.

Levi-Strauss, Claude. 1970. *The Raw and the Cooked*. London: Cape.

———. 1973. *From Honey to Ashes*. London: Cape.

———. 1978. *The Origin of Table Manners*. New York: Harper & Row.

Lindenbaum, Shirley. 1986. "Rice and Wheat: The Meaning of Food in Bangladesh." In R. S. Khare and M. S. A. Rao, eds., *Food, Society, and Culture: Aspects in South Asian Food Systems*. Durham, NC: Carolina Academic Press, pp. 253–275.

Mann, Mary. 1959. "Women's Homecraft Classes in Northern Rhodesia." *Oversea Education* 31(1): 12–16.

Mintz, Sidney W. 1986. *Sweetness and Power: The Place of Sugar in Modern History*. New York: Penguin Books.

Mpashi, Stephen A. 1969. *Betty Kaunda*. Lusaka: Longmans of Zambia.

Muntemba, Dorothy C. 1987. "The Impact of the IMF/World Bank on the People of Africa with Special Reference to Zambia and Especially Women and Children. "Unpublished paper presented at conference of the Institute for African Alternatives on the Impact of the IMF and World Bank on the People of Africa, held at City University, London, September 7–10.

NAZ (National Archives of Zambia)/NR 2/27. 1944–54. African Welfare, General Correspondence.

NAZ/NR 2/512. 1949–59. Native Education, Female.

Nshila. 1963. "Ministers Wives Find Big Houses Cost Big Money—but Love Them." 132 (February 12): 40–41.

Packard, Randall M. 1989. "The 'Healthy Reserve' and the 'Dressed Native': Discourses on Black Health and the Language of Legitimation in South Africa." *American Ethnologist* 16(4): 686–703.

Powdermaker, Hortense. 1962. *Copper Town: Changing Africa*. New York: Harper and Row.

Republic of Zambia. 1985. *1980 Population and Housing Census of Zambia*. Analytical Report vol. III. Lusaka: Central Statistical Office.

Raikes, Philip. 1988. *Modernising Hunger: Famine, Food Supplies & Farm Policy in the EEC & Africa*. London: James Currey.

Richards, Audrey I. 1969. *Land, Labour and Diet in Northern Rhodesia: An Economic Study of the Bemba Tribe*. London: Oxford University Press.

Taylor, John V., and Dorothea Lehmann. 1961. *Christians of the Copperbelt: The Growth of the Church in Northern Rhodesia*. London: SMC Press.

Thomson, Betty Preston. 1954. "Two Studies in African Nutrition: An Urban and a Rural Community in Northern Rhodesia." *Rhodes-Livingstone Papers*, no. 24.

Wilson, Godfrey. 1942. "An Essay on the Economics of Detribalization in Northern Rhodesia," Part II. *Rhodes-Livingstone Papers*, no. 6.

Woodruff, H. W. 1955. "The African Native Market." In *The Federation of Rhodesia and Nyasaland: Economic and Commercial Conditions in the Federation of Rhodesia and Nyasaland*. Overseas Economic Surveys. London: Her Majesty's Stationary Office, pp. 67–73.

Woman's Exclusive. 1984a. "Cookery Corner." 3: 22–23.

———. 1984b. "Cookery Corner." 4: 26–27.

———. 1989. "Cookery Corner." 1: 31.

4. CHANGING PATTERNS OF FOOD CONSUMPTION IN CENTRAL KORDOFAN, SUDAN

Joachim Theis
Save the Children Federation,
P. O. Box 20243, East Jerusalem, Israel

INTRODUCTION

This article describes the economic and environmental changes that took place in central Kordofan during this century, analyzes the coping strategies farmers adopted to deal with these changes, and examines the impact these changes have had on the farmers' food consumption patterns.

Central Kordofan, which has an environment and economy that are typical for the Sahel, lies in the 200 to 400 mm rainfall zone known as the gum belt, an area where *Acacia senegal* grows and is tapped for gum arabic. The major food crops cultivated are millet, grown mainly on sandy soils, and sorghum, grown predominantly on clay soils.[1] Other crops grown are sesame, groundnuts, hibiscus, and watermelon.

The area is inhabited mainly by Arabic-speaking sedentary farmers or former nomads who settled at the end of the last century after losing their livestock due to famine and civil strife during the Mahdia (1881–1898). Today the people living in the rural areas of central Kordofan gain income from agriculture, animal husbandry, labor migration, gathering of wood or herbs, wage labor, remittances, and petty trade.

The semi-desert that lies to the north of central Kordofan is largely unsuitable for rainfed cultivation and is inhabited by camel nomads. South of central Kordofan rainfall increases to more than 400 mm annually, and sorghum becomes the main cereal crop. The population consists of various groups of sedentary Nuba farmers and of partly sedentary, partly nomadic Baggara cattle herders.

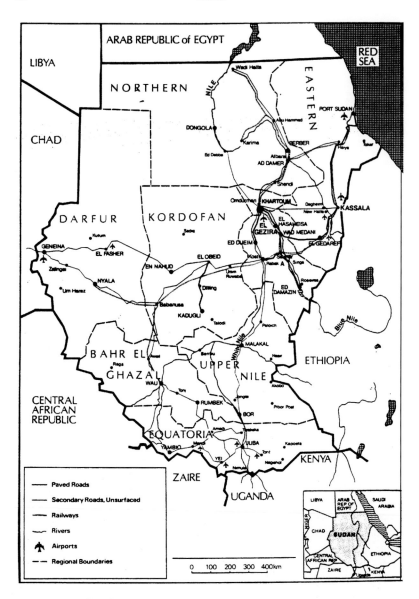

Figure 1   Sudan (from Cater 1986).

Information collected during various surveys carried out under the auspices of the Save the Children Federation's relief and development program in Um Ruwaba district forms the basis for this article. A review of secondary sources and interviews with villagers and Save the Children staff provide additional insight.

TRADITIONAL FOOD CONSUMPTION PATTERNS

Until the middle of this century millet was the main staple cereal in central Kordofan and was eaten year round. Even today, farmers of central Kordofan prefer millet over sorghum because of its taste and the higher nutritive value they ascribe to millet. Especially in the northern parts of central Kordofan, which are too dry to grow any cereal crop except millet, sorghum is not highly valued as food for humans.[2] It was used in the past only as animal feed or as food in years following a bad harvest.

The traditional staple dish in rural Kordofan consists of a porridge (*asida*)[3] made from either millet (*dukhun*)[4] in the northern part of the province, or sorghum (*dura*) in south Kordofan. This porridge is served with one of many different sauces (*mulah*). Most commonly the sauce consists of dried meat with fried onions, water, and some dried okra powder, or of sour milk. Depending on availability and the purchasing power of the consumers, fresh meat or fresh vegetables may be added to the sauce.

Traditionally, hot milk with tea and sugar was the only thing consumed before breakfast. During most of the year farmers obtained milk from their own cows or goats. A large breakfast eaten around 9:30 A.M. consisted most commonly of millet porridge with a sauce of sour milk with clarified butter. Breakfast was followed by sweetened tea. For lunch (around 3:00 P.M.) porridge was eaten with a sauce of vegetables and meat. This meal was also followed by tea. The only food consumed in the evening was a cup of hot milk, sometimes with a thick layer of clarified butter on top. Millet or sorghum beer constituted an important supplemental food, prepared primarily for work parties.[5]

The farmers' consumption patterns changed according to the season. During the rainy season they consumed mainly millet (in the form of porridge and beer), milk, and fresh vegetables from their own fields. Very little meat was consumed because cash was short during the rains. In the harvest season, the time of plenty, farmers ate the new millet crop and consumed meat more regularly than they did the rest of the year. In the dry, hot season, milk and meat became scarce and were consumed only rarely.

URBAN TASTES AND MECHANIZED FARMING

War and famine had depopulated central Kordofan during the Mahdia, but subsistence farmers resettled the region early in this century. Their main economic activities were rainfed cultivation of millet as a staple cereal for home consumption, animal husbandry, and gum arabic tapping to cover cash expenses.

Until World War II agricultural production in central Kordofan was primarily subsistence oriented, and cash cropping was largely confined to areas with good transportation systems that linked them to the main marketing centers in Sudan. Under colonial rule the towns of El Obeid, Um Ruwaba, and Er Rahad developed into major regional centers, which marketed local produce and which gradually drew the subsistence farmers into the market economy.

The rapidly increasing urban population in these marketing centers consists largely of immigrants from various parts of northern Sudan who came as traders or as government employees. The consumption habits of these immigrants differ greatly from those of the local farmers. The immigrants prefer wheat and sorghum over the locally grown millet, and this preference explains why no significant urban market could develop for the millet crop produced in central Kordofan. Additionally, the urban population has a large demand for edible oil, mainly sesame and groundnut oil. During the last fifty years dozens of mechanical oil mills have been set up in the major towns to process the locally grown oilseeds. The promotion of oilseed cultivation, which accompanied the establishment of oil extraction factories, led to an increase in the production of sesame and groundnuts in the traditional rainfed areas at the expense of gum arabic and millet.

The other major reason for the shift toward cash crops in rainfed agricultural production is the establishment of large-scale mechanized farms in the fertile clay plains that stretch across the Sudan, along the 600 mm isohyet, which borders the gum belt to the south. The government of Sudan encouraged the expansion of mechanized sorghum farms into areas occupied by traditional rainfed agriculture, as part of the attempt to turn Sudan into a major grain exporter, the "Breadbasket of the Middle East." "With money for loans and subsidies from the World Bank and other agencies, businessmen were encouraged to buy leases on large tracts of land, import tractors, and plant crops, mainly sorghum for export" (Cater 1986: 22). Most of these businessmen were not indigenous to the area but were northern Sudanese immigrants who lived in the marketing centers.

These enterprises mainly produce sorghum for the urban areas, but since this mechanically produced sorghum is transported to many parts of the country, it is no longer necessary for farmers in central Kordofan to be self-sufficient in cereal production and to meet their grain requirements from their own production of millet alone.

As a result of the growing demand for oilseeds and the availability of a cheap cereal crop as a substitute for millet, the farmers of central Kordofan developed new cropping strategies. They now cultivate large amounts of cash crops (sesame, groundnuts, and hibiscus), which they sell after the harvest to cover their consumption needs and to buy sorghum, which is cheaper than the locally produced millet.

Sorghum has become the rural population's main cereal food. It is estimated that at least half of the grain consumed by farmers in central Kordofan is sorghum imported from mechanized enterprises in south Kordofan (Reeves and Frankenberger 1982: 72). This figure may exceed 80 percent of total grain consumption in bad years.

As farmers in central Kordofan regard millet as having higher nutritional value and as they prefer its taste to that of sorghum, they try to save the millet crop in underground storage pits for the rainy season to give them more strength for the work on their fields.

> The ideal, which only the wealthier households satisfy, is to eat millet throughout the year either from the family's own stocks or from purchases from village merchants. Farmers that are less well off are compelled to buy *feterita* [sorghum] at least for the dry season in order to save their millet for rainy season consumption. The general belief is that *feterita* is "light" (*khafiif*) and "cold" (*baarid*) making it an undesirable food for the rainy season, a time when farmers are engaged in the heavy labor of weeding their fields. For this work they need a "heavy" (*tagiil*), "hot" (*sukhun*) staple, which millet is, to give them the strength to work hard. During the rainy season, too, when meat is not affordable due to the farmer's low purchasing power, millet *asida* can be eaten with oil rather than a meat sauce because it is filling, high in fiber, and good tasting. *Feterita*, on the other hand, is so bland that villagers prefer to eat it with a meat sauce for flavor. (Reeves and Frankenberger 1982: 75)

During winter, which follows the harvest season, farmers continue to eat millet porridge, but in the hot dry season from February to June, farmers consume more sorghum than millet. They say millet sits heavily in peoples' stomachs (Reeves and Frankenberger 1982: 133).

Farmers try to buy several sacks of sorghum after the harvest when prices are low and when they have cash from the sale of their sesame crop. But due to lack of capital, many farmers have to buy sorghum in small quantities throughout the year at increasing prices. They consume their cereal stocks before the new harvest and have to borrow grain from the village shopkeeper when grain prices reach their peak. To repay loans and to cover other urgent household expenses, these farmers often have to sell not only their sesame crop but also part of their millet immediately after the harvest.

During the dry season farmers and their families often pursue economic activities that take them away from their villages to places where they find only sorghum and wheat and have to do entirely without millet, their preferred staple. In the rainy season, when they return to their villages to cultivate their fields, they revert to the old ways and eat their own millet, provided they managed to store some of the grain from the previous year's harvest. Through their contacts with people from other parts of Sudan the farmers of central Kordofan have adopted a variety of new dishes such as *kisra*, a crepe-like bread,[6] rice, and lentils which supplement the traditional porridge. Many village households now eat porridge only for breakfast.

Until the 1950s it was not uncommon for rural households to eat only one proper meal per day, as is still the case in some parts of southern Sudan. An important supplemental food was *merisa*, a thick, gruel-like and nourishing beer made from sorghum (or millet) which was prepared mainly for communal work parties. Much of the hard work on the fields (namely, planting, weeding, and harvesting), the building of houses, and occasionally the tapping of gum arabic trees (Josten 1988: 59) was done through this reciprocal exchange of labor known as *nafir*. After completing the work the participants drank beer together, and the host of a communal work party was expected to reciprocate his or her guests' labor by working in turn at their *nafir*.

The increased production of cash crops and the integration of the rural society into the market economy has made wage labor more widespread. As a consequence *nafir*, as an integral part of the subsistence economy, has generally declined, and the consumption of *merisa* has declined along with it. *Nafir* and wage labor mutually exclude each other; farmers who have their fields cultivated by wage laborers do not go to the *nafir* of their neighbors (Josten 1988: 61).[7] Increased market production has contributed to socio-economic stratification, and rich farmers are less likely to take part in *nafir* than poor farmers.

The decline of beer consumption may reflect the reduced cultivation of cereal crops in central Kordofan, as a result of various economic and environmental factors. Although sorghum or millet beer is not necessarily lower in nutritional value than porridge, it is generally consumed in larger quantities than porridge and is, therefore, a less economical way of turning grain into food. As evidence from other parts of Africa shows, in times of grain shortages beer is the first item to disappear from the farmers' diet, as beer is produced to feed large groups of people and not just for the consumption of the individual household.

The increase in labor out-migration has also contributed to the decline in the consumption and production of beer, since young men used to be the main consumers of sorghum beer in the village. The introduction of Islamic *sharia* law in the Sudan in September 1983 did not have a signifi-cant impact on the consumption and production of alcoholic beverages in the remote rural areas which lie on the fringe of government control. Nonetheless, popular support for fundamentalist Islamic ideas in northern Sudan has in recent years reduced the social acceptability of beer drinking and of beer parties. Nowadays a meal of *asida* or *kisra* may be served with tea and sugar at communal work parties rather than beer.

Wheat and wheat flour are among the food commodities rapidly gaining importance in central Kordofan.[8] The main urban staple food is bread with broad beans (*ful*), a dish that found its way into the Sudan from Egypt and that is now served in restaurants along the main truck routes in the Sudan. With the building of a modern infrastructure, itinerant traders and educated strangers such as teachers and health workers have come to the rural areas of central Kordofan, and the urban foods they prefer have found their way into the province along with them. Villages with a health post, school, mechanical water pump, and weekly market often have a bakery where wheat bread is produced. Wheat bread is normally fed to the school chil-dren in villages with bakeries and is also increasingly used in the homes of school children and labor migrants, who have become accustomed to eating bread with beans. So far the distribution of wheat bread is con-fined to larger villages where bakeries have been established, but with the availability of fast food, people's tastes are also changing and the demand for bread and bakeries is increasing.[9]

All bakeries and most restaurants are run by men, whereas it is invariably women who prepare more traditional dishes such as *kisra* and *asida*. Women in rural Kordofan shoulder all economic activities inside their home, includ-ing fetching water, cooking, tending the children, and making handicrafts, as well as a large part of the agricultural labor. Women experience a constant conflict in the allocation of time among their diverse activities, and they spend long hours preparing food. Much of this time is spent grinding and cooking the staple millet or sorghum dish, and fetching water and fire-wood. The availability of commercial cereal processing facilities such as bakeries and flour mills frees the women of some of their domestic chores and allows them to devote more time to cultivating their own land and to spend less time fetching water and firewood and preparing meals.[10]

With the spread of wheat and wheat bread a wide variety of new dishes have found their way into the diet of farmers in rural Kordofan. Bread may be eaten with salad, beans, sauce without dried okra, a handful of dates or groundnuts, or just by itself. A snack can be prepared in short time by making donuts (*legemat*) dipped in sugar and eaten with sweet tea. In some rural households, especially those of farmers who have been exposed to formal education and urban employment, wheat flour is mixed with sorghum or millet in the preparation of porridge which gives the dish a smoother texture. Occasionally, thick pancakes (*gurrasa*)[11] are prepared from wheat flour, but it is rare for uneducated farmers to eat these pancakes unless there is a shortage of millet or sorghum.

It is not just the consumption patterns of staple foods that have changed. Until the 1960s meat was available only on special occasions, such as weddings or circumcisions or when a sick animal had to be slaughtered. Most villages did not have a butcher who slaughtered regularly for sale, and meat purchased in the market was dried at home and stored for later consumption.[12] With the commercialization of the rural economy butchers are now commonplace, at least in the larger villages, and farmers can purchase fresh meat in small quantities whenever they have the necessary cash.

Sugar consumption has considerably increased during the last decades in the rural areas of northern Sudan, and sugar can now be considered a staple.[13] The average person in Kordofan and throughout northern Sudan consumes an estimated one to two kilos of sugar per month, if it is available and affordable. When in 1989 sugar became scarce and sugar prices skyrocketed, farmers in many villages in central Kordofan stopped consuming sugar and even sold their precious sugar rations in order to buy grain.

ENVIRONMENTAL CHANGE

The transformations in the rural economy of Kordofan have been accompanied by far-reaching environmental changes, which have led to the general decline in the region's economic and environmental situation over the past twenty-five years. This area, once self-sufficient in terms of food production, now depends on subsidies and donations. The steady growth in population (2.5 percent annually) over the last decades has led to a rapid increase in household consumption and cash requirements which has not been matched by increases in production.

Improvements in the infrastructure, such as schools and health posts, the drilling of boreholes, and the digging of wells, contributed to the growth of the population and to the increasing pressure on the land.

Economic and Environmental Change in Central Kordofan

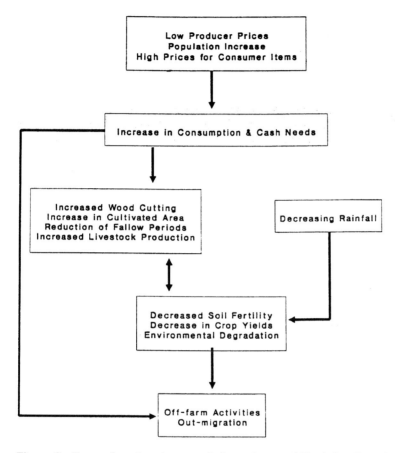

Figure 2   Economic and environmental change in central Kordofan. From Save the Children Federation 1988: 3.

During the 1960s and 1970s the government of Sudan launched several extensive well-drilling programs to open up new areas to agriculture and livestock production. The newly drilled waterpoints attracted large populations to regions that had thus far been waterless and therefore unsuitable for permanent settlement.

Since the early 1960s rainfall has been consistently below the long-term yearly average, and this shortage has led to a decrease in crop yields.[14] In order to compensate for the reduction in yields and income brought about by continuously low producer prices and steadily increasing prices for essential consumer goods, farmers adopted a number of strategies: they expanded the area under cultivation,[15] reduced fallow periods, and increased the size of their animal herds. Seeking an additional ready source of income, the population cut trees for sale as building materials, firewood, and charcoal, thereby further decreasing soil fertility and crop yields and continuing the vicious circle of overexploitation of the land and environmental degradation.

As a result of these adverse economic and environmental conditions, farmers have increasingly sought off-farm activities to supplement their income and to cover their expenses. An estimated 20 to 25 percent of the rural population, including women and children, migrates permanently or seasonally to agricultural schemes in the central Sudan and south Kordofan or to the urban centers along the Nile. This contact with other parts of the Sudan has contributed to the change in consumption patterns and the introduction of new foods into rural Kordofan.

Due to the chronically low rainfall in the area during the last twenty-five years, early maturing millet varieties have gained in popularity among the farmers. Although they yield less, have smaller seeds, and do not taste as good as the traditional late-maturing varieties, they produce a crop even in years with relatively low rainfall when the long-season varieties would never reach the maturity stage.

Two consecutive years of complete harvest failure accelerated these developments and brought about the collapse of central Kordofan's already vulnerable economy. High cereal prices and low livestock prices characterized the drought years. Whereas the price of one camel equalled fifty sacks of sorghum before the drought, at the height of the famine a farmer could buy only one sack of grain with his camel. The heavy loss in animal wealth led to a sharp increase in livestock prices after the drought, making it difficult for livestock owners to replenish their herds.

Until the famine of 1983–85, milk constituted an important element in the diet of the sedentary farmers who kept herds of sheep, goats, camels, and cattle. The importance of dairy production in the Um Ruwaba district is indicated in its name—literally, Um Ruwaba means "place of sour milk starter."[16]

Since 70 to 90 percent of the livestock died, were sold,[17] or were consumed during the drought, milk and milk products (sour milk, clarified butter) have largely disappeared from the diet of rural households, and hardly any fresh milk has been available for sale in Um Ruwaba town since the recent drought.[18] Given the present environmental conditions (lack of rain and poor pastures) in north Kordofan, most farmers now invest their scarce capital in goats rather than in sheep or cattle. Goats are hardier and reproduce more quickly than sheep or cattle, but they give little surplus milk for human consumption since most of the milk goes to the kids. The restocking strategy of the farmers therefore focuses on the short-term build-up of a herd as a savings fund for hard times, rather than on providing milk and meat.[19]

FAMINE AND RELIEF FOODS

During the 1983–85 drought food was in very short supply, and the prices for the staples millet and sorghum rose to levels far beyond the purchasing power of the impoverished farmers, who took to eating wild seeds.[20] In response to the emergency, large quantities of relief food, such as wheat flour, bulgar wheat, dry skim milk, corn soy milk, sorghum, and soybean oil were donated by the United States and Western European governments to alleviate the worst effects of the famine.[21]

Together with wheat flour, a mixture of vegetable oil and dry skim milk was given out as high-energy and high-protein food during the relief agencies' feeding programs.[22] To ensure that the relief food was prepared properly, oil and milk were mixed at the food distribution centers to prevent mothers from mixing the milk powder with contaminated water, which can cause diarrhea, dehydration, and death in small children.[23] The mixture had to be cooked before being consumed. By adding wheat flour, the women made it into a dough, which they either fried as donuts or pancakes or cooked into a porridge. Alternatively, they diluted the mixture with water and boiled it into a beverage that substituted for the traditional drink of fresh milk with clarified butter. The women of rural Kordofan used the new and unfamiliar relief food commodities as substitutes for traditional foods, which were unavailable during the famine, and they integrated the new commodities without difficulty into the diet of their families.

As the mixture had a much lower market value than the dry skim milk and soybean oil would have had if these commodities had been sold separately, the mixing of milk and oil prevented the food recipients from selling the relief food in the market to purchase other needed food items, such as sugar, tea, salt, and hot pepper. In some cases, however, dry milk found its way into the market, where it was bought by cheesemakers who made it into feta cheese.

During the drought years wheat flour came to be known as famine food and as the food of the poor. The rural population generally disliked wheat flour, which they believed to have low nutritional value and to cause malnutrition among children. Most households lacked the facilities and knowledge to make leavened wheat bread and preferred to sell some of their wheat flour rations to bakeries than to eat bland homemade pancakes. Whereas wheat bread was appreciated, pancakes were not. In this way the distribution of wheat and wheat flour as part of the relief food rations contributed to the popularization of wheat bread among the farmers of central Kordofan.

American sorghum was also imported during the famine. The red American sorghum differed from the locally known varieties in color, size, and taste. The "Reagan sorghum" (*eish reagan*), as it was called, was accepted, but as soon as the worst effects of the famine had been overcome, its popularity dropped quickly, and some of the grain was used to brew alcoholic drinks, fed to animals, or sold.

Whereas many educated Sudanese felt uneasy about the large-scale relief operation and its possible consequences for economic and cultural dependency on western nations and the United States in particular, in the folk culture of Kordofan Ronald Reagan became something of a hero. The rural population thought of him as a rich American farmer who sent some of his surplus food to the starving population in Africa. Children made up rhymes and songs praising Reagan and his people (*nas reagan*, the foreigners). Here are some examples:

1. Reagan, good man, brought the people out of the drought
   reagan, wad el hana al marag lena min as-sana

2. Reagan, good man, brought sorghum and milk
   Reagan, good man, gives life to the folk

3. If Reagan is here I don't fear two years of drought
   lau reagan fi ana ma bakhaf lau tabaga sanaten jafaf

A few people, however, raised doubts about the motives of the American government in providing free food handouts. These feelings were expressed particularly by some religious men who saw a Christian conspiracy to weaken their Islamic society. Questions were asked about the origin of dry skim milk and soybean milk and whether it was permitted for a Muslim to consume it. For a while rumors circulated that dry skim milk made women infertile. Since food distributions ceased in late 1986, the famine, Reagan, and the food relief program have faded into oral lore.

Some farmers tried planting the American sorghum, not realizing that second-generation hybrid sorghum is not suitable for seed. When the American hybrid sorghum performed poorly, the farmers interpreted it as a sign that American sorghum was infertile. The rumor spread, by analogy, that women who ate American sorghum would become infertile. Moreover, as Americans were not known to consume sorghum, people in Kordofan concluded that Americans grew this grain as animal feed and that the United States government had sent animal fodder to feed the starving population of Africa.

During the emergency food distribution in central Kordofan people became familiar with dry skim milk, corn soy milk, bulgar wheat, soybean oil, and "Reagan sorghum." These new food commodities, on the whole, did not have a lasting impact on consumption patterns, mainly because they disappeared from the market and from the farmers' diets as soon as the relief food distributions ended. The food was widely appreciated because it was free, but given a choice, the majority of the population would prefer millet porridge, sesame oil, and fresh cow's milk.

FOOD PRICES

Agricultural prices greatly affect the production and consumption of food in central Kordofan. The farmers respond quickly to any changes in crop prices by expanding or reducing the areas cultivated in various crops to take advantage of prevailing market conditions. During the drought years lack of food led to high grain prices, to which farmers reacted by increasing the areas planted in cereal crops. A fair harvest in 1986 coincided with the handout of free relief food during the emergency feeding program launched (1985–86) by non-governmental organizations, causing a sharp drop in cereal prices.

> With the prospects of a good harvest and the continuing rise of production costs there is concern over sorghum pricing policies. The current sorghum market price does not offer adequate return for the smaller producers. This could offer a serious threat to future cultivation. (Relief and Rehabilitation Commission, Government of Sudan, 15 October 1986: 3)

Farmers responded by reducing the areas cultivated in millet and sorghum and by increasing the production of sesame and other cash crops the following season. The year 1987 produced a poor harvest, and grain prices again rose sharply. This rise was followed by a renewed increase in the area planted in cereal crops in the 1988 season, which in turn caused grain prices to fall.

Sorghum Price Fluctuations
El Obeid Market

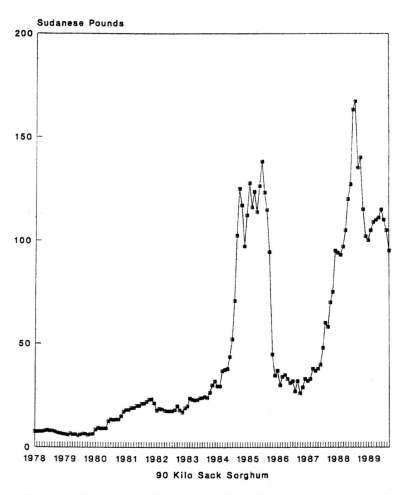

Figure 3   Sorghum price fluctuations at El Obeid market 1978–89.

Small farmers are consistently hurt by unstable cereal prices. When their own stocks are low and they have to buy grain, prices are high; when their grain reserves are high, prices are low and they cannot reap the benefits of a good harvest. Those who profit from the price fluctuations are merchants, middlemen, and parastatal grain purchasers, such as the

Agricultural Bank of Sudan, who understand and control the market and who have the capital to store grain until the selling prices are favorable.

As in most developing countries, the government of Sudan's food policy is geared primarily toward satisfying the consumption needs of towns and cities. The cultivation of sorghum on mechanized farms, the promotion of sesame and groundnut production, and the import of American PL-480 wheat are the main elements in the government's program to feed the growing urban population. This urban bias is a consequence of the fact that most politicians are themselves townspeople and that urban professionals, students, and workers are able to put pressure on the government in times of food shortages. The food riots in late 1988 in Khartoum demonstrate this clearly. Farmers in the provinces, on the other hand, usually do not have the means to express their needs and demands or to put pressure on the government to alleviate their problems. Their lack of political and economic power became apparent during the famine.

During the last few years many food items have disappeared from the market or have become too expensive for most farmers to buy, such as cow's milk, sour milk, dates, and sugar. The farmers, however, are experienced in dealing with hardship situations and have been better able to cope with these shortages than many town dwellers.[24]

CONCLUSION

The shift from subsistence farming to market production, urban migration, population increase, environmental degradation and prolonged periods of drought, and a food and agriculture policy that favors the urban economy, have fundamentally altered the economic situation of the village population in central Kordofan. As a consequence of these factors, the food consumption patterns of the rural population have changed dramatically over the past thirty years.

Among the long-term and permanent changes are a shift from the subsistence production of millet to the market production of sesame and an increasing reliance on the market to meet basic consumption needs, including the purchase of sorghum on a regular basis. As environmental conditions for the cultivation of millet have deteriorated (lack of rain and abundance of pests) and the population has increased, millet is not likely to regain its place as the main staple in central Kordofan. Today only rich landowners can afford to eat millet throughout the year. Most people consume millet mainly during the rainy season and at harvest time, whereas the rest of the year, from February to June, sorghum and wheat form the main staple.

Integration into the market economy has altered the impact of, and the farmers' response to, drought and famine. The rural population has become more vulnerable to food emergencies, as agricultural production is geared toward the market. Farmers no longer satisfy their consumption needs from their own production, and grain is no longer stored for several years to provide for times of drought or poor harvests.

Famine and the distribution of relief food did not leave a lasting impression on the farmers' consumption patterns and did not create a demand for or dependency on new food commodities. To a certain extent, the feeding programs of 1985–86 took the place of wild foods during previous famines. However, food relief programs exposed the farmers of central Kordofan to a variety of new food commodities and contributed to the process of dietary innovation, which over the last decades has changed food consumption patterns as the population's contact with the outside world has increased through labor migration, formal education, and market transactions.

The drought has dealt a heavy blow to the farmers' livestock wealth. They have opted against restocking their cattle herds in the face of high market prices for cattle and severe environmental constraints to cattle rearing. Goats are the preferred animals in which farmers invest their post-drought savings with the aim of regaining a minimum level of economic security. Goats reproduce faster and are better adapted to the present environmental conditions than cattle, but they do not give large amounts of milk. The days of plentiful milk and millet belong to the past.

In the face of increasingly adverse environmental and economic conditions, the farmers have responded flexibly and creatively in integrating available food resources into their diet. Food consumption patterns in central Kordofan are likely to diversify further, and to a large degree the availability and price of food commodities in the market will determine what farmers eat. Millet porridge with sour milk will remain, however, the favorite dish of the rural population in central Kordofan.

NOTES

The author lived in Sudan for a total of six years during which time he carried out ethnographic field research among the Koma in the Blue Nile Province and worked in the relief and development program of the community development organization Save the Children Federation/U.S. in the Um Ruwaba district of North Kordofan Province. During this period the author was in charge of a district-wide emergency food distribution program and coordinated a Baseline Survey of the Um Ruwaba district. I would like to thank my colleagues Mohammed Ali Idris, Amna Ahmed, Awatif Abdalla, and Farouq Mohammed El Amin El Murad for their help and advice in the researching of this paper

1. Millet (*Pennisetum typhoideum*) requires a minimum of 200 mm annual rainfall on sandy soils and sorghum (*Sorghum vulgare*) as much as 400 mm on clay soil, provided the rainfall is evenly spread over a three-month period.
2. *Mareg* (*Sorghum verticilliflorum*) is the main locally grown variety of sorghum.
3. "This is a porridge made from fermented millet or sorghum flour. It is prepared by boiling water in a medium container and gradually adding the flour with continuous stirring for a half an hour or more. This porridge is then placed in large bowls and eaten with various types of sauce" (Reeves and Frankenberger 1982: 128).
4. The farmers of central Kordofan call millet *eish* (literally, life, i.e., staple). *Eish* always refers to the staple grain. Depending on the area of Sudan, this may be millet, sorghum, or wheat. Farmers in central Kordofan refer to sorghum by the name of the variety (e.g., *mareg, feterita*) rather than by its generic term. Millet plants cross-pollinate easily, and few distinct varieties exist. In this respect it differs from sorghum for which the farmers distinguish dozens of different varieties.
5. These food consumption patterns represent an ideal situation. In case of a drought these patterns might change considerably, and poor families might eat only one proper meal a day.
6. *Kisra* is "made from fermented flour (usually sorghum) [and] it resembles a crepe. It is prepared by pouring the batter onto a hot, flat metal surface (*saaf*). After spreading the batter out very thinly and allowing it to cook for 15 to 30 seconds, the *kisra* is peeled off the hot surface and ready to be eaten" (Reeves and Frankenberger 1982: 128).
7. This observation is supported by evidence from other parts of Africa where market and subsistence production have come into contact.
8. The increasing popularity of wheat bread is reflected in the fact that five out of the sixteen bakeries in Um Ruwaba, a town with about 35,000 inhabitants, were built only during the last eight years. Each bakery prepares an average of 1,000 loaves of bread per day, provided there is a steady supply of wheat flour.
9. However, bread production depends largely on the import of wheat flour from the United States, and recent shortages in wheat imports have forced bakeries all over Kordofan to close down.
10. Flour mills are widely used in central Kordofan to grind millet, sorghum, and wheat. The following example may illustrate the increasing demand for wheat bread even in the more remote areas. In Samandia, a village of about 1,100 inhabitants in Um Ruwaba district, a group of young women formed a cooperative to build and operate a bakery. During the agricultural season the women preferred to spend their time cultivating their fields or working on the field of a large landowner for money than preparing food. It is more time consuming to cook a meal with millet or sorghum, which takes hours to grind and cook, than with wheat bread.
11. *Gurrasa* "is a bread made out of wheat flour which is unfermented. It is much thicker than *kisra*. This bread is prepared the same way as *kisra* on a hot flat surface. It is usually covered with clarified butter and sugar and is eaten by itself. However, sometimes it is eaten with *mulah* [sauce]" (Reeves and Frankenberger 1982: 130).
12. Sun-dried meat (*sharmut*) from wild animals, such as gazelle, was sold in every market in central Kordofan until the early 1970s, but due to deforestation and a sharp increase in the number of domestic animals during the 1970s and early 1980s wildlife has virtually vanished from the area.
13. In Sudan the government rations and sells sugar at the official subsidized price of LS 0.85 ($0.20) per pound of sugar (in late 1989). Depending on availability, the government sells 3 pounds of sugar per family member every month.
14. Millet yields in North Kordofan declined from 640 kg/ha in the early 1960s to 377 kg/ha in the 1970s to 210 kg/ha in the early 1980s (Reeves and Frankenberger 1982).
15. The area under cultivation in Kordofan and Darfur increased from one million *feddan* (0.42 ha) in 1960 to seven million *feddan* in 1980 (el-Sammani 1985: 156).
16. The town used to be famous for the sour milk (*rob*) that was brought to the market by nomads. Women produce sour milk and liquid butter (*samin*) by pouring milk in a gourd

(*bukhsa*) or an animal skin (*siin*) and fermenting it with *rawab*. By shaking the container the milk is separated into *rob* and *samin*. (Save the Children Federation 1988: 93).

17. Rich merchants in the marketing centers benefited in various ways from the famine by selling grain at inflated prices, buying livestock cheaply for the urban meat market, and buying gold from the starving farmers. The severity of the drought affected virtually the entire rural population in central Kordofan and did not spare the wealthier landowners and traders in the villages.

18. The drought affected not just the herds of the farmers, but also those of the nomads, who now cross the areas of the farmers during the rainy season in much smaller numbers and with many fewer animals than before. As recently as 1982 it was observed that "aside from millet, more milk products are consumed which are obtained from migrating nomads" (Reeves and Frankenberger 1982: 133). As a reminder of the times when nomads passed through the area on their annual migrations and exchanged milk and milk products with the sedentary population for grain, people still refer to buying and selling milk as exchanging milk (*baddil laban*), even if it is sold for cash.

19. Since the loss of animal wealth, especially in villages that had relied on livestock as a primary source of income, farmers have followed alternative economic strategies. After the famine a number of village communities built schools for their children, as they see education, which is closely linked to labor migration, as an economic career for children who prior to the drought were needed to tend the large animal herds.

20. In times of severe food shortages women and children supplement the household diet by gathering wild fruits, herbs, and seeds, such as *tebeldi* (*Adansonia digitata*), *nabag* (*Ziziphus mauritania*), *aradeb* (*Tamarindus indica*), *mulukhia* (jewsmallow), and *lalob* (fruit of *Balanites aegyptiaca*). Some of the famine foods used in drought years in Kordofan are: *heskanit* (*Cenchrus biflorus*), *diffra* (*Echinochloa colonom*), *kursan*, *mukhet* (*Boscia senegalensis*), and *koreb* (*Aristida pubifolia*).

21. In the Um Ruwaba district Save the Children Federation distributed 50,000 metric tons of food to 400,000 people between August 1985 and December 1986. SCF handed out locally produced sorghum after the initial consignment of American sorghum had been distributed, and the 1985–86 harvest in the Sudan had created a food surplus in some parts of the country.

22. In the Um Ruwaba District supplemental food rations of milk, oil, and wheat flour were targeted toward severely malnourished children and their families, whereas basic rations of sorghum were distributed to all families based on the harvest ratings of their village. Villages whose harvest had failed in 1985–86 received more food than those who had harvested a better crop.

23. Relief agencies provided nutrition training to women of malnourished children. Nutrition surveys carried out during the drought showed that malnutrition rates of girls were generally higher than those of boys. This observation appears to be the direct result of the traditional division of food in the households where women give the best food to men and boys, who eat by themselves before women and girls eat what is left over. Men are also more mobile and generally find more food and a larger variety of foods than women or children.

24. At least in towns, wheat bread is less expensive (in 1988) than *kisra* due to the high prices for sorghum and charcoal. Preparing *kisra* is also more time consuming than buying ready-made bread. An increasing number of families no longer make their own *kisra* and they no longer own the flat metal pan (*saj*) needed to prepare this leavened sorghum bread. In times of wheat shortage, however, as in 1989, town dwellers revert to a diet of sorghum *kisra*. Since the military coup in Sudan (30 June 1989), the new government has tried to control prices with the effect that many food commodities disappeared for weeks or months at a time. The urban population was hit more seriously by these shortages than the rural communities. In the towns and cities professionals reverted to eating *kisra* and *asida* or made *gurrasa* if they could find a few kilos of wheat flour in the market, as most bakeries closed down after the government imposed the new prices.

BIBLIOGRAPHY

Abdelmajid Khogali Mohamed Ahmed, 1984. *Desertification and Low Productivity in the Traditional Agriculture of North Kordofan, Sudan.* Reading.

Born, Martin, 1965. *Zentralkordofan.* Marburg: Universität Marburg, Geographisches Institut.

Cameron, Margaret, and Yngve Hofvander, 1983. *Manual on Feeding Infants and Young Children.* Oxford: Oxford University Press.

Cater, Nick. 1986. *Sudan: The Roots of Famine.* Oxford: Oxfam.

Coughenour, C. Milton, and Saadi M. Nazhat, 1985. *Recent Changes in Villages and Rainfed Agriculture in Northern Central Kordofan: Communication Process and Constraints.* INTSORMIL Report No. 4. Lexington: University of Kentucky.

Josten, Siegmund, 1988. *Leben mit der ökologischen Krise: Fallstudie bei den Shiwyhat in El Graiwyd, Nord Kordofan, Sudan. Auswertungsbericht für das ASA-Projekt "Kulturvergleich," Sudan, 1987.* Berlin.

Lipton, Michael, 1975. "Urban Bias and Food Policy in Poor Countries." *Food Policy* (November 1975): 41–51.

Reeves, Edward B., and Timothy Frankenberger, 1981. *Farming Systems Research in North Kordofan, Sudan.* INTSORMIL Report No. 1. Lexington: University of Kentucky.

Reeves, Edward B., and Timothy Frankenberger, 1982. *Farming Systems Research in North Kordofan, Sudan.* INTSORMIL Report No. 2. Lexington: University of Kentucky.

Reeves, Edward B., and Muhammed Majzoub Fideil, 1984. *An Indigenous Marketing System in North Kordofan, Sudan.* INTSORMIL Report No. 3. Lexington: University of Kentucky.

Relief and Rehabilitation Commission, Government of Sudan, August 1986–September 1989. *Early Warning System Bulletin.* Khartoum: RRC.

el-Sammani, Mohamed Osman, ed. 1985. *Kordofan Resource Inventory.* Khartoum: Institute of Environmental Studies.

Save the Children Federation, 1988. *Baseline Report: Um Ruwaba District, North Kordofan Province, Sudan.* Khartoum: SCF.

Sukkar, Mohammad Yusuf, 1985. *Human Nutrition for Medical Studies and Allied Health Sciences.* Khartoum (distributed in the U.K. by Ithaca Press).

Technoserve, 1987, *KORAG Credit Component Baseline Study.* El Obeid: Technoserve.

USAID, Office of Food for Peace, 1988. *Commodity Reference Guide.* Falls Church: The Pragma Corporation.

USAID, Africa Bureau, 1988. *FEWS Country Report—Sudan (October 1988).* Washington.

Yagoub Abdalla Mohamed et al., 1982. *The North Kordofan Rural Water Supply Baseline Survey.* Khartoum: Institute of Environmental Studies.

5. FOOD AID IN PERU: REFUSAL AND ACCEPTANCE IN A PEASANT COMMUNITY OF THE CENTRAL ANDES

Leticia Delgado

Centre d'Etudes Comparatives sur le Développement (CECOD)
Centre St-Charles, 162 rue St-Charles, 75740, Paris,
Cedex 15, France

INTRODUCTION

Today's Andean food style[1] is a prominent example of the responses Andean societies have developed toward changes imposed upon them by successive dominant societies (Herrera 1987; Sánchez 1987). Thus, in recent years one could observe a food behavior in Peru that keeps the Andean matrix but is, at the same time, modified by the influence of both the urban social classes and the food industries linked to transnational companies. Since the 1940s the policies of successive Peruvian governments relied on imports of foodstuffs to the detriment of Andean production, which enabled this "urban-industrial" food style to spread throughout the country. This led to "national food dependence" and to the deterioration of the food situation of the petty food producers, particularly in the Andes. These petty producers are now considered the sector of the Peruvian population most disadvantaged by the changes occurring on a national scale in the patterns of consumption (Lajo 1986).

In order to reverse this situation of "food dependence," the Peruvian government developed toward the end of 1985 a plan of action, whose main objective was to reduce imports, in the medium and long run, through the reorientation of production and consumption. At the same time, the plan incorporated the existing Food Aid programs and proclaimed the need to expand them in order to improve the immediate situation of the low-income

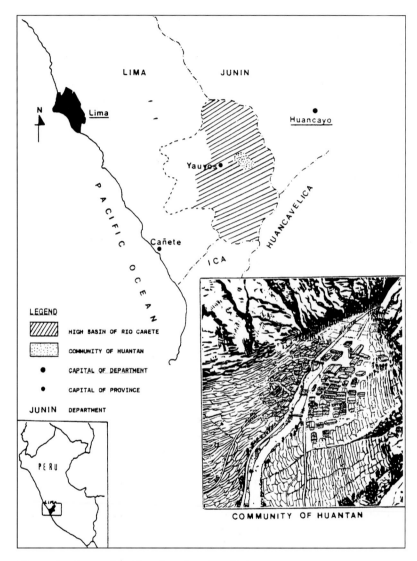

Figure 1   Geographical location of area studied.

groups. The Andean rural population was selected as a priority group to benefit from these programs (*Plan Nacional de Seguridad Alimentaria* 1986: 32). However, the government's declarations were contradictory, even when considered from the perspective of consumption alone, because not all the food items used in the Food Aid programs promote the reorientation of consumption that was supposedly the plan's long-term objective.

Governments and institutions appealing for international Food Aid base their arguments on the well-known nutritional needs of Peru's rural population. The political and ideological interests of these official actors, however, and the negative effects of the aid have been widely commented upon in the Food Aid literature, again with special reference to Peru's rural areas (*Rimanakuy* 1986: 231–243; Häbig 1988) and to Lima's slums (Degregori et al. 1986: 194–207). But this did not prevent an increase in the food donations that Peru has received continuously since 1959: from 1976 to 1986, the volume of cereal, powdered milk, and vegetable oil given as Food Aid to Peru increased by 544 percent, 405 percent, and 1144 percent, respectively (Griffin 1978; FAO 1983; 1987). Since 1979, the food donations have been partly incorporated into "Food for Work" programs (Amat y León and Curonisy 1981), which at present constitute one of the preferred channels of distribution for international Food Aid: 16 percent of all aid is given out in exchange for work (Erard and Mounier 1984: 99). Some authors find the "Food for Work" system preferable to the free distribution of foodstuffs (Fryer 1981: 55), whereas others consider it an ultimate form of slavery (Schuftan, cited by Erard and Mounier 1984: 103). The system does indeed seem to present a number of drawbacks: the programs provoked, for instance, the disappearance of some forms of self-consumption (Erard and Mounier 1984: 102) and allowed landowners to appropriate the benefits of the "food-earners'" work (Fryer 1981: 81).

The populations benefiting from "Food for Work" programs have frequently expressed refusal toward the food supplies they receive. While this fact has been acknowledged in the literature, it has not been studied carefully enough up to the present, particularly in Peru. In this paper, I want to analyze the attitudes of a social group that benefits from Food Aid in the "Food for Work" modality. I shall try to establish the factors that induce expressions of acceptance or refusal toward Food Aid and the food it supplies, by studying from a sociocultural perspective the relationship between Food Aid and changes in food behavior. My analysis is based on field research in the peasant community of Huantan (Yauyos Province, Lima Department) on the western slope of the Central Peruvian Andes and deals with "Food for Work" programs carried out between 1982 and 1987.

SOME CONCEPTUAL ELEMENTS AND METHODOLOGY OF THE ANALYSIS

The study of food practices has distinguished between real metabolic need and felt need (Chombart de Lowe 1956: chap. 7) and shown that individuals react mainly to the latter, subject to multiple cultural influences. More recently, it was suggested that "what is perceived as necessary is actually some form of order, rules and criteria, reliable principles for behavioral organization" (Fischler 1986: 962). Without denying the existence of metabolic or economic need, I shall consider that in a sociocultural dimension people's ideology frames the notion of need with respect to food, with normative and arbitrary elements specific to the food styles they produce. It is well known today, for instance, that the value that is attached to food assumes an essential and determining role in the attitudes of individuals or groups toward it.[2] These attitudes are manifest in food behaviors, ranging from the selection of foods to be consumed to the qualities subjectively bestowed on food and the quantities required for consumption. Over wide ranges, these food behaviors are expressed in terms of acceptance (tendencies, attractions, tastes, appetites) or, on the contrary, in terms of refusal (repugnance, aversion, contempt, repulsion, or even horror) (Brunault 1981: 3). By the various expressions of acceptance or refusal, societies or social groups assess their food style and recognize or differentiate themselves in relation to other groups (Calvo 1982: 388–389).

Food style and practices, like other social expressions, are not static but dynamic, and their transformations result from a complex and dynamic interplay of various factors. In this paper, I shall consider the relationships between the group subject to change and the other social actors, and I shall pay particular attention to the way in which the state mediates these relationships (Haubert 1985, 1988). I shall also take into account external factors or "impersonal forces" (Mirsky 1981), such as commercialization and culture contact, as well as internal factors, such as the cognitive structure of family members (Lewin 1943) and the values and "taste" specific to the peasant style of consumption (Grignon and Grignon 1980).

The present study is based mainly on interviews with peasant domestic units[3] and participant observation during 1986–87. It also draws on food consumption and market surveys which I conducted at the communal level. Information concerning the donor institutions (objectives, programs, assigned rations) is drawn mainly from documents produced by the organizations intervening in Huantan and from interviews with their officials.

The interviews with eleven domestic units of the Huantan community revealed that while there was a general attitude of refusal toward foodstuffs received via Food Aid, certain differences exist between the domestic units concerning the notions of help and need, the perception of the foodstuffs, and their effective use. The domestic units studied could be divided into two groups, namely, a refusal and an acceptance group. In order to explain the different behavior of these families, several variables regarding their household cycle, economic situation, and food practices were considered. In general, the following questions guide my study: (1) What are the logics of the different actors (the state, the donor institutions, the peasant community, and the domestic units) in the implementation of Food Aid in Huantan, and how are they related? (2) Does Food Aid change the food behavior of Huantan families?

THE STATE, THE NATIONAL FOOD PROGRAM, AND THE FOOD AID ORGANIZATIONS

From 1986, the Peruvian state has become one of the main actors in Food Aid action, by integrating the Food Aid programs into the National Food Security Program (*Plan Nacional de Seguridad Alimentaria*) and by granting private donor institutions the status of "development agents."[4]

In Huantan, both the Seventh Day Adventist Welfare (OFASA, *Obra Filantrópica Social Adventista*) and the Peruvian section of CARITAS International, the two main private donor institutions in Peru, have worked and employed the modalities of "Food for Work" programs since 1979. The State organization that intervened in Huantan, the National Office of Food Aid (ONAA, *Oficina Nacional de Apoyo Alimentario*), was originally created to centralize information and coordinate the Food Aid actions of private institutions. My interviews with officials revealed, however, that in actual practice the actions of private donors are not coordinated, except in cases of food emergency, and that each organization has its own "supported population" and its "work area." Nevertheless, the state does control the action of the private organizations to a certain extent. Although the donor countries determine the types and quantities of food items sent to Peru, the Ministry of Health is supposed to supervise the rations established by the local organizations to ensure that "the food items are likely to be replaced by national products" in the future.[5] Moreover, state institutions (Ministries of Health, Education, or Agriculture) and governmental organizations such as *Cooperación Popular* and the Development Cooperation (CORDES, *Cooperación para el Desarrollo*) control the implementation of Food-Aid programs. In fact, state control of Food Aid concerns the peasant population in particular. Communities are granted Food Aid, in its "Food for Work" modality, only when the work to be performed is agreed upon, financed, and supervised by a state institution or a governmental organization to ensure that the rations are even and the work is done. This system allows for state presence in the life of the communities, and enables the political party in power, present mainly through CORDES, to attract more sympathizers, willingly or by force of circumstances.

Although the state intervention in Food Aid action lowers transport and staff costs for the private donor organizations, OFASA and CARITAS accept ONAA's interference only reluctantly, considering it "one actor more" and even a "competitor"; and they feel the same about the Ministry of Health's control of the rations. Despite this control, however, the rations vary according to the institutions involved and to the projects. In the rations that ONAA assigned to Huantan in 1987, for instance, wheat was the only cereal, and it had been increased at the expense of corn, which had made up the previous rations; fish, introduced for the first time, replaced canned meats and green peas, which had not been accepted. SCM, a soycorn-milk mix which forms a regular component of urban projects of Maternal and Child Health, was used in Huantan in 1982 by OFASA in order to "round out the rations."[6]

This "multi-actor" system is often a source of conflict. Tensions arise, for instance, because the action is not coordinated between Adventist and Catholic donor organizations (Degregori et al., 1986: 203) or because the work modalities imposed by the intermediary institutions are poorly accepted by the peasant population, which leads to the interruption of communal work and hence of Food Aid. Furthermore, CARITAS and OFASA are reluctant to accept a role as instruments for the realization of the government's social and political objectives, which do not necessarily coincide with their own aims. By acknowledging them not as "charity trusts" but as "development agents" integrated into a national program, however, the state grants them an official status and thus enables them to deal with other "institutional social agents" on equal grounds.

THE RELATIONSHIP BETWEEN HUANTAN AND THE FOOD AID ORGANIZATIONS

The peasants' negative perceptions of Food Aid projects and their conflict-ridden relationships with the donor organizations were brought to the fore by the 1986 meetings between the head of the state and the representatives of 3,200 peasant and Indian communities. From the proceedings of these meetings, it becomes clear that the criticism concerned the practical aspects of the projects as much as their ideological contents. "Under the pretext of Aid, they deceive the peasants with donations from foreign countries and doctrines that belong neither to our reality nor to our identity" (*Rimanakuy* 1986: 165). Notably, the peasant representatives considered that the Food Aid projects encouraged paternalism and damaged their traditional systems of reciprocity "through the introduction of new modalities of compensation which provoke conflicts between the community and its members" (ibid.: 231, 241). Conflicts with the intervening organizations in Huantan revealed similar attitudes of refusal, for which I identify three levels of explanation: the social organization of work in the communal projects, the conditions imposed for receipt of the food items, and the nature of the contact with the donor institutions.

The accustomed social organization of work in communal projects in Andean communities is often at the root of conflicts between the community and the external institutions involved in the "Food for Work" programs. Traditionally, the community distributes work among its members by rotation, according to the planned working time and the number of participating households, whereas the intervening institutions insist on a stable and less numerous labor force for the whole duration of the project. For instance, for the construction of the Paria-Cayuna irrigation channel in 1987, ONAA specified that 80 food rations should be distributed among 10 workers who would work the whole time, while the community preferred to distribute them among 80 families who would work one day each.

The reception of aid is defined by a given set of conditions: the community must have an adequate storage place for the supplies, a sketch of which (with exact measurements) must be submitted before food delivery may begin. Furthermore, the community must elect a commission (consisting of a president, a secretary, and four members) to oversee the storage and distribution of the food, according to the modalities prescribed by the donor institution. Finally, the community must present a list of the laborers to whom the work will be assigned and an estimate of the time needed. To comply with these conditions requires a considerable effort on the part of the community, and the peasants view the implicit necessity to write, read, and manage written documents as a difficult responsibility and a constraint.

The communal representatives prefer a direct contact with the donor institutions, which enables them to know their interlocutor and expose their needs as they feel them. However, direct contact with the Food Aid organizations is very costly in money (travel, stay in town) and time. As a consequence, the peasants are forced to communicate their needs through an intermediary, who transmits their requests to one of the Food Aid organizations, and the answer and the food supplies generally reach them through the same channel. Sometimes, however, several agents interfere in this process. For example, the construction of the community road that connects Huantan with the provincial main road took over two years, and for twelve months of the time Food Aid from OFASA and ONAA was received through the intermediary of the Ministry of Transport. A few years later, in July 1987, the Ministry of Agriculture supplied technological know-how for the construction of the Paria-Cayuna irrigation channel, while CORDES acted as an intermediary that supervised the work and ONAA was in charge of Food Aid.

This complex network of actors causes some confusion among the recipients of the aid who do not know the identities, roles, and affiliations of the various organizations involved. They consider them all food donors and distinguish only between "the state" and "the foreigners." Nevertheless, their expressions are more precise when referring to the reasons for which they think Food Aid is granted. Certain domestic units consider that they receive food "because we work," while others believe that they are helped "because we need it." These different perceptions correlate with the internal differentiation between poor and well-to-do households that can be observed in Huantan. The attitudes of households differ even more when referring to the food supplies received.

HUANTAN: A FOOD STYLE IN EVOLUTION

The communities of the High Basin of Cañete have, like many other Andean communities, their origin in the *reducciones* (administrative units for Andean people) instituted by the Spanish administration. Most of their inhabitants descend from Yauyos and Kaukes peoples, settled in the area since the pre-Inca and Inca period. Today, they are mainly Spanish-speaking and, with a few exceptions, keep vestiges of their cultural heritage only in some elements of clothing.

The food style currently observed in Huantan reflects the changes in the life of these communities, particularly from the 1940s (De la Cadena 1980: 49; Velasquez 1985: 9–10). According to my surveys, more than half of the food consumed by the 130 domestic units of Huantan (which occupies a vast territory between 3,200 and 4,500 m of altitude) derives from the households' own production. As cash revenues increase, however, the purchase of foodstuffs has gradually become more common, whether from other households of the community for meat and other local goods, or from communal shop-keepers and the traders who periodically serve the community by truck, for salt, sugar, oil, wheat flour, noodles, rice, etc.

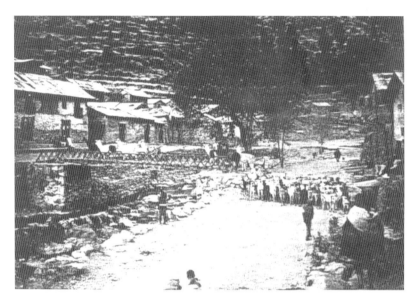

Figure 2 A view of Huantan village.

Barter remains a widely exercised practice, but today it is quantitatively less significant than purchase.

Nevertheless, the foodstuffs that derive from one's own production and from barter continue to rank at the top of the food hierarchy, well above those purchased on the market. These foods are typical of the Andean food style,[7] belong to both daily and festive activities, and play an important role in age-old Andean relationships of mutual help (*turnas*) and labor compensation in food (*minga*), as well as in modern relationships of wage labor (*peón*). Consumption needs alone do not determine the productive strategies of domestic units. These units also consider the roles their products assume in these social practices, roles that express the status of the families within the communal system of values. The foods correspond to these values according to a hierarchy based on a number of age-old elements to which other elements, more recently introduced, are added (Amat y León and Curonisy 1981: 60–66). High ideological value attaches particularly to rainfed tubers and maize, for which people refuse to use chemical fertilizers and modern technology. Rainfed tubers, that is, various traditional varieties of potato, as well as *oca* (Oxalis tuberosa) and *olluco* (Ollucus tuberosus), are all communal symbols of cohesion, not the least because their production involves interhousehold cooperation. Maize already occupied a privileged

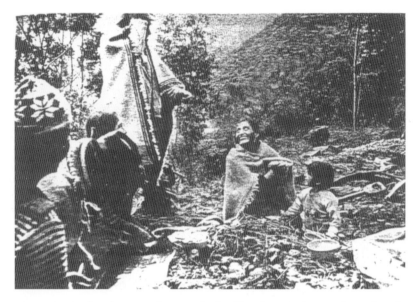

Figure 3 During the potato harvest, the families share the *huaytia* (a meal made of potatoes, cooked in a hole in the ground) with the *peones* and the *mingados*.

place in the symbolic system of the Inca Empire, where it is thought to have constituted the basis of food (Horkheimer 1973: 81–91). Despite the fact that in Huantan alfalfa has slowly displaced maize and that maize *chicha* (beer) has almost disappeared from the festive drinks, it still represents the highest value in the local food hierarchy. Maize and rainfed tubers bear the image of *food* per se and are considered essential to the practices of reciprocity between households in the community.

Wheat, barley, and fava beans, introduced by the Spanish in the sixteenth century, are important mainly in social practices within the domestic sphere. Cheese, finally, which has become the most important source of revenue for Huantan's families, and, more recently, improved varieties of potatoes (produced with modern technology and irrigation) are considered "modern": they allow an articulation with the market and, concomitantly, an increase in prestige within the community that seems to be greater even than the probable accumulation of capital. Furthermore, cheese, which bears the image of communal know-how, participates in the relationships of reciprocity between outsiders and community members.

The Huantainos' perception of the economic differences between the community households illustrates the close relation that they construct between food and social hierarchy. A first group are "those who have a lot" (*los que tienen harto*). They are assessed according to the importance the articulation with the market acquires in their household economies, whereas "those who have little" (*los que tienen poco*) are perceived according to their food needs. This second group can again be subdivided into two categories. Firstly, there are those caught between economic and social needs: at certain times of the year, for instance, they may be forced to take food items (commonly cheese) from the "family share" and sell them in order to cover economic needs, instead of consuming them within the family or using them in social practices of exchange between households. Secondly, there are those who have to work in exchange for food (*minga*) in order to feed themselves. The households in this study that constitute the "refusal" group in relation to Food Aid belong to the first group of this social hierarchy, while those that can be considered the "acceptance" group belong to both categories of the second one.

THE ATTITUDES TOWARD FOOD AID

The Refusal Group

The communal population that expresses contempt or refusal toward Food Aid is represented by six of the eleven domestic units analyzed in the present study. They are evenly distributed among all age groups and share a common characteristic: they are relatively well off economically. They figure among the important cheese producers and also grow improved varieties of potatoes in the irrigated area of the community, and they sell the surplus (after self-consumption) in the community and in the towns. The domestic units of this group that are most well off are local shopkeepers and/or traders in cheese and animals, whose business puts them in close contact with regional merchants and urban commercial activities. These links partly define their place and role within the community: as informants of the outside world within the community they are bestowed with social prestige. They always attend communal assemblies, and those to whom "civic" values or managerial capacities are attributed are called upon to take on responsibilities. At the same time, they can mount a strong opposition to communal plans, whenever the interests of the majority go against their own commercial interests. A level of education higher than the communal average (especially among the younger families, who moved to town to attend secondary schools) and close links with towns (repeated trips to Lima or Huancayo, where some of their children have settled) also

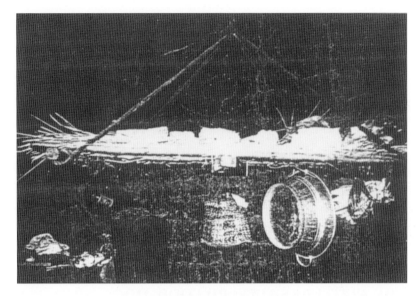

Figure 4 "Rich family's grid": several kinds of goat and cow cheeses, used fresh, dried, or smoked for various dishes.

reflect their more comfortable economic situation. Nevertheless, in public or private demonstrations of their lifestyle (clothing, furniture, domestic dwelling), they display no external signs of wealth that could harm the image of homogeneity which the community intends to maintain.

Most of the food that these households consume comes from their own production, except for wheat, for which substitutes in the form of flour and noodles can be bought on the market. Instead of adopting a strongly market-integrated and urban-oriented food style, the well-to-do house-holds modify, rather, the peasant food style: they follow the community's general pattern but consume more meat than the average, buy "wholesale" salt, sugar, and wheat flour (in 50 kg bags) and oil (in 5 liter barrels), and prefer the truck dealer to the small communal trader.[8]

The way these domestic units behave toward Food Aid programs shows that the principle of aid is well considered by most of them ("They help us because we work"). Nevertheless, four out of six regard Food Aid itself with detachment and mistrust: "Who knows them? They may be foreign-ers" (R. R., 74 years old); "It is some help even if we have enough to eat" (M. H., 57 years old); "It helps a bit, especially for those who do not have animals" (O. J., 32 years old); "Sometimes it is necessary" (R. H., 62 years

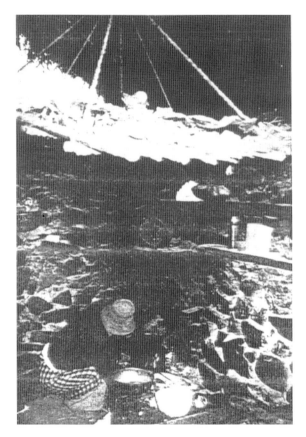

Figure 5 "Poor family's grid": bones and dried meat
(*charqui*) used for the soup.

old). And two young families refused Food Aid completely: "We do not
need it; the land gives us all we need, the rest, we get from our shop."

Concerning the aid foodstuffs, attitudes vary from suspicion and contempt to selectivity: "They are old: there are spider webs in the flour bags:
they are not good, except Trigor" (R. R.); "We have to be careful, they
may be old. We give them to pigs. The milk, we don't use it because we
have good milk here" (M. H.); "The oil and the flour are good; the rest is
for the dogs" (O. J.).

With respect to the actual use the six households make of Food Aid
items, two singular practices must be noted. When they do not consume
the foodstuffs themselves, they can always either use them to feed their

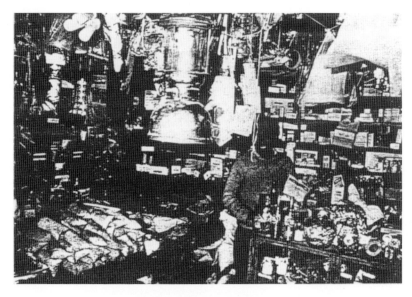

Figure 6   The most important grocery in Huantan.

animals or add them to the food offered in exchange for work (*minga*). This second practice is hidden and difficult to observe, but seems to be quite widespread and is criticized by those who work as *mingados*. Only one household declared that it used all the foodstuffs given, but in reality it employed them mainly to compensate a family taken on *minga* to weave a blanket. Likewise, the two households that expressed a total refusal of Food Aid had themselves replaced in the last "Food for Work" program by *mingados*, who then received the aid foodstuffs. In both cases, however, the aid foodstuffs formed a complement to the compensation, not its basis.

The Acceptance Group

The five domestic units in this study who have accepted Food Aid consist of three young households, still in their formative period, and two households with family heads of 35 and 65 years of age who failed to strengthen their economic situation in the second stage of the domestic cycle. All share a common characteristic with the other families of low economic position in the community: the household heads offer their labor as *peón*. The five domestic units of the "acceptance" group have, on average, less land in the irrigated area of the community than those of the "refusal" group. They

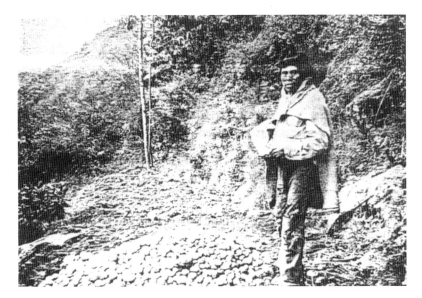

Figure 7   The old men are hired as *mingados* during the harvest and receive a portion of the harvest as well as daily meals and some coca.

produce small amounts of every item they consume and grow proportionately more of their own wheat than the former group. Some of them raise animals, mostly goats, but the sale of kids and cheese provides extra income only to the two older households, which managed to build up a herd of thirty to forty animals. The other households, which have no more than two to four heads of cattle, produce cheese and curdled milk for their own consumption and for various social uses, and only occasionally sell on the communal market.

Among the younger domestic units of the "acceptance" group, secondary education is the exception rather than the rule and, if begun, is seldom completed. Nevertheless, these households are conscious of their role in the communal relationships of power between the "old people" (the rearers) and the "younger people" (the farmers) and fulfill their civic obligations in the community with less reluctance than members of the economically better-off group. With respect to national politics, they vote "on the left," as opposed to most of the "refusal" group who choose right wing candidates or, in the end, "those who have most chances to be in power."

The households of the "acceptance" group often need to combine work on their own farm with extra-domestic modalities of work: the man works as *peón*, the woman as *mingado*, and both, at some time of the year, ask for and return mutual help (*turnas*), since social support is essential in their strategies to obtain food. With the money acquired from *peón* work, women buy necessary foodstuffs (sugar, salt, oil, etc.) at the communal grocer, by 100 g or by the "handful." The families of this group consume more rice, noodles, and grain or ground wheat than those of the "refusal" group, particularly when their own production is not sufficient, due to a bad harvest, or during the period of scarcity that precedes the next harvest. These purchased foodstuffs, however, are also consumed year-round, because they reduce the time required to prepare meals—an advantage that is especially important when the labor migration of the head of the family puts an extra strain on the woman's already tight time budget.[9]

The households of the "acceptance" group tend to appreciate Food Aid much more than do the households of the "refusal" group: "It is a blessing from God; it is very good, it should be increased" (B. A., 60 years old); "It helps us a lot" (T. C., 45 years old). Nevertheless, the young domestic units express a critical attitude toward the "Food for Work" modality, because of the physical and economic efforts they have to make to receive such aid. "Now they give us less, there is no more soya, semolina, ... and we have to pay for transportation from the road to here: 50 Intis per person. It is a lot for us!" (E. O., 28 years old); "I was there for the building of the bridge. It was very hard work; the women carried stones. My husband had gone to work in Satipo. They were going to give us foodstuffs, they said. So we carried a lot, it hurt the back and the stomach" (G. J., 32 years old). But although these younger families have a clear sense of the inequality involved in this exchange of work for food, they often agree to replace another family in communal work partly in return for Food Aid foodstuffs.

The attitudes of the "acceptance" group toward the foodstuffs received vary from total acceptance to selectivity and a differentiated appreciation of the quality of the products. "The food items are very good; we use them in different ways; we like soya, powdered milk ... everything very much" (B. A.). "Some of them have a good taste, but we eat them all" (T. C.). "Some of them hurt, such as powdered milk and Trigor which cause diarrhea; they must be old. With imported goods, who knows when they were produced? Some others are good: soya, oil" (E. O.).

From an analysis of the two groups, it becomes evident that their different attitudes toward Food Aid correlate with their economic differentiation and with the different roles they occupy in the community, much like the Sherifs (1968) pointed out. The range of attitudes toward Food Aid have, however, one point in common: a selectivity toward the foods received. Economic categories cannot explain this common attitude, which relates, rather, to the group's culture or, more specifically, to cognitive elements of Huantan's food style. Now, "peasant culture" (like other cultures) is not a homogeneous entity but one that members of a group internalize according to their position in the social structure (Mintz 1973: 95–98). Similarly, Food Aid foodstuffs are used in practices common to the whole community (culinary and commensality practices), as well as in specific practices related to the families' economic and social position (animal feeding, *minga*, family support). An analysis of the whole of these practices, whether common or specific, will better identify the factors most relevant to the families' behavior toward Food Aid. Nevertheless, one must remember that the elements intervening in a "food fact" are multiple and simultaneous (Calvo 1983). In the appreciation and the use Huantainos make of the aid food supplies, factors such as access to the market and sociocultural contact interact with cognitive factors.

FOOD PRACTICES AND FOOD AID ITEMS

On the whole, when used for human consumption, the foodstuffs from Food Aid programs receive no specific preparation, but are incorporated into the accustomed daily dishes, just like other industrially produced food items introduced via the market. Grain wheat is used for soups, or ground into flour for the preparation of *tortillas*, a kind of salty fritter made from wheat flour and water and fried in oil. With the soy-corn-milk mix, the women prepare a thick porridge, similar to the *sango* (made from barley grains roasted and ground and mixed with milk) that is eaten for the morning meal. Oil has been available through the market for a few years and today has almost completely replaced animal fat which was customarily used; frying, a coastal urban culinary practice, is now usual in Huantan. The oil received from the Food Aid programs is used for frying trout, potatoes, eggs, and sometimes cheese or cassava slices. Powdered milk, whether bought or received as Food Aid, is not reconstituted to be consumed as "milk," but is used in the morning meal mixed with infusions or as an ingredient of *mazamorra* (sweet porridge made from corn or wheat flour and milk), or is used in *pan con leche* (a snack of bread, soaked in milk, for children). Canned fish (sardines and tuna), bought or received from Food Aid, is eaten mainly along with rice, as are the trout that were introduced into the rivers and lakes of the area several years ago.

Other canned products like green peas and pork are unanimously rejected. Huantan, like other Andean communities, consumes many more cereals and tubers than vegetables. Vegetables brought by the traders (most commonly tomatoes, onions, lettuce, and pumpkin) are appreciated only if they are fresh, and they are used as ingredients of stews and soups "to give some taste." Similarly, pork meat is not consumed as such: pigs are reared not for family consumption but for sale: if the animal dies by chance, the fat is used as bacon or for frying (*chicharrón*). The regularly consumed meats (sheep, beef, llama), fresh or dried (*charqui*), are used as ingredients of soups or stews.

Wheat grain, oil, milk, and canned fish from Food Aid are used as ingredients of daily culinary practices and seem to be well accepted at this level. Canned pork and green peas, however, do not fit into the culinary practices of Huantan food style. One important reason for this difference is the fact that the former food items have been available on the market for several years, while canned pork and green peas have not and are therefore still unfamiliar to the Huantainos. This explanation suggests that by facilitating a "prior knowledge," the market is the main external factor determining the refusal or the acceptance of Food Aid items, especially since the rejected food items are not ones the Huantainos know through contacts with "urban-industrial" food styles.[10] It must also be noted that the daily dishes in Huantan, such as soups, *tortillas*, and *mazamorras*, are "dishes of encounter," whose elements come from both Andean and Creole cultures and whose ingredients have undergone many transformations over the centuries. It is likely that the "mixed" origin and previous transformations of these dishes culturally predispose the households to accept the new ingredients, namely those Food Aid items whose tastes resemble local products or their industrial substitutes, which are bought on the market.

By contrast, Food Aid items were not used in the dishes of highest value playing an important role in the relationships of cohesion in the community, such as *pataska* and *carapulka* (stews made from various kinds of potatoes and meats, and from whole or cracked wheat) which are prepared for the great moments of work and sharing (e.g., *Herranza* livestock branding, *Limpiacequia* irrigation-canal cleaning, and maize seed-time) and for family events like funerals, the nomination of a boy's godparents (*cortapelo*), or important visits. Even the poorest domestic units put some wheat aside for the preparation of these dishes, which are common in all the communities of the Cañete Basin but display culinary variations that are invoked to enhance group identity. All this suggests that the cultural value of a particular new food is determined not only in relation to the value of food items already known, but above all in relation to the whole sociocultural context into which it has to be incorporated (Delgado 1990).

An observation of specific non-culinary practices supports and broadens this hypothesis. Two families of the "acceptance" group criticized certain food items (powdered milk and Trigor) when they were obtained via Food Aid but appreciated them when they were received from the extended family or bought from the local shops. Thus, it seems that these foodstuffs become acceptable when "reconverted" or re-appropriated through specific actors (the extended family or the local shopkeeper) and social practices (mutual family aid or purchase) integrated into the community's system of sociocultural representation. In the "refusal" group, some families incorporated scorned products through two different practices: animal feeding and the *minga*. The fact that certain foods are considered inedible for humans but good for animals must be viewed within the context of the Andean food system in which each part of a product has a specific function. The parts of some products like leaves and stems, for instance, which are not consumed by humans, are integrated into the domestic economy through animal feeding. Similarly, even though contempt toward specific Food Aid items prevents the households from using them for human consumption, they integrate the items into the domestic economy through practices of reprocessing, recycling, and transformation, which are characteristic of the "behavior of self-sufficiency structures" (Raybaut 1981: 404).

The fact that Food Aid items appear in the *minga*, a traditional relationship of production that normally favors local food, must be considered a notable change. In the *minga*, the employer is customarily expected to prove his status by giving his *mingados* some of his own produce, and his prestige is at stake if he does not comply with these norms. But as sectors of Huantan's population are increasingly integrated into the national society, the communal notion of prestige and its relationship with food are undergoing a process of transformation (see Orlove 1987). Hence, the norm of compensating *mingados* with one's own produce may gradually weaken. Still, the fact that Food Aid foodstuffs only complement and never completely replace the customarily offered food items, shows continuity rather than radical change in this social relationship.

CONCLUSION: ACTOR LOGICS AND FACTORS OF CHANGE IN FOOD AID ACTION IN HUANTAN

One may summarize schematically elements of analysis from the present study, although in the food reality these elements compose a series of complex and dynamic relationships.

The symbolic and concrete transfers that Food Aid action effects intensify the relationship of inequality between the state and the donor institutions with their divergent but complementary interests, on the one hand, and the peasant community, on the other. At the same time, the aid action transforms social relationships in the latter. One can wonder, then, why the Huantan community asks for Food Aid, when it seems to be so full of conflicts and surrounded by negative connotations? It is the destitution experienced by Huantan's low-income households in particular, that motivates the community to ask for Food Aid in the event that communal works are scheduled. The relatively well-off families who do not actually need Food Aid foodstuffs themselves can either use their rations as partial compensation for *minga* work or choose not to participate in the project and be replaced by families who then recieve the rations in their place. This is how the principle of the *minga*, in the context of "Food for Work" programs, develops into a social instrument aptly used by the community to ease the economic situation of the poorer households and by members of the better-off sector of the community to enhance further their social position. In this sense, the Food Aid action is a power relationship: the state and the donor institutions produce an ideological deviation from the customary social content of the Andean practice of food for work and, at the same time, indirectly force a sector of the Andean population to transform its system of values and become actors of change.

The transformation of the system of values is, of course, difficult to apprehend, particularly in the food sphere, where facts are a matter of economy, social relations, and politics, as well as of culture and even of religion. Nevertheless, food practices remain a sphere of manifestations of "identity" in areas where a language, clothing, and religion different from the national society have long since disappeared or been greatly modified, as has been the case in Huantan and generally in the Peruvian Central Andes. To determine fully the role of new values in food practices and behavior would require a long-term study. This paper has a much more limited objective: to highlight the different factors playing a role in the Food Aid action in a peasant community and to contribute some empirical and conceptual elements to the analysis of processes of dietary transformation.

Factors that influence the peasants' perceptions of Food Aid include the often conflict-ridden relationship between the community and the intervening institutions; the peasants' misunderstandings about the donor organizations; and the fact that the food items are not chosen voluntarily but are assigned to the population. These factors form the "ideological background" (Bruneton Gouvernatori 1984) that explains why the people of Huantan are predisposed to an attitude of global refusal of Food Aid. The market—or rather the "voluntary" innovations it has effected in the Huantainos' diet—is another important factor shaping acceptance attitudes toward Food Aid items. "Food for Work" projects are indirectly a factor of change in food behavior, or they at least intensify ongoing processes of change, when their rations resemble in characteristics and imported origin foodstuffs introduced through the market.

Within this global disposition, behavior toward Food Aid foodstuffs is as diversified as the population itself. Socioeconomic differentiation is the main factor explaining the behavior of different domestic units toward the projects and the food supplies. It is mainly sociocultural factors, such as the cognitive structure of domestic units, the values and the taste specific to their own peasant food style, that determine whether the group will validate the Food Aid ingredients by incorporating them into their sociocultural practices.

NOTES

The data presented here are based on field research in Peru, 1986–87, and form part of a PhD project on the social dimensions of food practices at the Centre d'Etudes Comparatives sur le Développement (CECOD), Institut d'Etudes du Développement Economique et Social (IEDES), Université de Paris I. For the research, I received a grant from the Institut Français de Recherche Scientifique pour le Développement en Coopération (ORSTOM), within the project "Políticas agrarias y estrategias campesinas" (UNALM/IFEA/ORSTOM).

I wish to thank the CECOD researchers and particularly Dr. Maxime Haubert for his contribution to the analysis of the actor logics and Dr. Manuel Calvo for his insistence on the relevance of ingredients and dishes as categories of analysis in the study of food practices. I would also like to express my gratitude to the ORSTOM team of the P.A.E.C. project in Lima and the L.E.A. laboratory in Montpellier for their comments.

1. Food styles are intellectual representations of food reality. They are built from an analysis of the food objects, the attitudes and behaviors toward foods, and the practices of food consumption, which are, in turn, an integral part of the total social activity of groups or societies. By definition, food styles are dynamic, heterogeneous, and multi-dimensional (Calvo 1983: 426–427).

2. Attitudes, internal states of the individual belonging to the domain of human motivations, are not directly observable but are necessarily inferred from behavior. The Sherifs (1968: 112, 135) have demonstrated that the concepts of "acceptance" and "refusal" (which are opposite latitudes within the structure of attitudes) differ for members of a group according to their roles and to the importance of the issue to that group. Close links exist between the individual attitudes and the sociocultural and ideological values of a group.

3. For purposes of briefness, I shall use the terms "domestic units," "household," or "family," instead of "community's peasant domestic units" which would be more precise. These notions refer to the family nucleus of production and consumption, which is considered the first level of social organization, the second and third ones being the extended family and the community, respectively.

4. Between 1959 and 1979, Food Aid given to Peru relied heavily on donations. Ninety percent of the donations were received from USAID, which through organizations such as the Church World Service distributed the food items to institutions with religious affiliation and charitable, humanitarian activities (in Peru, mainly to CARITAS and OFASA). The latter also received foodstuffs from their respective U.S. homologues (Catholic Relief Service and Seventh Day Adventist Welfare). All foodstuffs had to be used in local programs with the approval of the respective U.S. organizations and USAID. From 1979,

"Food for Work" partly replaced free donation and the Peruvian state started to intervene more directly.

5. For instance, wheat, which is the main imported foodstuff, had a consumption-dependence coefficient (indicating the percentage of imports of the whole quantity of a specific foodstuff offered on the internal market) of 90.8 in 1986 (Lajo 1986: 12), and made up 93.5 percent of the cereals received as Food Aid in 1985–86 (FAO 1987: 48). It turned out to be the main food item in the rations allocated to the peasant communities by the Peruvian organizations in "Food for Work" programs.

6. Each ration is calculated on the basis of 360 grams per working day; a family receives 1,800 grams of food items each working day.

OFASA ration (1982)

Trigor (cracked wheat)	150 g
SCM (soy-corn-milk mix)	100 g
Green peas	30 g
Skimmed powdered milk	40 g
Vegetable oil	40 g

ONAA ration (1982)		*ONAA ration (1987)*	
Wheat grain	150 g	....	250 g
Corn flour	100 g	....	0 g
Skimmed powdered milk	40 g	....	40 g
Canned chicken or pork	40 g	Canned fish	30 g
Vegetable oil	40 g	....	40 g

7. Ferroni (1982: 853) describes the Andean dietary pattern as largely vegetarian, characterized by a large proportion of starchy staples, and very low contents of sugar and fat. Consumption of fruits, eggs, and dairy products is infrequent. The key elements are potatoes, maize, barley, quinoa, canihua, and beans. Variations within this basic dietary pattern mainly reflect differences in altitude.

8. Although this "wholesale" supplying could be considered simply a consequence of their more prosperous economic situation which allows them to take advantage of economies of scale in foodstuff purchases, there seems to exist another dimension as well: practiced within the peasant food style, "wholesale" supplying on the market practically and symbolically replaces self-supplying through one's own production (see Grignon and Grignon 1980: 536).

9. The families of the "refusal" group can cope with the lack of time by paying an extra worker and hence rely on home-grown foodstuffs which require more time-consuming procedures of preparation all year round. Nevertheless, families from both groups use industrially produced products because it allows them to "diversify the dinner meal."

10. Canned meat and canned vegetables have no part in the food style of the urban low-income population, with whom most of the Huantainos migrating or traveling to towns come into contact, nor are they consumed by well-to-do towndwellers, whom Huantainos working as traders, apprentices, or domestics may get to know. These products are not generally commercialized in the urban or rural markets, but instead seem to remain part of the temporary quotas of Food Aid.

REFERENCES

Amat y León, Carlos, and Dante Curonisy. 1981. *La alimentación en el Perú.* Lima: Centro de Investigaciones de la Universidad del Pacifico (CIUP).

Benavides, Marisela, and Robert Rhoades. 1987. "Socioeconomic Conditions, Food Habits and Formulated Food Programs in the Pueblos Jóvenes of Lima. Perú." *Archivos Latinoamericanos de Nutrición* 37, 2: 259–281.

Brunault, Jean. 1981. *Le Choix alimentaire: Emprise psycho-sociale et régulation*. Paris: Université de Paris V.

Bruneton Gouvernatori, Ariane. 1984. "Alimentation et idéologie: le cas de la châtaigne." *Annales: Economies, sociétés, civilisations* 6: 1161–1185.

Calvo, Manuel. 1982. "Migration et alimentation." *Information sur les sciences sociales* 21, 3: 383–446.

Calvo, Manuel. 1983. "Des Pratiques alimentaires." *Economie rurale* 154: 44–48.

Chombart de Lowe, Pierre. 1956. *La Vie quotidienne des familles ouvrières (Recherches sur les comportements sociax de consommation)*. Paris: Université de Paris. Faculté des Lettres.

Degregori, Ignacio, C. Blendet, and N. Lynch. 1986. *Conquistadores de un nuevo mundo. De invasores a ciudadanos en San Martin de Porres*. Lima: Instituto de Estudios Peruanos (IEP).

De la Cadena, Marisol. 1980. *Economía campesina, Familia y Comunidad en Yauyos*. Lima: Pontificia Universidad Católica del Perú (PUCP).

Delgado, Leticia. 1991. "Blé, savoir et saveurs: Alimentation et transition dans les Andes centrales péruviennes." In *Savoirs paysans et développement*, ed. G. Dupré. pp. 155–179. Paris: Karthala-ORSTOM.

Erard, Pascal, and Frédéric Mounier. 1984. *Les Marches de la faim. L'Aide alimentaire en questions*. Paris: La Découverte.

Ferroni, Marco. 1982. "Food Habits and the Apparent Nature and Extent of Dietary Nutritional Deficiencies in the Peruvian Andes." *Archivos Latinoamericanos de Nutrición* 32, 4: 851–866.

Fischler, Claude. 1986. "Learned versus "Spontaneous" Dietetics: French Mothers' Views of What Children Should Eat." *Social Science Information* 25, 4: 945–965.

Food and Agriculture Organization (FAO). 1983. *Food Aid in Figures*. Rome.

Food and Agriculture Organization (FAO). 1987. *Food Aid in Figures*. Rome.

Fryer, Jonathan. 1981. *L'Aide alimentaire, un marché de dupes*. Genève: Centre d'Etudes du Tiers Monde (CETIM).

Griffin, Philip. 1978. "L'Aide alimentaire au Pérou." In *L'Aide alimentaire pour le développement*, ed. Hartmut Schneider, pp. 98–119. Paris: Centre de Développement de l'Organisation de Coopération et de Développement Economiques (OCDE).

Grignon, Claude, and Christiane Grignon. 1980. "Styles d'alimentation et goûts populaires." *Revue française de Sociologie* 21: 531–569.

Häbig, Manfred. 1988. "Hilfe gegen die Selbsthilfe. Zehn Thesen zur Nahrungsmittelhilfe." *Der Überblick* 3: 59–61.

Haubert, Maxime. 1985. "Quelle autosuffisance?" In *Politiques alimentaires et structures sociales en Afrique Noire*, ed. Maxime Haubert et al., pp. 13–63. Paris: Institut d'Etudes du Développement Economique et Social (IEDES), Collection Tiers Monde.

Haubert, Maxime. 1988. "Coopératives de réforme agraire et sécurité alimentaire dans la sierra équatorienne." Mimeographed. Paper presented at the 7th World Congress for Rural Sociology. Bologna, Italy, 26 June–2 July.

Herrera, Nelson. 1987. "La racionalidad campesina andina y la alimentación. El caso de la comuna de Yanaturo en la Sierra Central del Ecuador." *Agricultura y Sociedad* 45: 183–227.

Horkheimer, Hans. 1973. *Alimentación y obtención de alimentos en el Perú prehispanico*. Lima: Universidad Nacional Mayor de San Marcos (UNMSM).

Lajo, Manuel. 1986. *La Reforma agro-alimentaria. Antecedentes, estratégia y contenido*. Cusco: Centro de Estudios Rurales "Bartolomé de las Casas" (CERA).

Lewin, Kurt. 1943. "Forces behind Food Habits and Methods of Change." *The Problem of Changing Food Habits. National Research Council Bulletin* 108: 35–65.

Mintz, Sidney. 1973. "A Note on the Definition of Peasantries." *The Journal of Peasant Studies* 1, 1: 91–106.

Mirsky, Richard. 1981. "Perspectives in the Study of Food Habits." *Western Folklore* 40, 1: 125–133.

Murra, John. 1975. *El "control vertical" de un máximo de pisos ecológicos en las economias de las sociedades andinas*. Lima: Instituto de Estudios Peruanos (IEP).

Orlove, Benjamin. 1987. "Stability and Change in Highland Andean Dietary Patterns." In *Food and Evolution*, eds. Marvin Harris and Eric Ross, pp. 481–515. Philadelphia: Temple University Press.

Plan Nacional de Seguridad Alimentaria. 1986. Lima: Instituto Nacional de Planificación (INP).

Raybaut, Paul. 1981. *Autoconsommation et société traditionnelle*. Paris: Ecole des Hautes Etudes en Sciences Sociales (EHESS).

Rimanakuy. Hablan los campesinos del Perú. 1986. Cusco: Centro de Estudios Rurales "Bartolomé de las Casas" (CERA).

Sánchez, Rodrigo. 1987. *Organización andina, drama y posibilidad*. Huancayo: Instituto Regional de Ecologia Andina (IRINEA).

Sherif, Muzafer, and Carolyn Sherif. 1968. "Attitude, Ego-Involvement and Change." In *The Social Judgment Involvement Approach to Attitude*, ed. Wiley, pp. 95–139. New York.

Velasquez, Benjamin. 1985. *Estudio Microregional de la Cuenca del Río Cañete*. Lima: Universidad Nacional Agraria La Molina (UNALM).

6. TASTY MEALS AND BITTER GIFTS: CONSUMPTION AND PRODUCTION IN THE ECUADORIAN ANDES

M. J. Weismantel

Department of Anthropology and Sociology, Occidental College,
Los Angeles, California 90041-3392, U.S.A.

The Quichua-speaking inhabitants of Zumbagua, a high rural parish of the Ecuadorian Andes, use a variety of indigenous terms to talk about the foods they cook and eat. Through a close reading of the parish discourses involving three of these terms, *mishqui, jayaj*, and *wanlla*, I argue that while they appear to operate in a sphere of consumption divorced from that of work, the terms contain implicit meanings derived from systems of production and exchange. Further, the deployment of these terms, apparently a symbolic rather than an instrumental action, is in fact a strategy for negotiating crises and hazards that originate in the larger economic system outside the parish. One could interpret the current use of these words in Zumbagua as showing a reluctance to conform to changing economic realities. But according to my interpretation, rather than reflecting a symbolic refusal to adapt to practical circumstances, the Zumbaguans' use of these terms reveals an accurate assessment of their situation and constitutes a realistic response to it.

These three terms are quite different: the opposed pair *jayaj* and *mishqui* (strong/bitter/hot and sweet/tasty) refer to physical taste sensations, while *wanlla* is one of a set of words that categorizes foods as appropriate to specific social contexts. In both cases, however, these terms place foods in a cultural context that shapes how people know them, creating implicit connections between sensory experience, cultural knowledge, and the political and economic structures of social life. The initial referents of the words in turn evoke other, more complex meanings. In the case of *mishqui* and *jayaj*, careful analysis of their uses reveals that for Zumbagua

Quichua-speakers, sensations of sweetness, saltiness, and hotness are sub-
tly related to issues of gender, of the social and productive roles of women
and men. Words such as *wanlla*, more explicitly social in their significa-
tion, refer to the role foods play in marking and maintaining relationships
between individuals and households.

The meanings of these words derive from the social relationships within
and between households that form the basic relations of production within
the parish. Analysis of the use of these terms thus reveals much about the
conflicts inherent in the Zumbaguan economy and also provides clues to
how the people of the parish experience, interpret, and respond to these
conflicts.

ABOUT ZUMBAGUA

Lying in a high valley of the western Cordillera of the Ecuadorian Andes,
the parish of Zumbagua is a very high, cold place whose population is
poorer and more Indian than are those of much of the Sierra.[1] Seen from
outside, Zumbagua appears to be a traditional Indian peasant society,
locked into a way of life centuries old. However, the people of Zumbagua
are facing changes and conflicts that are both profound and uniquely contemporary. It is not the case that Zumbagua, once a subsistence economy, is
only now becoming integrated into the national economy; rather, changes
in the nature of its centuries-old articulation with the world economic
system have presented this generation with a different set of problems than
those their parents faced.

From the 1600s until the mid-1960s Zumbagua was a hacienda run by a
series of white, urban-based owners and managers, ecclesiastic, state, and
private. Initially a tremendously lucrative property producing quantities of
wool for the Latacunga *obrajes* (textile workshops), as centuries of heavy
exploitation with no investment rolled by, the hacienda gradually sank
into poverty and obscurity, which its peons inherited when the Agrarian
Reform of 1965 made them its owners.

According to De Janvry (1981), in areas where the hacienda was previously the basic institution of agrarian tenure, a new dominant pattern of
social relations has emerged, characterized by semiproletarianization. This
term aptly describes the situation in which young men and women in
Zumbagua find themselves, living suspended between the rural homestead
and the urban workplace. Neither economy can fully support the household, and so women, children, and the old eke out a meager living on the

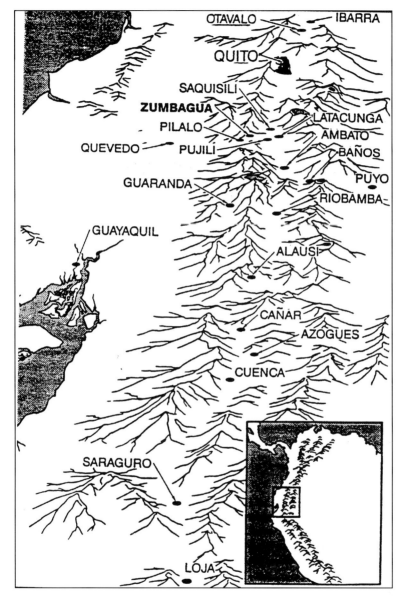

Figure 1 The Ecuadorian highlands. Adapted from *Republica del Ecuador: Mapa físico* (Instituto Geografico-Militar del Ecuador, 1978); used by permission. With map showing area of detail, from *Physical Map of South America* (National Geographic Society, 1972).

farm, with their monetary needs being partially met by the husband's wages, while he in turn is supported by both his wages and the farm.

The resulting dietary transformations in Zumbagua are unsurprising; trends include increasing poverty and reliance on purchased foods. The importance of manufactured items such as enriched flour and packaged noodles is rising and in some households has come to rival the role played by subsistence foods such as barley, potatoes, and fava beans. Mass-produced sugar and salt are replacing older forms; refined white sugar has become a food of some importance in the diet, and its significance is growing. Inadequate meals are "bolstered" by the addition of white sugar in poor households, while working men who cannot afford staple foods from the city bring home candies instead.

The expanding role of sugar in the diet highlights the fact that for impoverished rural families, the move away from farming is not always a sign of increasing prosperity. In the outlying rural areas of the parish, one finds that many of the families and individuals whose involvement in the cash economy is the heaviest and whose cultural traits are far less "Indian" than their fellows', are in some ways poorer than their neighbors. Their comparative poverty clearly shows in the nutritional inadequacy of their diet. Orlove (1987: 482) suggests that for the Andean area as a whole, "replacing locally produced native foods with purchased Western-style foods [is] accompanied by a decline in nutritional status," as cheap processed foods are substituted for the grains and vegetables of the agrarian diet.

Within Zumbagua, there are alarming signs that the diet of the parish as a whole is worsening and that the inhabitants are increasingly impoverished. Foods such as maize and vegetables, which cannot be grown in the parish but which parish residents commonly used to acquire through barter or purchase, are out of most peoples' reach today. In addition, apparently as a result of decreasing soil quality due to erosion, many farmers find themselves unable to grow potatoes, one of the three major subsistence crops in the parish. The lack of potatoes in the diet is keenly felt; families who can afford to buy them do so, using funds they would once have used to buy fruits from the lowlands or maize from the valley lands, foods increasingly defined as exotic or luxury foods.

The primary staple food in the parish today is not potatoes but barley. In some households day follows day with nothing cooked and eaten in the kitchen except barley gruel. In fortunate households sugar or salt or a lump of fat may flavor the potage. However, I have frequently shared meals consisting solely of ground barley and water; as I shall discuss below, such meals are most frequently eaten in households where husbands are absent doing wage labor in the city.

PRODUCTION AND CONSUMPTION

These changes in consumption are obviously related to changes in the economy as a whole and especially to changes in the realm of production, as an overdetermined cycle of ecological, economic, and social decline continuously weakens the subsistence economy and as dependence upon wage labor through male temporary migration steadily increases. Although the relationship between these changes and the way people in Zumbagua cook and eat is clear, the actual process by which changes in production transform consumption is not.

Marx emphasized the dialectical relationship between production and consumption: "Production creates the material as outward object of consumption; consumption creates the want as the inward object, the purpose of production" (Marx 1973. 93). Consumption is driven not only by material constraints, or what is possible, but also by the immaterial, culturally shaped definition of what is desirable.

What people eat represents the meeting-point between the desirable and the possible; as the latter changes, so must the former. In Zumbagua, for an older man who remembers other times, every month without a maize-based meal to break the monotony of barley is a month of lacking and hardship; but for his grandchildren the same regimen represents a state of unsurprising normality. For them, dietary variation means occasional indulgences in hard candies and a shared cola, rather than eating meals that contain different kinds of agricultural products.

The cultural concepts ruling the making of meals are far more complex than the simple definition of foods as desirable and undesirable. Scholarly discussions of diet have too often focused simply on quantities and types of food consumed, but this kind of treatment reveals little about how people decide what to eat and what to buy, judgments that are based on a complex structure of categories that define foods as appropriate for specific uses. Analyses of changes in consumption, if they are to reveal the processes by which economy affects culture, must also consider how these categories are altered. What needs to be explored is the process by which new products, perhaps initially perceived as novelties and luxuries, become, to borrow Mintz's succinct formulation, "transformed into the ritual of daily necessity and even into the images of daily decency" (Mintz 1979: 65).

In Zumbagua, potatoes are no longer a necessity but a luxury, while manufactured foods that were once a novelty have become commonplace. The changes are more subtle, however. As the productive structure of the Zumbagua economy changes, social relations between women and men, as well as relations within and between households, alter accordingly. These shifts in turn produce a transformation of the elaborate rituals of exchange that are intrinsic to Andean economy and society, a transformation that encompasses ongoing dietary shifts and makes them part of a less visible but more profound alteration in the very categories by which foods are defined, understood, and enjoyed. These cultural categories reflect the economy and society in which they arise: both rituals of consumption and the organization of production inform them.

For example, in Zumbagua a contrast is made between *caldo de cuy* (guinea-pig and potato stew) and a simple barley and cabbage soup, the former being a luxurious, special-occasion dish and the latter a mere everyday meal that meets the basic necessity of eating and living. These categories of the luxurious and the necessary, the special-occasion and the everyday, serve to distinguish foods that can be served to guests from those deemed appropriate for consumption within the household. These categories exist because a household has two kinds of needs: the need simply to maintain itself in the physical sense, and the need to maintain itself as a social entity interdependent with other entities. Changes in these definitions of foods or other consumer goods reveal the alteration of household consumption patterns to conform to changing productive strategies and capacities.

As is true throughout the Andes and in much of Latin America, a category of fictive kin or *compadres*, a relationship between adults established through the idiom of the Catholic "godparent" (Bolton and Mayer 1977; Dávila 1971; Foster 1953; Mintz and Wolf 1950; Ravicz 1967), enlarges the network of kin upon which each household in Zumbagua depends. Foods— cooked and raw, as gifts and as shared meals—are of paramount importance in establishing and maintaining these relationships of *compadrazgo*. While liquor, eggs, bread, and other foods may play a role at various points in the unfolding of a *compadre* relationship, one food, the *cuyes* or guinea pigs raised in every household, is so strong a symbol of the social networks that bind households that the animal simply cannot be conceptualized apart from its role in sustaining these relationships: "Why do we have *cuyes*? Because we have *compadres*."

Now, however, new strategies for survival make rich, white *compadres*, who may have influence at a bank, a school, or a politicians office, more valuable than a neighbor who unfailingly comes to help with the harvest. Indigenous Zumbaguans hesitate to serve *cuy*, an "Indian" food, to white *compadres*; one must serve them chicken and rice. This, in turn, affects household productive strategies, for while *cuyes* are raised outside of the market economy (in Zumbagua they are never bought or sold, and are fed gathered wild grasses), chickens and rice must be purchased with cash.

This sequence shows the intimate and dialectical relationship between production and exchange: because agriculture has become less important, the definition of a desirable *compadre* changes. The new relations with white *compadres*, in turn, make subsistence activities even less important, since they can no longer be used to support the *compadre* relationship.

The role of foods in the rituals that establish and maintain *compadre* relationships has often been commented upon (see, for example, Mayer 1974). But the meanings categories of consumption give to foods pertain not only to the exchanges in which foods are consumed but also to the social relationships involved in their production.

Peasant economies are marked by heterogeneity. By its very nature the modern peasant household is involved in a variety of productive activities, each implying a different type of articulation with the outside world. Subsistence agriculture, wage labor, petty commodity production; buying, selling, trading: no single economic practice characterizes the rural household. Rather, the very multiplicity of their endeavors defines contemporary peasants.

It is not a single peasant but rather the peasant household as a whole that is involved in all these activities; individuals are typically somewhat specialized. The family assigns productive roles to its members according to age and sex or other social criteria. Children may be the primary shepherds, for example, while adults concentrate on agriculture, or women may be the exclusive agents in the petty commodities market while men are engaged in primary production. As a result, of the products that the household receives as the fruits of its collective labor, specific family members contribute certain categories of things.

These productive roles in turn inform the roles assigned to certain foods as consumables. The productive origins of foods affect their categorization in consumption, and, as part of this process, the social roles of the producer become part of the meanings foods carry. These social variables can influence even the sensory experience of eating.

TASTY INSIDES AND BITTER OUTSIDES

Thus in Zumbagua, the taste of certain things is characterized as *jayaj*, bitter or strong. The basic *jayaj* product is the hot red pepper or *uchu*, but the symbolic referents of *jayaj* are many, and I can summarize only a few of them here: a *jayaj* food is eaten raw, and it is associated with males, with the hot *yunga* (cloudforest) zone that lies below the parish, and with suprahousehold networks of production and exchange. In its symbolic associations, it is related to other lowland products such as tropical fruits, to rock salt, to cane alcohol, and to tobacco. All of these products share origins outside the parish, involvement in spheres of suprahousehold consumption especially during rituals, and a role in consumption defined by an absence of cooking and by use either as a condiment superfluous to the body of a meal (rock salt in some cases, and *uchu* always) or as a product consumed outside the structure of meals (fruit, tobacco, and alcohol).

These characteristics can be compared with those of *jayaj*'s contrasting term, *mishqui*. Modern Ecuadorian Quichua dictionaries (see, for example, Stark and Muysken 1977: 256; Moreno Mora 1955: 295; Guevara 1972: 336) translate *mishqui* as "sweet" or "*dulce*," with a secondary meaning of "*sabroso*," "tasty." These brief definitions do not capture the polysemous and seemingly contradictory nature of the word, however. For example, *mishqui* foods may be either sweet or salty: the two items for sale in the markets that Zumbagua women refer to as *mishqui* are candy (although in Zumbagua the Spanish *caramelos* is more common than the Quichua *mishqui*) and the package of instant flavoring for soups, of which the predominant ingredients are salt and monosodium glutamate. However, in Zumbagua *mishqui* is most commonly used in speaking not of things for sale in the market, but of foods cooked at home: starchy, boiled, and (to my palate) typically bland dishes are referred to as *mishqui* when the intent is laudatory.

As with the term *jayaj*, epitomized by the hot *yunga* product *uchu*, the best way to grasp the essential meaning of *mishqui* is to begin with its central, most basic usage. Among all the foods adjectivally described as *mishqui*, there is one that is simply named *mishqui* and so may be considered to be the quintessential *mishqui* food. This is the simple gruel made of sweetened ground barley without other ingredients.

The meaning of *mishqui* becomes clearer if we contrast the manner in which this food is produced and used with that of *jayaj* foods. Whereas *jayaj* evokes a masculine realm of exotic foodstuffs acquired beyond the parish, this plain barley gruel is of all the foods eaten in Zumbagua most purely the product of household labor and of subsistence agriculture. Similarly, when many other foods are described as *mishqui*, such as soups, stews, and gruels, the word seems best glossed as "tasty" or "well cooked"; the word then points to the nature of these foods as cooked, nourishing, and made within the home, to be eaten by the members of the household alone. The contrast to *jayaj* foods, with their strong or bitter tastes, their exotic origins, and their role in extrahousehold ritual, is clear. *Mishqui* has a definite sense referent of tastiness, whether sweet or savory, and it thus applies to sugars, salts, and other seasonings used in cooking, and hence to the candies that are as sweet to the taste as raw sugar or *panela*.[2] But the central significance of *mishqui* resides in the warm, comforting, sweet cooked gruel that is perhaps the food most closely associated with family life, with childhood, and with motherhood.

Not only is *mishqui* the first solid food a woman gives her babies and the food she first feeds her family on many days; it is also the food that is most purely the product of women's labor. Cooking is, of course, the fundamentally feminine task, but in Zumbagua the production of a barley-based meal involves women's labor on a much greater scale, from the initial sorting of seeds, to planting, weeding, harvesting, threshing, storing, and grinding, and to the final stages of toasting and boiling. As male labor is increasingly withdrawn from agriculture and becomes wage labor, all of these tasks, not just the final processes, are coming to be defined as feminine (Deere 1976).

The burden of labor placed on women has thus become more onerous, and at the same time, as agricultural yields decline because of the region's degraded ecology, their labor produces progressively smaller portions of the family diet. *Jayaj* and *mishqui*, with their referents of male-raw-outside and female-cooked-inside, may have once referred to an agricultural economy in which both women and men worked in the fields (for the hacienda as well as on their own plots or *huasipungos*) and in which the task of going outside the parish to acquire exotic products was a male enterprise, while the final processing and cooking of agricultural products were feminine ones.[3] Now, however, the division of labor is changing and so is the composition of the cookpot. Subsistence agriculture is increasingly feminized, but not all of the staple foods used in cooking are the products of that subsistence labor.

Women still cook *mishqui*, but for the most part young men do not go down to the *yunga*, nor are the foods they acquire jungle products. They work in Quito, the capital, and the products they bring home are largely manufactured goods. Like jungle products, some of them are not essential to the meals a household shares; if he meets with a windfall, a man will purchase tropical fruits. And some of the foods men buy, such as breads, crackers, cookies, and candies, play a part in the flow of *fiesta* and special-occasion foods that link households. But many of the processed foods brought home from the city take the form of bags of flour and noodles and Quaker oats, staples that are used in cooking and feeding the family.

Ideally, men would like to return to the parish each weekend bearing all of these foods: a flashy display of candies and cookies, big bags of bread and lush fruits for immediate enjoyment, and beneath it all a substantial amount of foodstuffs for the week ahead. Breads and fruits, however, are expensive;

for most men on most weeks, a few bags of the cheapest noodles and flour and a handful of penny candies must suffice. But whatever the actual composition of the groceries brought home, the term that is used to describe them is not *jayaj*, but another, quite different indigenous concept, *wanlla*. And on Saturday morning when he takes his family down to the weekly market, the foods he buys there will also be described as *wanlla*. The use of this term to describe the staple elements of a man's contribution to the household diet, however, seems to contradict the widely accepted meanings of the term.

WANLLA: THE GIFT

Wanlla is anything that is not part of a meal. In this sense, it can be translated as "snack," "treat," "junk food," or "dessert food," and *wanlla* can be all of these. There are four types of foods that are always *wanlla*: bread, fruit, sweets, and cooked food bought in the market. But just as *uchu* epitomizes the word *jayaj*, or sweet barley gruel *mishqui*, bread is the *wanlla* par excellence. It is the universally appropriate gift, the favorite treat. The distribution of bread is critically important in many social and ceremonial contexts. Large amounts of bread are necessary for certain formal gift-giving exchanges: between bride's and groom's families at weddings, for the dead on *Finados* (All Saints' Day), when asking a formal favor.

In Zumbagua minds, bread has none of the qualities of a staple. It is truly a *golosina*, a treat, a luxury. Although people express greed for bread, it is not thought of as something to satisfy hunger. Unlike staple foods, the amount of bread a household consumes depends directly on the family's disposable cash income. It is the one special food that everyone would like to have on hand all the time, while at the same time it is agreed that no one ever "needs" bread. Potatoes and barley are necessities; bread, like fruit and sweets, is for enjoyment.

In the same way, food that is bought in the market is seen as *wanlla* rather than as an actual meal, even when it is similar to food that is prepared at home. Many people bring cooked food from home to eat at the market, being unable to afford to buy lunch there; eating at the food stalls is a pleasure and an indulgence.

The function of these kinds of treats is obviously more social than dietary. The social uses to which *wanlla* foods are put defines, in fact, the whole category, whether those foods are animal or vegetable, expensive or cheap. *Wanlla* can be defined as treats or snacks, but a more exact translation is "gift." One buys *wanlla* foods primarily in order to redistribute them, but the motive is less altruism than the exercise of power. Giving *wanlla* is a critically important social and political action in Zumbagua; no one can be a successful social actor without understanding how to give and to manipulate others into giving. *Wanlla* is double edged. When done informally, the giving of *wanlla* expresses a relationship of superiority/ inferiority: men give *wanlla* to women, parents to children, rich benefactors to the humble poor. To give *wanlla* to a social equal, such as a sibling, is both to offer them pleasure and to gain a slight advantage in prestige over them; to offer this type of *wanlla* to persons who consider themselves one's social superior is to insult them.

Whereas men spend their Saturdays exchanging toasts of cane alcohol at the *trago* shops, marketday for women is distinguished by gifts of *wanlla*, *golosinas* as they say in Spanish: little food treats shared among sisters or friends, but especially among persons with blood bonds. It is at the marketplace, among other women and girls, that the giving of *wanlla* becomes a women's affair. A woman gives her *comadre* a two-sucre sweet bread; it is divided in half to be shared with the *comadre*'s sister, who breaks it again to split between her two children. Some *wanlla*, once received, can be tucked away to be redistributed later; not the least of the pleasures it gives its recipient is the possibility of using the treat as a gift for someone else.

In other contexts, *wanlla* expresses respect and the acknowledgement of an ongoing relationship. A woman's siblings bring *wanlla* when she bears a new child. Adult children who have established their own household bring *wanlla* when they go to share festive meals with their parents. *Wanlla* of this sort, while it may be embellished with fruit, cookies, or the like, usually takes the form of uncooked staples. Noodles, flour, rice, or other purchased foods are the preferred form.

Intrinsic to the tradition of *wanlla* is the idea that whereas it is a necessary aspect of social interactions and, hence, is necessary for households in their social reproduction, it is not essential to the simple everyday maintenance of the household in an economic sense. *Wanlla* foods are not part of a meal; they play no part in the sustenance of family members; such a role would be antithetical to the concept of *wanlla* itself.

Wanlla is necessary to the household, but only because according to Zumbagua thinking the household depends upon the goodwill of other households. In the Andean agrarian economy, no household can survive without ties of kin and *compadrazgo* to support it (Alberti and Mayer 1974; Bolton and Mayer 1977). These ties, which primarily provide access to labor and mutual aid, are created and maintained largely through the ritualized exchange of food and drink. The movement of foods between households is also the mark of ongoing exchanges of labor: families that share food share agricultural tasks as well.

Wanlla plays an extremely important role in interactions between members of a household, as well as between households. At the market on Saturday, husbands who work in the city make a point of buying cooked food for their wives, and this is thought of as *wanlla*. So, too, are the little bags of *mote* (hominy) or lupines topped with chopped vegetables, toasted maize, bacon bits, and hot sauce; fried fish; portions of pork; sweet breads; even cooked potatoes with hot sauce are wrapped up in scraps of cloth, paper, or plastic and taken home as *wanlla* for household members who stayed home to care for animals and children. In order to understand why these little food treats that parents bring home from the market, or that husbands and fathers bring back from the city, are defined by the same term as is used to describe formal prestations of food between households, it is necessary to grasp the internal social and economic structure of the household. Unlike the Western family, the indigenous Andean marriage is not based on the principle of the merging of property. Rather, the household is a union of members, each of whom owns certain resources, inalienably theirs, and contributes labor and products to the household in exchange for the labor and products of other household members. The sheep penned behind the house are individually owned but jointly tended; land holdings are similarly individually owned and jointly worked.

When a husband goes to work in the city, the wages he earns are his own; his wife has no right to them. The Western model of the wife as dependent is utterly alien to Zumbagua minds, although changing circumstances may make it familiar. A man comes home from the city bearing gifts because it is incumbent upon anyone returning from a trip to re-enter the house with *wanlla*: gifts, treats, luxuries, exotic products from distant places.

But while the symbolic role of *wanlla* remains that of snacks and treats, frivolous little elaborations to a diet that depends upon the basic sustenance provided by the family farm, the realities of household economics are quite different. As subsistence farming's ability to support the family erodes, groceries bought with wages are of ever-increasing importance. The *wanlla* a man brings home from the city includes not only the readily consumable items typically referred to by that term—bread, fruits, candies—but also raw ingredients for cooking, such as noodles and Quaker oats, that require a woman's labor to become edible. These items serve as *wanlla*, gifts, like any foodstuff, when the newly arrived family member presents them to his fellow household-members. But they will be transformed into the *mishqui* soups and gruels his wife serves later, although, as Zumbaguans emphasize, only a meal made of ingredients that are home-grown as well as home-cooked is truly *mishqui*.

Why do the people of Zumbagua continue to refer to noodles, flour, wheat, and rice destined for the cookpot as *wanlla*? The answer to this question lies not in the realm of culture and symbol, but in the precarious economic situation of the parish.

POVERTY AND WEALTH

The dietary changes occurring in Zumbagua reveal several related processes: the increasing inability of the land to provide a basic subsistence, so that cash is being used not only to purchase luxury foods but also to provide part of the basic caloric intake; a move on the part of many young males to seek wage-labor jobs instead of remaining in the agrarian economy; and a concomitant interest in abandoning "Indian" ethnic markers of language, dress, and culture in order to compete more successfully for jobs. At the same time, however, there is a great deal of political turmoil and social conflict within the parish over whether to abandon agricultural work and indigenous lifeways. Opposition derives not so much from innate conservatism as from the perception that, to date, few men from Zumbagua have found more than transient employment outside the parish.

Superficially, young men often seem to be better off than their parents. Not only do they speak Spanish and converse easily of the big cities and national current affairs, topics of which their elders profess ignorance; but they have jobs and money, wear shoes and wristwatches, live in tin-roofed houses, and travel around the parish by bus, while their parents trudge barefooted back and forth from their fields to thatched huts. Young men also seem to have long periods of leisure, while their wives and parents must leave home before dawn to work in the fields.

To the indigenous way of thinking, however, neither idle hours nor small change for bus fares counts as wealth. Wealth consists of land, livestock, and access to labor—things the old have and the young do not. Land and animals one acquires very gradually over a lifetime (Lambert 1974: 8–17); the lifelong partnerships of the *compadrazgo* system, which provide one with business partners, loan services and agricultural labor, accumulate even more slowly.

The money that young men earn is enough to buy some of the trappings of whiteness: a cassette tape player, a radio. It is not enough, however, to buy land or livestock; nor do these men earn enough to live solely on purchased foodstuffs like true proletarians. Young adults remain dependent on their parents for their daily sustenance and for their long-term survival as well, through the property they will eventually inherit. At the same time, however, they cannot afford to invest in an agricultural future.

The semiproletarianized local economy, coupled with the steadily deteriorating national economy, creates tremendous strain for young adults in Zumbagua. Women and men experience the problem differently, but its roots are the same. For men, the experience of seeking work in the city, which for young boys holds a tremendous glamour and appeal, quickly deteriorates into a grueling battle for scarce, badly paying, temporary jobs. Among the psychological traumas involved is the need to hide one's indigenous heritage. Physically, the five- or twelve-day sojourn in Quito is an exile, lived out in cramped quarters shared among a dozen men and boys, eating lunches of Coke and bread and suppers of noodles and salt. Despite every effort to economize, constant inflation erodes one's scant earnings as the week goes by. Bus fares to and from Zumbagua alone may eat up one or two days' wages. As his family grows, a man's return home is met with increasing demands for shoes, clothes, groceries, medicine, and school supplies; for while a Zumbagua wife is not a dependent, children nevertheless are.

Many women, in the meantime, live a feast-or-famine life. They subsist on barley and water during the week, awaiting the return of a husband who takes the whole family to the market on Saturday morning and treats everyone to sodas, potato pancakes, pieces of pork, mutton, and fish, oranges and bananas, and bread, only to disappear again on Sunday afternoon.

Under these circumstances the category of *wanlla* comes to have a meaning reciprocal to the *almuirzu*, the full home-cooked meal. Wives anxiously prepare the best meal they can on Friday or Saturday, knowing that their husbands have eaten scantily and poorly during the week. And in the days before his arrival, thoughts and conversation turn repeatedly and anxiously to speculation over what *wanlla* he may bring.

As foods bought with wages continue to grow in importance, even the meal a woman prepares to welcome her husband may use flour paste rather than ground barley as its base. Nevertheless, both partners de-emphasize the total economic importance of the man's contribution; just as they continue to treat his travels to Quito as a temporary phenomenon, maintained only until he can resume his real life as a full-time subsistence farmer.

ECONOMIC FACTS AND CULTURAL FICTIONS

Zumbagua ideologies continue to emphasize the primacy of the agricultural and domestic world and its ability to maintain the family, and it is men as well as women, the boys who work in the city as well as their elders, who subscribe to these views. For the people of Zumbagua not only the economic primacy of farming, but the social hierarchy within the family that the relations of production in the domestic mode demand, are centrally important to their cultural identity.

Like the Zumbagua valley's isolation from the outside world, the self-sufficiency of the farmstead is a necessary fiction, a self-image contradicted by practice. Describing contributions that come from the urban, cash-based economy and are acquired through wage-labor as *wanlla* allows the household to maintain the image of itself as an agrarian unit, surviving on its own local resources of land, animals, and traditional labor patterns.

The only dependency the household acknowledges as absolutely necessary to its survival is the network of kin and neighbors sustained through the giving of *wanlla*. According to this way of thinking, the Saturday market is significant primarily as a site for small exchanges of cane alcohol and *wanlla* between members of different households.

The market thus serves as a major playing field for weekly games of giving and receiving that reinforce rural economy and society. But this fabric of interactions is a thin overlay adorning without concealing the main economic movement of the market. While interaction between locals sustains a network of kin and neighbors, the significant movement at the market is the transfer of sucres from the hands of local people into those of the petty commodity sellers who come up from nearby towns and urban areas. The market people who come to a high rural area like Zumbagua charge inflated prices to cover their long trip and the cold and discomfort they must endure there; if they did not make a profit, they would not come at all.

Although the ideology of reciprocal gift-giving is still strong in the parish, narrow economic ties with the anonymous market system are steadily supplanting these relationships. As dependence on purchased goods produced outside the parish increases, the rural household draws less and less support from its web of personalized thick relations with kin and *compadres* and becomes instead an isolated unit of consumption and production interconnected more with the economy outside the parish than with its neighbors.

Ironically, the demands of the gift-giving relation between households aggravate the need for cash. Increasingly, food produced in the parish is not used in prestations between households. Barley, fava beans, onions make very poor *wanlla*; the only really acceptable *wanlla* foods are those sold in the cities or in the market. Thus, the demand for cash has permeated even the social and affective ties that bind household and parish together.

Similarly, the bond between husband and wife is increasingly predicated on the gift of manufactured and purchased *wanlla*. Although the women of Zumbagua spend their working lives involved for the most part in the subsistence economy, they fill their hours with reflections on things only money can buy. Sifting ground barley, peeling potatoes, singeing a *cuy*, women frequently turn thoughts and conversation to the deployment of precious Quito-earned sucres.

For men, while the first adventure of going to the big city may have made home seem shabby and unimportant, as years go by these same men are capable of spending almost all their days and nights in the city and yet never faltering in their assertion that they *live* in Zumbagua: Quito is just where they temporarily work. It is very important to them that their home life and the subsistence agriculture on which it is built remain intact, for it is their only security when ill, unemployed, or in their old age. It is the only haven they can offer their children and elderly parents, whom their wages cannot possibly support. And, in fact, although the subsistence economy is weakened, it remains crucial for Zumbagua survival. Only a tiny percentage of the households in the parish could survive on wages alone; most would starve without the barley gruels and potato soups that make up many meals.

Life in Zumbagua today, then, is based upon a strategy of involvement in two economies in which the distinction between male and female deploys individuals as producers, while the institution of marriage unites them as consumers. The need all household members share for the rural farmstead to remain intact and economically viable keeps alive a strong ideology of agrarian self-sufficiency and indigenous isolationism. Ecological degradation, overpopulation, and the lack of a market for rural products makes the peasant lifeway less and less tenable, yet it remains indispensable for the survival of Zumbagua residents.

Because of this situation, family members unite in their insistence that the farmstead is the center and home, while urban wage-labor is a temporary and peripheral aspect of modern life. The category of *wanlla*, applied to consumer goods purchased in the city or market, enables Zumbagua households to maintain this ideology whatever the actual financial and nutritional significance of these contributions. The use of this category reveals a determined insistence on a definition of purchased foods as treats, snacks, luxury foods, and frivolous gifts. By defining starch foods purchased with wages as *wanlla* even when they are destined for simple everyday consumption, Zumbagua consumption terminology asserts that the subsistence farm, not wage labor, is the fundamental, dependable locus of household economic activity.

The category of *wanlla* refers to foods only as consumer items; it says nothing about how they are produced or, indeed, about the substances of which they are made. In this it differs from the *mishqui/jayaj* categories, yet, like them, *wanlla* contains implicit meanings about the social and economic structures that make consumption possible. The immediate referents of the term *wanlla* and its use as a label for products that originate in the market economy, suggest a commitment to an ideal of agrarian self-sufficiency and indigenous identity. This ideal does not stem from a system of cultural values that ignores economic realities; rather, it relates directly to the household's productive strategy. As long as wage labor does not offer a permanent and stable alternative to subsistence farming, Zumbagua households remain wary of endorsing it as central to their survival: men's contributions to the diet from their wages are fundamentally just *wanlla*.

Mishqui and *jayaj* are terms whose immediate meaning is a sensory experience of taste, but they also refer to the relations of production through which foods are made or acquired. Likewise, to call a bag of Quaker oats *wanlla* is to refer production both directly and indirectly. Directly, the term refers to the male purchaser's role of bringing manufactured goods acquired through wage labor into the household to complement the subsistence crops produced by his wife; indirectly, the term reflects an ideological insistence on preserving an "Indian-farmer" identity. Far from existing *despite* the household's increasing involvement in urban wage-labor, this ideology is, in fact, maintained *because* of it.

The use of the indigenous categories *jayaj*, *mishqui*, and *wanlla* to describe foods is not a residual or traditional aspect of Zumbagua culture, unrelated to current economic transformations. These categories of consumption have a complex relationship to spheres of production and exchange: they not only reflect or react to changes in the latter, but actively speak to them. In describing a food bought with wages as *wanlla*, household members express their experience that wages are inadequate and intermittent. Furthermore, using the word is part of an active strategy, based on this perception, that tries to contain their growing dependence on those wages. Words are not charms: calling manufactured foods *wanlla* will not grow more potatoes from exhausted soils or change the economic crisis of the Andes. But naming foods and, in so doing, naming the crisis and defining a strategy for surviving it, is an act, and such acts are part of the active role Zumbagua people play in making their own history.

NOTES

This paper is based on twenty-four months of research done between 1982 and 1985. Funding came from a Fulbright-Hayes grant and from several smaller grants from the University of Illinois. My primary debt of gratitude is to the people of Zumbagua and especially to the Familia Chaluiza, but the support of the Instituto del Patrimonio Cultural del Ecuador also made my work possible. For the elaboration of the map, thanks are due to Mark Stone. For further development of the ideas presented here, see Weismantel (1988).

1. Zumbagua is a civil parish located in Cotopaxi Province, Canton Pujilí. It lies just west of the parish of Tigua, with which it shares many cultural traits, and is bisected by the Latacunga–Quevedo highway. The parish encompasses some 10,000 hectares of land, divided more or less evenly between high *páramo* grasslands used in sheep-llama pastoralism and lower agricultural lands. Elevations range from slightly above 3,200 meters to well above 4,000. Population estimates indicate a figure above 15,000.

2. It will not have escaped the attentive reader's notice that salt and sugar are inherent parts of the cooking process, yet both have origins outside the parish and would seem to fall outside the definition of *mishqui* that I give here. The full implications of these contradictions lie beyond the scope of this paper, but I interpret them as reinforcing an Andean ethic that insists on the reciprocal dependence of outside and inside, male and female, self-dependence and interdependence, as economic and moral imperatives. Thus at the very heart of the woman's labor in cooking is an ingredient (whether sugar, salt, MSG, or other purchased seasoning) that, while nutritionally irrelevant to the task of feeding the family, is nevertheless imperative for its aesthetic and sensory success; and this ingredient is precisely that which must come from the masculine, extra-household sphere.

3. Again, some contradictions which the argument I am pursuing does not permit me to expand upon: In previous centuries Zumbagua was not a subsistence economy, so earlier economic arrangements did not involve a simple production for use, but rather production for the hacienda. Additionally, in preceding decades men went to the *yunga* zone not only to acquire exotic goods but also to earn money through what is laconically referred to in the parish as working *michitiwan*, "with a machete": wage labor on small sugar *fincas*. This type of labor still contributes to the economies of some households today.

REFERENCES

Alberti, Giorgio, and Enrique Mayer, eds. 1974. *Reciprocidad e intercambio en los Andes peruanos*. Perú problema 12. Lima: Instituto de Estudios Peruanos.

Bolton, Ralph, and Enrique Mayer, eds. 1977. *Andean Kinship and Marriage*. Special Publication of the American Anthropological Association, no. 7, Washington, D.C.: American Anthropological Association.

Dávila, Mario. 1971. "Compadrazgo: Fictive Kinship in Latin America." In *Readings in Kinship and Social Structure*, ed. Nelson Grayburn, pp. 396–406. New York: Harper and Row.

Deere, Carmen Diana. 1976. "Rural Women's Subsistence Production in the Capitalist Periphery." *Review of Radical Political Economics* 8, 1: 9–7.

De Janvry, Alain. 1981. *The Agrarian Question and Reformism in Latin America*. Baltimore: Johns Hopkins Press.

Foster, George M. 1953. "Cofradía and Compadrazgo in Spain and Spanish America." *Southwestern Journal of Anthropology* 9, 1: 1–28.

Guevara, Dario. 1972. *El castellano y el quichua en el Ecuador*. Quito: Casa de la Cultura Ecuatoriana.

Lambert, Bernd. 1974. "Bilaterality in the Andes." In *Reciprocidad e intercambio en los Andes peruanos*, ed. Giorgio Alberti and Enrique Mayer, pp. 1–27. Lima: Instituto de Estudios Peruanos.

Marx, Karl. 1973. *Grundrisse der Kritik der politischen Ökonomie*. Trans. Martin Nicolaus. New York: Random House.

Mayer, Enrique. 1974. "Las reglas del juego en la reciprocidad andina." In *Reciprocidad e intercambio en los Andes peruanos*, ed. Giorgio Alberti and Enrique Mayer, pp. 37–65. Lima: Instituto de Estudios Peruanos.

Mintz, Sidney W. 1979. "Time, Sugar and Sweetness." *Marxist Perspectives* 2: 56–73.

Mintz, Sidney W., and Eric R. Wolf. 1950. "An Analysis of Ritual Co-Parenthood (Compadrazgo)." *Southwestern Journal of Anthropology* 6, 4: 341–368.

Moreno Mora, Manuel. 1955. *Diccionario etimológico y comparado del Kichwa del Ecuador*. Vol. 1. Cuenca: Casa de la Cultura Ecuatoriana, Nucleo del Azuay.

Orlove, Benjamin. 1987. "Stability and Change in Highland Andean Dietary Patterns." In *Food and Evolution: Towards a Theory of Human Food Habits*, ed. Marvin Harris and Eric B. Ross, pp. 481–515. Philadelphia: Temple University Press.

Ravicz, Robert. 1967. "Compadrinazgo." In *Handbook of Middle American Indians*, ed. M. Nash, 6: 238–252. Austin: University of Texas Press.

Stark, Louisa R., and Pieter C. Muysken. 1977. *Diccionario Español-Quichua/Quichua-Español*. Guaya-quil: Museo del Banco Central del Ecuador.

Weismantel, Mary J. 1988. *Food, Gender, and Poverty in the Ecuadorian Andes*. Philadelphia: University of Pennsylvania Press.

7. ALCOHOL CONSUMPTION BETWEEN COMMUNITY RITUAL AND POLITICAL ECONOMY: CASE STUDIES FROM ECUADOR AND GHANA

Carola Lentz

Institut fuer Historische Ethnologie, University of Frankfurt, Germany

"Drinks construct the world as it is," "drinking constructs an ideal world," "alcohol entrenches the alternative economy ...": Mary Douglas summarizes her anthropological perspective on alcohol consumption in these three statements. Anthropologists should study not only the social role of alcohol in the construction of communities (and hierarchies) and the ritual–symbolic (religious, ecstatic) aspects of alcohol consumption, but they should also examine the economic basis of the production and distribution of alcohol—a dimension which remains largely unexplored in many anthropological studies.

Whether alcohol actually helps found an "alternative economy", as Douglas suggests, or whether it stabilizes the ruling economic and political power structures, is an empirical question. As I will show in this chapter with examples from Ghana and Ecuador, alcohol can do both; it can strengthen the economic position of women in the village society (northern Ghana), but it can also secure the rule of Mestizos over Indians (Ecuador). However I would like to emphatically underline Douglas' plea that anthropological studies of alcohol should combine aspects of both the political economy and the ritualism and symbolism of alcohol consumption. Through the examples mentioned above, I hope to demonstrate the usefulness of such a combined approach. As suggested in the introduction to this book, it is precisely the study of the historical changes in alcohol consumption (and consumption in general) which requires the consideration of both the symbolic–ritualistic and the political economic aspects.[1]

Before I proceed with my examples from the Ecuadorian highlands and northern Ghana, I would like to briefly review the history of anthropological research on alcohol consumption.

THE HISTORY OF THE ANTHROPOLOGICAL RESEARCH OF ALCOHOL CONSUMPTION

More so than many other fields of anthropological research, alcohol consumption has been and continues to be a highly controversial topic. One of the reasons for this is the fact that long before anthropologists took up the topic, it was already being examined by other disciplines such as medicine, epidemiology, psychology, psychiatry, sociology and economics. But more important, since the nineteenth century, in Europe and the United States, alcohol has increasingly become the subject of public controversies between supporters and opponents of the temperance movements, different medical schools, pastors, politicians, middle-class social reformers and leaders of the workers movement. In these debates, alcohol consumption was mainly considered a "problem". Alcohol consumption was observed under the perspective of "excessive drinking", and scholars as well as politicians searched for the definition of this problem and its causes. While in the eighteenth century, excessive alcohol consumption was considered by and large a moral problem, nineteenth century physicians defined it as a sickness, which was manifested in a loss of self-control and had its roots in the alcohol itself. Starting in the 1930s, people searched for the cause of the sickness known as "alcoholism" in the human body and then later, in the drinker's personality.[2] This paradigm continues to influence our popular views of alcohol problems to this day and has also influenced the anthropological perspectives on alcohol consumption, at times directly, and at other times indirectly.

A good example of the "alcohol as a problem" perspective is one of the first anthropological dissertations on alcohol consumption, the work of Donald Horton, published in 1943 as *The Function of Alcohol in Primitive Societies,* by the Yale Center of Alcohol Studies, which was founded a few years before this publication. Drawing on data from the Human Relations Area Files, Horton compared drinking patterns in fifty-six societies across the world and came to the conclusion that alcohol was above all used for the "reduction of anxiety." Alcohol, Horton argued, makes it possible to overcome culturally learned inhibitions that forbid the open show of aggression. Thus, alcohol consumption can help to overcome stress resulting from, for example, economic uncertainty, war, sexual restrictions or conflict-ridden processes of acculturation. The proximity of Horton's study to the "alcohol consumption as a problem" paradigm is obvious.

The first observations of alcohol consumption in non-Western societies did not occur in anthropological studies, however, but in reports from nineteenth and early twentieth century explorers, traders, missionaries and colonial officials. They often categorized alcohol consumption as "problematic", especially when it took the form of ostentatious public feasts. Many felt that what they saw as "excessive drinking" should be regulated through the prohibition of the importation and sales of foreign spirits as well as the rigid control of the local production of alcohol. Whether gin increased the working morale of the migrant laborer or was detrimental to discipline was a hotly contested question, on which mine managers, local African consumers, distillers of hard liquor, bar owners and government officials in South Africa at the turn of the century had opposing views, according to their respective interests.[3] However, the emphasis on the destructive effects of alcohol on the social structure, as reflected in these early reports, was not unconditionally and exclusively the expression of a Eurocentric perspective. In many places, the reporters raised their critical voices against the commercial strategies of the European colonial alcohol producers and traders who primed local consumption and wanted to use it as another lever of exploitation.[4]

The 1950s and 1960s saw a clear shift in the emphasis of anthropological studies; there was now more of an emphasis on the aspects of enjoyment, taste and the positive functions of alcohol consumption for the social order of the society being studied. Well into the mid-1970s, however, very few anthropologists were working explicitly on the subject of alcohol consumption. Most observations were made as a sort of by-product of studies focusing on other subjects. It is this methodologically unplanned and unsystematic approach to the subject of alcohol consumption and the observation of only a particular aspect of the reality of alcohol, namely social drinking, that the epidemiologist Robin Room (1984) holds to be responsible for the underestimation of alcohol related problems by anthropological studies. Room criticizes that anthropologists, because of their functionalist perspectives on society and culture, tend to overemphasize the social integrative aspects of alcohol. He suggests that anthropologists, in their efforts to counterweigh the problem-inflating perspective of missionaries, government officials and physicians, are throwing out the baby with the bath water. In fact, anthropologist Dwight Heath, in his review of the anthropological and culture-studies literature on alcohol consumption, comes to the conclusion that, viewed worldwide, alcohol consumption poses no problem, "even in many societies where drinking is customary and drunkenness common place" (1987: 18–9). Room considers such a statement naive and asks for a more thorough reflection of culture-specific versus universal definitions of "alcohol problems", a demand that several studies have now lived up to.

But even Room does not contest that the anthropological study of "normal" alcohol consumption has revealed many aspects that epidemiologists and psychologists often overlooked. The anthropologists' interest was and is mainly directed toward the social embeddedness of alcohol consumption and the cultural rules guiding it. In a 1965 article, David Mandelbaum summarized the anthropological perspective: "When a man lifts up a cup, it is not only the kind of drink that is in it, the amount he is likely to take and the circumstances under which he will do the drinking that are specified in advance for him, but also whether the contents of the cup will cheer or stupefy, whether they will induce affection or aggression, guilt or unalloyed pleasure. These and many other cultural definitions attach to the drink even before it touches the lips" (1965: 282).

Anthropologists consider alcohol consumption as regulated behavior. In part explicit, in part implicit culture-specific norms determine what is considered "normal" and what is considered "problematic" alcohol consumption. Norms affect the amount and type of drinks consumed, according to the occasion and frequency of the consumption. Norms regulate the participation in drinking rounds and the course of drinking invitations, the pouring out, toasts and many other aspects of drinking rituals. Finally, norms also affect the "time out", the stage of drunkenness which is universally differentiated from normal consciousness but is manifested in quite different ways.[5]

Anthropologists are interested in alcohol consumption as a symbolic activity. Social status and rank can be expressed through the rules of drinking and the drink itself. Alcohol is used to mark time and plays an important role in many religious rituals. In addition, alcohol consumption signals group belonging, through the exclusion or inclusion of certain groups: one can think of the so-called German *Damenlikör*, the "lady's sweet liquor". Finally, alcohol consumption can also build social networks, for example, through a type of credit system of reciprocal invitations or through beer feasts accompanying communal agricultural work. Anthropologists are interested in alcohol consumption, because it can give information about hard to observe social networks and cultural ideals. Changes in alcohol consumption are often an important indicator of wide-reaching transformations of the society being studied. I will address this aspect in more detail below, using the examples of Ghana and Ecuador.

To conclude this brief foray into the history of research on alcohol, I would like to emphasize that the production and distribution of alcoholic drinks and the power strategies with which they are often associated remained marginal to most anthropological studies of the topic. These aspects have been authoritatively addressed by social historians. However, both sides of alcohol consumption, the economic-political and social-symbolic dimensions, as was discussed earlier must actually be integrated into the study of alcohol.

ALCOHOL CONSUMPTION IN INDIAN ECUADOR

All the above mentioned aspects of alcohol consumption—alcohol as part of religious ritual, as an expression of community and social hierarchy and as a facilitator of economic networks—can be graphically analyzed in the example of Indian alcohol consumption in the highlands of Ecuador. I will look at a village south of Riobamba, Shamanga, which was a part of a hacienda, a large estate with a quasi-feudalistic structure, until the 1960s. When the hacienda was finally broken up, few villagers received sufficient land to farm. Because of this, most of the villagers have to complement their meager harvests with income from labor migration to the coast, a strategy of survival which for some families dates back as far as the 1920s.[6]

In Shamanga, communal drinking strengthens both the horizontal, reciprocal inner-village networks of solidarity and the hierarchical (vertical) social relations, earlier with the patron of the hacienda, and today with the Mestizo *compadres* (godfathers) of the parish. Whether it is communally drunk on the spot or stored for a later round of drinking, alcohol, especially in the form of *trago* (sugar cane liquor), is the most important gift for establishing new social relationships and strengthening existing social ties and obligations. Every visit of a *compadre*, the meeting of one's future in-laws, the search for relatives and friends, who will support the *prioste* (the host of a village festival) economically and socially in the organization of the festivities, is accompanied by a gift of *trago*. Alcohol is part of a wide-ranging net of credit relationships: who receives a bottle of sugar cane liquor or a pail of Indian corn beer is precisely remembered, and an adequate gift is expected in return, and, if necessary, called into memory by more or less subtle means.[7]

During family and village festivals, drinking can continue for several days. Special events such as the purchase of a piece of land, communal work or the return of a migrant worker are also occasions for communal alcohol consumption. No one drinks alone: even those in the village labeled as notorious "drunks" look for drinking companions. Whoever

drinks on a daily basis or drinks outside the sanctioned drinking occasions
is considered *vicioso* (vicious, profligate) or *enfermo* (sick). However,
such a stigmatization is always the result of bargaining and power relationships. It is very rare for a man from an affluent influential family who is
known to be generous among his male friends to be declared a "drunk,"

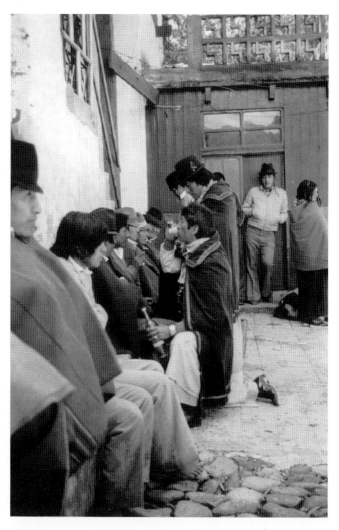

Figure 1 Formal toasts during an Indian wedding, Shamanga
(Ecuador) 1985.

even if he drinks a lot and is criticized as *vicioso* by his wife and children. Those known in the village as "drunks" are normally older, poorer, and relatively isolated men and women.[8]

All of the drinking rounds begin with the pouring of the drinks—during communal work, by members of the village council, during festivals by the host. He goes around with a bottle of sugar cane liquor or a pail of home-brewed corn beer[9] and, using a single glass, offers everyone a drink. The participants must finish the drink in one gulp and give the glass back to the host. Refusal to participate is tantamount to a serious insult.

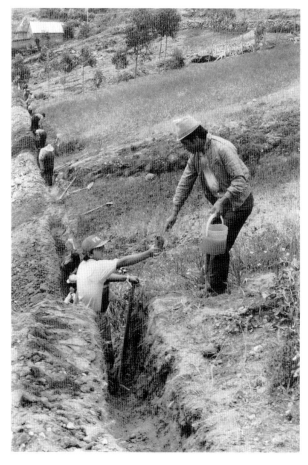

Figure 2 Offering *chicha* during communal labor, Shamanga (Ecuador) 1989.

Acceptance is not just considered as honoring one's relationship to the host, but also obligates the participant to reciprocate at a later date.

Drinking sprees usually proceed in two phases. First, drinking is expected to stimulate one's spirit and infuse one with strength and warmth. In this way, the task at hand or the special event, such as the communal cleaning of the irrigation canals, can be successfully tackled. The second phase, after the work is finished, is to explicitly get drunk. "We are not satisfied to just sip. When we drink, we drink properly...," the Shamanga villagers explained to me. For this reason, high-percentage alcoholic drinks are often preferred and beer is mostly drunk in combination with liquor. The fact that the drinking round usually ends only when most of the participants are so drunk that they are overcome by sleep, can be explained not only by the cultural desirability of this stage of drunkenness, but also by the specific rules of pouring and offering the drinks and, more generally, the economy of prestige. During most drinking sessions, more than one person offers drinks, and whoever accepts a glass from the first giver finds it harder and harder to refuse a glass from the following hosts. Each giver of drinks can demonstrate his economic prestige and his generosity by offering drinks until everyone is completely drunk.[10]

This second phase of drinking is characterized by gradual disintegration of the hierarchical etiquette. At the beginning of a drinking round everyone pays close attention to the hierarchically ordered succession of drinking and toasting. But as drinking progresses, social distances are crossed over, gender roles are broken through and fantasies of omnipotence, wishes of brotherhood, fears and aggression are often loudly expressed.[11]

Ritual drinking rounds ending in complete drunkenness were already an integral part of the Indian way of life before the Spanish conquest and the Spanish chroniclers complained that more corn was being used to make *chicha* than was being eaten. It is interesting to note that the alcohol consumption of the North American Indians seems to have followed a similar dynamic, although many of these Indian groups obtained alcohol only from the Europeans. Some anthropologists interpret these obviously pan-Indian drinking patterns as an expression of a specific spirituality, which through alcohol and drug use seeks unity with the cosmic powers.[12] Whether the Shamanga villagers are attempting to get closer to *Pacha Mama*, Mother Earth, through intoxication, remains an open question. But there is no question that alcohol plays an important role for the Indians in Catholic festivals and rituals, allowing them to communicate with the souls of the dead. On All Souls Day, for example, they never visit the gravesites of their relatives without their favorite foods and *trago*, which is poured on the graves while murmuring salutations.

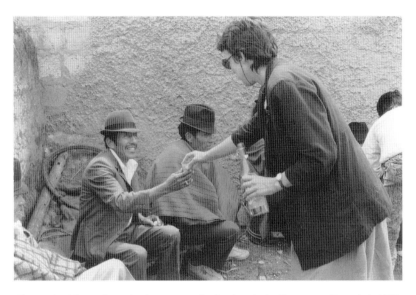

Figure 3   The anthropologist as *comadre* (godmother), Shamanga (Ecuador) 1989.

Let us take one more look at non-religious drinking. It is interesting that the Shamanga villagers who migrate to the coastal plantations adopt the drinking rituals customary among their coastal work mates. Just as in the highlands, no one orders and pays for himself alone. However, the purchaser buys not only a single bottle, but a bottle for everyone; everyone gets his own glass, pours his drink and toasts the one who invited him, and then drinks his drink in the same tempo as the other participants of the drinking round. The drinking ritual in the highlands, which involves pouring and toasting, celebrates the community as a complex weave of individual interactions. The ritual practiced on the coast embodies other social assumptions. For one thing, the financial burden is greater here than in the village ritual. One cannot begin a round of drinking by just buying a single bottle, but the generous host must buy a bottle for every participant, and it is no coincidence that these rituals experience their culmination on pay-days on the plantations. On the other hand, there is no celebration of the hierarchical order of the offering of the drink, as characterizes the village drinking. The coastal pattern of collective drinking stresses a community of equals and is a ritual which especially expresses the solidarity of co-workers. The difference between the different ways of life, between village life and life on the coastal plantations and in the cities, becomes tangible through the various drinking rituals.[13]

SORGHUM BEER IN NORTHERN GHANA

Before addressing the economic and political dimension of the alcohol consumption of the Shamanga villagers, I will look at millet or, to be precise, sorghum beer in northwestern Ghana.[14] Here, inebriation is not the aim of drinking rounds. On the contrary, drunkenness is regarded as a sign of a lack of self-control and defective sociability. Everyone drinks from his own calabash at his own pace, and the pouring is not the responsibility of the buyer, but of the brewer or her daughter. After the first courtesy sip there is no obligation to continue drinking and the available beer is often exhausted before anyone can get seriously drunk. However, this control of beer consumption through the limited amount of available beer no longer operates everywhere. On remote farms and locales, the old mechanism is still valid. But because, since the 1950s, an increasing number of women are brewing beer for sale, beer has become more available, at least in market places and small towns—provided one has enough money to pay for it. In addition, other drinks, such as local gin, with a higher alcoholic content, a smaller amount of which can inebriate much more rapidly than beer, are now available. Today, then, the cultural norms of moderation and preservation of self-control are no longer supported through the absence of supplies, but have shifted more to the personal responsibility of the drinker. Indeed, the earlier normal pattern of social drinking until the supplies were finished (freshly brewed beer can only be kept for one or two days) has now turned into an instrument undermining moderation, which has become difficult to maintain in an environment where the only limits to the supply of fresh beer seems to be one's purchasing power. In reality, there are more than a few men who are said to be "drinkers." However, it is not abundant drinking that is being criticized, but the effects of drinking, such as uncontrollable, impolite and aggressive behavior and especially the neglect of work and care of one's household.[15]

In spite of the growing availability (and rising consumption) of alcohol, there are differences in the drinking norms between the Ecuadorian highlands and northern Ghana. Drinking a lot is perhaps more tolerated but definitely not expected and not socially rewarded in northwestern Ghana. However, the greater room for individual drinking styles does not mean that sorghum beer would not play a central role in the social, economic and religious life in northwestern Ghana the way Indian corn beer and sugar cane liquor do in Indian Ecuador. Beer is considered food in northwestern Ghana—even as the best food—and as an energizer. During the agricultural season beer is often the only foodstuff that is consumed by the farmers during the day. Chemical analysis has indeed proven that sorghum beer contains more valuable nutrients than the porridge prepared from the same grains or from millet. Last but not least, beer, which is cooked for many hours, is a healthier thirst-quencher than water from ponds or open wells that are often polluted.[16]

Beer not only used to quench thirst and satisfy hunger, but also to build social relationships. This is evident in the sociability associated with beer drinking in family compounds and more importantly in the village bars where all new developments in local and national politics are exchanged. During beer drinking, marriages are planned and one is reminded of the brideprice not yet paid; returning migrants drop in with news of the well-being of relatives in the south of the country. Beer is itself a constant topic of conversation. Which woman from which house is presently selling beer, whose beer tastes best, which young man has reserved a mug for the neighbor's daughter, who should be avoided because he is a bum—the entire social network of a village can be discussed over beer and in its relationship to beer.[17]

Beer is also a tool used in making networks. Every group of neighbors must be entertained with beer, when they were invited to take part in the work on the fields of one of the group members. A mug of beer starts the work in the morning, and, in the course of the day, the work turns into a

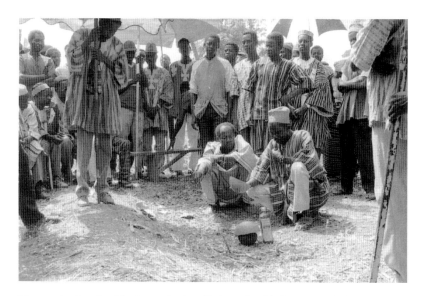

Figure 4   Pouring libation at the installation of a chief, Panyaan (Ghana) 1996.

beerfeast, which then often leads to a communal meal. Because the "work beer" and the communal meal can become quite expensive, many farmers attempt to recruit their work force with cash, especially when they are harvesting cash crops. Finding workers willing to work for cash exclusively, however, is by no means easy, and most often at least one mug of beer must be served in addition to the wages.

Beer not only plays a central role in work but also in all festivals and social events. It is the object of credit relationships and gift exchanges. It expresses social hierarchies and offers an arena for the competition for prestige. For example, the evening before a wedding the groom and his friends and relatives must visit the house of the bride who, with the help of her friends and relatives, has brewed a large quantity of beer which must now be purchased by the groom. Through the haggling over the price of the "beer of the bride," one can determine, in a playful way, the "worth" of the bride and the seriousness (as much as the economic strength) of the desires of the groom.

The circle of consumers—above all, of participants in the daily social drinking in the compounds and in the bars—has grown since the 1950s. In earlier times only older men enjoyed the privilege of beer drinking because only they had the grain necessary for brewing or the cowries (the local currency) to purchase the beer. With growing labor migration and new, local income, more young men—and also women—have access to money necessary to produce or buy beer. Because of this, the accessibility of beer was switched around. Previously, depending on their mood, the older men would ask the younger men (and older women) to join them for a drink; today it is not uncommon for young men to have the means to obtain beer while older men often do not have the money to purchase it. When the older men on market day or after church service by chance pass a bar where their younger relatives are having a round with their friends, they naturally expect to be invited to a calabash. With such more or less frequent and emphatic wishes to take part the young men have had to learn to cope, especially when corresponding return invitations in the long range are highly unlikely. They have to find the middle ground between the norm of respecting their elders and sharing their income, and the aversion to constantly caring for the "bums." A possible and evidently quite successful strategy has been the young men's attempt to differentiate neatly between different drinking situations; while beer carried to one's home is necessarily always shared more or less evenly among the inhabitants, the public drinking spot has become a place where expectations of the older men are more easily (tacitly) ignored.[18]

Beer does not taste good only to the people of northwestern Ghana but also to their ancestors, spirits of the bush and gods. The production of beer is explained in the *bagr* myth, the grand narrative about the origins of mankind and the travels of the forefathers. During the *bagr* initiation ritual, the initiated dies symbolically by the consumption of poisoned beer.[19] Hence, beer is not only the giver of life but it can also cause sickness and death. The central stages of the funeral, the most important social and religious celebrations in northwestern Ghana, are even named after the beer that is brewed for the special occassion.[20]

Different from Ecuador, where the everyday and the ceremonial beer can be differentiated by the grains used to produce it (corn v. barley), sacrificial beer in northern Ghana is made from sorghum exactly like the beer that is drunk during work in the fields or the beer that is sold and animates the social drinking. But there is a difference: ideally, the sorghum for the sacrificial beer should come from the granary of the house whose inhabitants offer the sacrifice, and should not be purchased. However, the beer that the women brew on their own account and which they sell in their own house or in the market, can be made from grain given as a gift from relatives or purchased at the market.[21] The requirements for sacrificial beer cannot always be met, and the separation between sacrificial beer and beer for sale is not as neat as the local actors like to maintain. But the fact that the market should be kept out of the sphere of the sacrifice is also evident from the fact that under no circumstances is industrially produced beer used for sacrificial drinking. Although labor migrants and the urban elite consume bottled beer (and gin as well as other high-percentage alcoholic drinks) since a number of years, in ordinary everyday as well as in more prestige related contexts in their consumption, and although bottled beer is available in many villages, this urban beer has still found no place in the ceremonial context. Regardless of how long a migrant has lived in the city and how much money he brings home, he is instructed that for all sacrifices a woman of his house must brew the sorghum beer from home-grown grain.[22]

THE POLITICAL ECONOMY OF BEER BREWING IN NORTHWESTERN GHANA

With the subject of sacrificial versus commercial beer, the second aspect of the analysis of alcohol consumption mentioned in the introduction is introduced, namely the embeddedness of the drinks and drinking within a larger economical and political context. This is precisely where one can see the greatest differences between the Ecuadorian and the Ghanaian examples of alcohol consumption.

In northwestern Ghana, the production and the consumption of sorghum beer has expanded greatly since the Second World War. A number of factors are responsible for this. First, because of an increasing crop yield and easier transportation, a flourishing regional sorghum market has developed. Due to this, more women were able to gain access to grain for brewing independently of their husbands and relatives, and the circle of women brewers has widened. At this time, it is no longer just the wives of rich farmers and chiefs who are brewing beer, but rather also widows, divorced women and younger girls (who borrow brewing equipment from other women until they have saved enough for pots and mugs of their own). Second, there is a greater availability of goods at the market and in the local shops, such as cloth, enamel pots and soap, which serve as incentives for the women to brew beer for sale and thus earn their own income, which allows them to buy the desired goods. Third, as previously mentioned, the demand for beer has grown, because the expanding labor migration and new local income opportunities have increased the amount of money in the hands of the young men which they can spend on the cherished drink. Whoever can pay buys and drinks beer, regardless of the old hierarchy of seniority, which in earlier times controlled alcohol consumption.[23]

With these three factors, a self-supporting growth spiral was set in motion. A growing demand for beer that increased even more quickly than

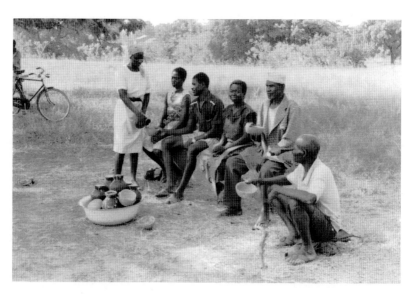

Figure 5   Drinking sorghum beer at the market site, Kulkyaa (Ghana) 1989.

the supply made brewing beer a more lucrative source of income for women. In northwestern Ghana, the growing integration of the local economy into the national labor and goods market thus has boosted beer production. In the 1960s and 1970s many popular and successful brewers were able to accumulate enough profit to purchase their own houses and expand their businesses. Admittedly, the sizes of the brewing operations and the amount of the sales differ widely: "the spectrum ranges from the intention to earn some extra pocket money to the purposeful accumulating of capital"(Göttke 1992: 141).

Since the 1980s, however, the brewers no longer enjoy the chances of accumulating spectacular wealth as they did in the past, which they like to conjure up in conversations. This is less because of the decreasing demand for homebrewed beer, and the competition of bottled beer, which has become available even in many villages, than for other reasons. Bottled beer now is certainly a symbol of prestige and is preferred by the local educated elite and some workers, but it is expensive and can be purchased only occasionally and as an addition to sorghum beer. The relation between the price of raw materials and the price of sorghum beer, which has certainly developed to the point of being unprofitable, is a more decisive reason for the decrease in the income potential of brewers. That the price of beer has not kept pace with the price of the raw materials is due to the cultural norms underlying the brewing of beer by women. Even when operated on a commercial basis, beer brewing is still guided by the ethos of the subsistence economy sticking to work beer and sacrificial beer. That women demand money for their beer is still somewhat disreputable in the eyes of men, and many strategies attempt to cover up the commercial character of beer-money transactions: one pays after the beer is drunk; the first mug of beer is often expected by the men to be free (and is also offered by the women free as a type of advertisement); if a woman brewer bluntly and boisterously demands payment of a debt, this is considered conduct unbecoming for a woman and can be punished by a bad reputation or even a boycott by the men.[24]

Moreover, the profits of the brewers, which could potentially be reinvested into the business, are often consumed by their own needs or more importantly, by the claims of relatives for a share of the brewers' income. The relatives and often the women brewers themselves, do not differentiate between gross and net profits. But not only these claims of income redistribution, the worsening relationship between raw materials and beer price, as well as the policies of male credit and free drinks curtail the margin of profit. It is also the success of the new branch itself which has been detrimental to the individual brewers: the competition waxes and wanes to such a point that the demand for beer can no longer be guaranteed and many women brewers can expect to earn no more than a small additional income. Nevertheless, still a good part of the monetary income which villagers earn away from home is appropriated by the local brewers.

FROM MESTIZO CONTROL OF INDIAN DRINKING TO THE PROTESTANT ABSTINENCE MOVEMENT

In Shamanga and other Indian villages in Ecuador the development of beer production went in the opposite direction: the production of alcoholic drinks has been less and less in the hands of the Indian women since the Second World War. Instead, Indian alcohol consumption has become a profitable source of income mainly for Mestizo brewing and bar businesses, the *chicherias*, in the parishes. Also in the relations between Indian peasants and the Mestizo or white owners of haciendas, alcohol became an instrument of exploitation.

Until the beginning of the 1970s, *chicha* was the most important alcoholic drink for the Shamanga villagers. During festivals the *chicha de jora* made from corn was drunk, while at everyday occasions, a different type of *chicha*, based on barley was drunk.[25] The production of *chicha de jora*, a beer with a higher alcoholic content, requires a special type of corn, which had to be obtained from the neighboring province Bolivar where some villagers from Shamanga worked for a short time during the harvest period for a corn farmer and were paid in corn. The major reasons why the *chicha de jora* was prepared only for important ceremonies appears to be the difficulty of obtaining enough high-quality corn of sufficient caliber for *chicha de jora* and the labor intensive production of the drink which make such manufacture worthwhile only if it is produced in large quantities. The issue is complicated further by the fact that the beer had to be quickly consumed because it spoils easily. Today the Shamanga villagers still produce it for Carnival and weddings, but sugar cane liquor and bottled beer have largely replaced *chicha de jora*.

The *chicha* consumed during agricultural work and everyday opportunities, and which has been almost completely substituted by Coca-Cola and bottled beer, was prepared from barley and had a low alcoholic content. It was not as much an inebriating drink as it was a refreshing and reinvigorating liquid, considered an indispensable element of every collective work effort. Whoever asked a group of relatives or godfathers for help during sewing or harvest had to offer *fuerza* (strength, in this case: *chicha*). This type of *chicha* also played an important role in the relationship between the villagers and the hacienda owner. Not during regular weekly work obligations of the tenant farmers but during the planting and harvest performed through unpaid *ayuda* labor (which was the "payment" for the use of hacienda pasture, water and rights of way), the patron had to provide *fuerza* for everyone. In the reciprocal exchange of labor services within the village, the one inviting the others to work gave out *chicha* in order to immediately "recompense" the help received, but was inevitably expected to reciprocate later by working in turn on the fields of his invited helpers. Communal drinking of *chicha* was an element that intimately connected work and sociability. The *chicha* given out by the hacienda owner, on the other hand, was an instrument to force the villagers to work on the hacienda owner's fields (without being compensated in cash or returned labor). Even before the task at hand had really started, the overseer would thrust a glass of *chicha* on reluctant villagers, and accepting the glass meant accepting an obligation to work. A traditional expression of horizontal reciprocity was thus transformed into a mechanism of stabilizing the power hierarchy, a strategy also used by the Mestizos of the neighboring parish who wanted to appropriate unpaid Indian labor.

Exactly when the Mestizos succeeded in bringing a good part of the Indian ceremonial as well as the everyday *chicha* consumption under their control is not clear. It is certain that, due to more money brought into circulation in the village economy since the 1920s, the business of selling illegally brewed *chicha* in the parish centers started to flourish. This business experienced its heyday in the 1950s and early 1960s.[26] The Shamanga villagers cite that in the 1930s they would spend at least part of the money which they earned as labor migrants on the coast or by selling eggs or barley on *chicha*. The Mestizo *chicheria* owners were not content with selling the Indians *chicha* for marriages, baptisms, funerals, Carnival and all other festivals taking place in the parish. They also encouraged the abundant consumption of *chicha* in a back room or in the courtyard of the bar owner during more regular occasions such as Sunday markets, visits to the parish offices and the departure or homecoming of the migrant workers.

Often the Mestizo brewers would force the first glass on the villagers for free, in order to ask for payment at the end of the drinking bout, when all were so drunk that they had lost track of what they drank. Many times they used physical force: they dragged passers-by into the bar or they stole a piece of clothing that would only be returned after *chicha* was bought and drunk. As a rule, however, the selling of *chicha* was interwoven into multiple social relationships. The same Mestizos who ran an illegal bar presented themselves as money lenders or as "clerks" or "writers" who backed up the illiterate during the recording of land purchases or during altercations with the police. Some were also buyers of the goods produced by Indians. Frequently, such relationships were ritually confirmed through *compadrazgo* (godparenthood, the Mestizo baptizing the Indian child). Drinking debts, in any case, had to be paid through free labor.

The *chicha* purchased from the Mestizos was often called *huagrachaqui* (Quichua: step of the cow) by the Indians and contained very little and sometimes no corn. It was a relatively strong alcoholic drink made from a base of *panela* (sugar) and water mixed with ammoniac to speed up the fermentation process. Whether it is truth or rumor, the Indians strongly maintain that the Mestizos also used animal bones, crushed agave leaves and even urine and human excrement. The production costs were, in any case, minimal, and the corresponding profit margin was exorbitant, and the villagers entangled themselves not only in a many-sided net of dependence, but also put their health in danger. Occasionally, state initiated campaigns tried to contain the illegal commercial *chicha* brewing, not the least because the state wanted to enforce its monopoly on the taxing of alcohol and did not want to relinquish such a lucrative source of income to the Mestizos alone. But for a long time, these campaigns were without worthwhile effect. The officials who were to control the parish took bribes from the *chicheria* owners and thus also profited from the consumption of alcohol by the Indians.

Why did the Indians allow the production and distribution of alcohol to be wrested from them? On the one hand, the Mestizos effectively transformed the traditional drinking rituals and built up patron–client relationships with individual villagers who then promoted excessive alcohol consumption among their kin and friends. On the other hand, the shortage of grains for brewing in the village and the amount of work required to produce *chicha* made a prepared, and comparatively cheap (though of low quality) drink seem attractive. This became even more important when due to the periodic absence of the migrating men, the workload of the women, who are responsible for brewing beer, increased considerably.

Since the 1970s, two developments have undermined the Mestizo control of Indian alcohol consumption. For one thing, an abstinence movement has grown among the many Indians who have converted to Christian evangelic fundamentalism. As a number of Shamanga villagers explained to me, they joined the Protestant churches specifically because they wanted to escape from the obligation of the mandatory, expensive (Catholic) festivals, which the Mestizos in the parish use to enrich themselves. But also, anyone who wants to get away from the village drinking rounds for a short time refuses the glass offered to him with the announcement *'soy evangelico'* ("I am a Protestant"). If he later feels like joining his friends

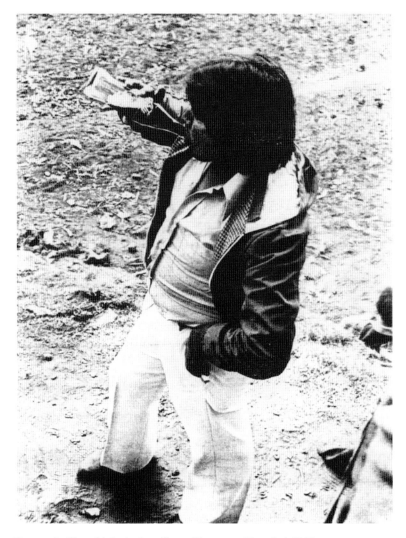

Figure 6 New drinks in the village, Shamanga (Ecuador) 1985.

in drinking, he "forgets" this conversion, a pragmatic back and forth process that the small group of convinced Protestants criticizes even more sharply than the Catholics.[27]

Among the Catholic villagers who continue to drink, the hold which Mestizo bar owners have over them has decreased due to the substitution of *chicha* by other alcoholic drinks. Already in the early years of labor migration, with cash obtained from salaried work on the coast, not only was *chicha* purchased from the Mestizos in the highlands, but also *trago* (sugar cane liquor). But it is only from the 1960s onward that the consumption of *trago* increased considerably, gradually displacing *chicha*.

As a prestigious and relatively expensive drink, sugar cane liquor first became an important part of ritual gifts during weddings and other festivals as well as gifts for the establishment of *compadrazgos*, godfather ties. Later it was also consumed more regularly during less ritualized drinking rounds. The increasing state controls of the illegal *chicha* businesses may have contributed to the gradual spread of the consumption of cane liquor. Because of the bribes mentioned above, the state officials were neither able nor willing to completely abolish the brewing of *chicha*, but forced many Mestizo bar owners to purchase a license and also to sell legally taxed bottles of *trago* in their shops. This meant, of course, that the Mestizos were also interested in propagating the new drink among their Indian clients.

In spite of the Mestizo involvement in the *trago* business, the shift to cane liquor allowed the Indians partly to escape from the control of their drinking rituals by the Mestizos and the concomitant relations of dependency. While *chicha* was served from big containers and had to be drunk on the spot, namely the Mestizo owned bars, the bottled cane liquor could easily be taken home to the village and be consumed in a social space relatively shielded from Mestizo incursions. In addition, many Indian labor migrants bought illegally brewed, cheap cane liquor on their way home to the village, from coastal producers or intermediaries with whom they maintained no personal and clientelistic relationships. Precisely because *trago* implied monetary aspects much more so than *chicha*, it made more anonymous forms of distribution possible. When in addition to cane liquor bottled beer also became more and more popular, drinking no longer necessarily forced the Indian villagers into local relations of dependency. Finally, the communal shop which was opened in Shamanga in 1980 and also sells alcoholic drinks, allowed the villagers to avoid completely Mestizo intromission into Indian drinking rituals. Nevertheless, in contrast to northwestern Ghana, the consumption of alcohol does not strengthen the local economy of the Indians. The recent developments merely shifted the profits to be earned from Indian drinking from the Mestizos in the parishes to the industrial producers of cane liquor and bottled beer. At best, Indians take part of the profits as intermediaries (traders), but trading in alcohol is a male trade, not a female business.

NOTES

A first version of this article was published in German, in *Sociologus* 1/1998.

1. A useful review of the development and the present discussion of consumption research is offered by Miller 1995.
2. For a history of the conceptualization of drunkenness and alcoholism, see Legnaro 1981 as well as Levine 1981 (with reference to North America) and Spode 1993 (with reference to Germany).
3. On the conflict-ridden history of alcohol consumption in South Africa, see the excellent studies of Van Onselen 1982 and La Hausse 1988. On similar conflicts around drinking patterns of the English lower classes, see Medick 1982; on the drinking behavior of industrial workers in Germany, see Roberts 1980 and Spode 1993.
4. An exhaustive overview of the early and recent literature on alcohol in non-western societies is provided by Heath 1976 and 1987. For an instructive case study on the complex interrelationships of the interests of colonial officials, missionaries, alcohol producers and African consumers which developed around the locally produced and imported gin in southern Ghana since the turn of the century, see Akyeampong 1994 and 1996.
5. For anthropological aspects of alcohol consumption, see the useful summaries in Schweizer 1981 and Feest 1988. It is only recently that questions of gender-specific consumption patterns started to appear in anthropological alcohol research; see Gefou-Madianou 1992 and McDonald 1994.
6. For more details on the history of Shamanga and its environment, see Lentz 1988 and 1991. I have conducted fieldwork in Shamanga and neighboring villages as well as the coastal destinations of the migrants in 1983–1985 and 1989.
7. See also Sanchez-Parga 1985.
8. See also the informative case study on an Indian village in southern Peru by Harvey 1994.
9. I will come back to the gradual displacement of home-brewed corn beer by sugar cane liquor and bottled beer since the 1950s and 1960s. For the symbolic placement of *trago* and *chicha* (corn beer) in a classificatory scheme of "bitter, hot" versus "sweet", or "hot" versus "cold", see Mangin 1957, Vasquez 1967 and the study by Weismantel 1988 of an Indian village about one hundred and fifty kilometers away from Shamanga. Weismantel also discusses the gender-specific categorizing of alcohol: *trago* = strong, therefore, a man's drink; to be drunk by the women only when they get older.
10. As early as the 1940s, Sandoval 1945, a priest, observed that rather sober Indians simulated full drunkenness on their way from the parish back to their home in the village. In Sandoval's opinion, they did this in order to demonstrate that they had sufficient money at their disposal to obtain enough alcohol to get drunk.
11. For the local discourses on the effect of alcohol ("warming the blood", "joyous heart") and the two phases of the drinking session, see Sandoval 1945, Sanchez-Parga 1985 and Harvey 1994.
12. Indian drinking to the point of unconsciousness was and continues to be interpreted differently: for example, Aguiló (1985:140–2) in reference to the Ecuadorian highlands reads it as a symbolic uniting with the *Pacha Mama* (Quichua: Mother Earth; essential to the Indian world view); Mencias (1962: 42) interprets it only as a periodic escape out of an impoverished living situation; Rohr (1981: 125ff) emphasizes, on the other hand, the role of alcohol for the reduction of normal physical control during specific rituals. On the history of Indian alcohol consumption in Ecuador, see Salomon 1980: 126–34, Flores 1935: 13ff, Burgos 1977: 194ff, 282ff and Aguiló 1985: 120ff. The literature on drinking rituals and problems of the North American Indians is very extensive; refer to, for example, Levy and Kunitz 1974, Waddell and Everett 1980 and Feest 1981. For a general view of the relation between alcohol and religious ecstasy, see Legnaro 1981.
13. On the Indian sub-culture on the sugar-cane plantation, see Lentz 1991: 78, 100–7.

14. The following observations are based on my frequent research stays in northwestern Ghana since 1987. In addition, I benefit from the research on beer brewers in Hamile, a small town on the Ghanaian-Burkina Faso border, conducted by one of my students in the winter of 1989–90 (see Göttke 1992).

15. See also the analysis of Akyeampong 1995 of drinking in southern Ghana and the extremely instructive case study by Colson and Scudder (1988: 108–15) who observed a similar phenomenon in Zambia.

16. See Voltz 1981 and Goody 1982: 72–7.

17. See also Hagaman 1977: 270–93 and Göttke 1992.

18. Very similar findings were observed by Colson and Scudder 1988: 103–8 in Zambia.

19. See also Goody 1972, 1982: 74–5, 96.

20. The ceremonies which take the form mentioned below are carried out only by non-Christian families; Christians rather integrate beer in a social remembrance of the forefathers after a mass for the dead, in the church. The non-Christian funeral-beer rituals are described in detail by Goody (1962: 45, 51, 213ff., 220ff., 235ff.). Three weeks after the burial, the *bobuur daa* is brewed, the soothsayer beer. It is expected that every participant in the divination round who may have had something to do with the death of the one who was buried, will get sick from this beer. The *ku daa tuo*, the bitter funeral beer which should be brewed from sorghum which the dead themselves have cultivated and harvested follows at the beginning of the next rainy season; at this beer festival, the inheritance is divided up and a temporary ancestral object (a wooden stick representing the ancestor) is produced. Finally, after the next harvest, the *ku daa baaro*, the cool funeral beer signals the end of the funeral ceremony and also the production of the final ancestral object.

21. See also Hagaman 1980 on these differences.

22. With respect to Zambia, see also Colson and Scudder 1988: 60–71. The use of gin from southern Ghana or imported from Europe in ceremonial contexts still needs to be examined more closely. For a long time gin has been the obligatory gift to the chief and gin is used as payment for diviners and healers who then use it themselves in the ceremonies. But I have only once observed a ritual offering to the earth god where first water, then sorghum beer and finally, also, gin were being used. For more details on the integration of gin in ceremonial contexts in southern Ghana, see Akyeampong 1995: 266–8.

23. For an almost identical dynamic of beer production in a rural region of Zambia, see Colson and Scudder 1988: 116–30. For northwestern Ghana, see Göttke 1992. Unfortunately, there is no reliable, quantitative study for northern Ghana, but the scale of beer production is probably similar to that of a neighboring region of Burkina Faso. For this area in the 1970s, there was a yearly per capita consumption of 236 liters of sorghum beer in the cities and approximately 360 liters in the countryside. In Ouagadougou alone, the capital of Burkina Faso with about a half million inhabitants, approximately 23 million liters of sorghum beer are consumed annually and 700 million liters of beer in the entire country are produced from 240,000 tons of sorghum. According to these calculations, about half of the harvested grain is used for beer. See Saul 1981 and Voltz 1981.

24. See the detailed observations and interviews with brewer women in Göttke 1992: 121–31.

25. For this difference between everyday and festive beer, see also Hartmann 1982 and Scheffer 1982.

26. See Vasquez 1967: 273, 277: the profit margin of *chicherias* in the province of Chimborazo was supposed to have reached 200%. See also Burgos 1977: 194ff, 316–25, on the asymmetrical Indian-Mestizo relationship.

27. For the history of Protestantism and its policy of prohibition in the province of Chimborazo, see Casagrande 1978 and Muratorio 1981.

REFERENCES

Aguiló, Federico (1985). *El hombre del Chimborazo*. Quito: Mundo Andino.

Akyeampong, Emmanuel (1994). "The State and Alcohol Revenues: Promoting 'Economic Development' in Gold Coast/Ghana, 1919 to the Present", *Histoire Sociale* 27: 393–411.

Akyeampong, Emmanuel (1995). "Alcoholism in Ghana—a Socio-Cultural Explanation", *Culture, Medicine and Psychiatry* 19: 261–80.

Akyeampong, Emmanuel (1996). "What's in a Drink? Class Struggle, Popular Culture and the Politics of Akpeteshie (local gin) in Ghana, 1930–67", *Journal of African History* 37: 215–36.

Burgos, Hugo (1977). *Relaciones interétnicas en Riobamba. Dominio y dependencia en una región indígena ecuatoriana*. México: Instituto Indígenista Interamericano.

Casagrande, Joseph (1978). "Religious Conversion and Social Change in an Indian Community of Highland Ecuador". In: Hartman, Roswitha and Udo Oberem (eds.), *Amerikanistische Studien—Festschrift für Hermann Trimborn*, Bd. 1, St. Augustin: 105–11.

Colson, Elizabeth and Thayer Scudder (1988). *For Prayer and Profit: The Ritual, Economic, and Social Importance of Beer in Gwembe District, Zambia, 1950–1982*. Stanford: Stanford University Press.

Douglas, Mary (ed.) (1987). *Constructive Drinking: Perspectives on Drink from Anthropology*. Cambridge: Cambridge University Press.

Feest, Christian F. (1981). "Alkohol bei den Indianern Nordamerikas". In: Völger, Gisela and Karin v. Welck (eds.), *Rausch und Realität. Drogen im Kulturvergleich*, Köln: Gesellschaft für Völkerkunde, Ethnologica Neue Folge Bd. 9: 162–8.

Feest, Christian F. (1988). "Trinken und Trunkenheit als kulturspezifische Phänomene", *Kulturjahrbuch* 7: 46–55.

Flores, Enrique (1935). *El problema del indio en el Ecuador. Aspecto religioso. El indio del Chimborazo y de Bolivar. Su catequización*. Riobamba.

Gefou-Madianou, Dimitra (ed.) (1992). *Alcohol, Gender and Culture*. London: Routledge.

Goody, Jack (1962). *Death, Property and the Ancestors: A Study of the Mortuary Customs of the Lo Dagaa of West Africa*. London: Tavistock.

Goody, Jack (1972). *The Myth of the Bagre*. Oxford: Clarendon Press.

Goody, Jack (1982). *Cooking, Cuisine and Class. A Study in Comparative Sociology*. Cambridge: Cambridge University Press.

Göttke, Edith Susanne (1992). "*In order to do business, you have to go against custom*": *Hirsebierbrauerinnen in Hamile (Ghana)*. MA Thesis, Institut für Ethnologie, FU Berlin.

Hagaman, Barbara L. (1977). "*Beer and Matriliny: The Power of Women in a West African Society*". PhD Thesis, Boston, Northeastern University.

Hagaman, Barbara L. (1980). "Food for Thought: Beer in a Social and Ritual Context in a West African Society", *Journal of Drug Issues* 10: 203–14.

Hartmann, Günther (1981). "Alkoholische Getränke bei südamerikanischen Indianern". In: Völger, Gisela and Karin v. Welck (eds.): *Rausch und Realität. Drogen im Kulturvergleich*. Köln: Gesellschaft für Völkerkunde, Ethnologica Neue Folge Bd. 9: 152–61.

Harvey, Penny (1994). "Gender, Community and Confrontation: Power Relations in Drunkenness in Ocongate (Southern Peru)". In: McDonald, Maryon (ed.): *Gender, Drink and Drugs*, Oxford: Berg: 207–39.

Heath, Dwight (1976). "Anthropological Perspectives on Alcohol: An Historical Review". In: Everett, Michael et al. (eds.), *Cross-Cultural Approaches to the Study of Alcohol*, The Hague: Mouton: 41–101.

Heath, Dwight (1987). "A Decade of Development in the Anthropological Study of Alcohol Use: 1970–1980". In: Douglas, Mary (ed.), *Constructive Drinking: Perspectives on Drink from Anthropology*, Cambridge: Cambridge University Press: 16–69.

Horton, Donald (1943). "The Function of Alcohol in Primitive Societies: A Cross-Cultural Survey", *Quarterly Journal of Studies on Alcohol* 4: 199–320.

La Hausse, Paul (1988). *Brewers, Beerhalls and Boycotts: A History of Liquor in South Africa*. History Workshop Topic Series 2, Johannesburg: Ravan Press.

Legnaro, Aldo (1981). "Ansätze zu einer Soziologie des Rausches—zur Sozialgeschichte von Rausch und Ekstase in Europa". In: Völger, Gisela and Karin v. Welck (eds.): *Rausch und Realität. Drogen im Kulturvergleich*. Köln: Gesellschaft für Völkerkunde, Ethnologica Neue Folge Bd. 9: 86–97.

Lentz, Carola (1988). *Von seiner Heimat kann man nicht lassen. Migration in einer Dorfgemeinde in Ecuador*. Frankfurt: Campus (spanish version: *Migración e identidad étnica: la transformación histórica de una comunidad indígena en la sierra ecuatoriana*. Quito: Abya-Yala, 1997).

Lentz, Carola (1991). *Buscando la vida. Trabajadores temporales en una plantación de azúcar*. Quito: Ediciones Abya-Yala.

Levine, Harry Gene (1981). "Die Entdeckung der Sucht—Wandel der Vorstellungen über Trunkenheit in Nordamerika". In: Völger, Gisela and Karin v. Welck (eds.): *Rausch und Realität. Drogen im Kulturvergleich*. Köln: Gesellschaft für Völkerkunde, Ethnologica Neue Folge Bd. 9: 118–24.

Levy, Gerold E. and Stephen J. Kunitz (1974). *Indian Drinking: Navajo Practices and Anglo-American Theories*. New York: Wiley.

Mandelbaum, David G. (1965). "Alcohol and Culture", *Current Anthropology* 6: 281–8.

Mangin, William (1957). "Drinking among Andean Indians", *Quarterly Journal of Studies on Alcohol* 18: 55–66.

McDonald, Maryon (ed.) (1994). *Gender, Drink and Drugs*. Oxford: Berg

Medick, Hans (1982). "Plebejische Kultur, plebejische Öffentlichkeit, plebejische Ökonomie. Über Erfahrungen und Verhaltensweisen Besitzarmer und Besitzloser in der Übergangsphase zum Kapitalismus". In: Berdahl, Robert et al., *Klassen und Kultur: Sozialanthropologische Perspektiven in der Geschichtsschreibung*, Frankfurt: Syndikat: 157–204.

Mencias, Jorge (1962). *Riobamba. Estudio de la elevación socio-cultural y religiosa del Indio*. Bogotá.

Miller, Daniel (ed.) (1995). *Acknowledging Consumption: A Review of New Studies*. London: Routledge.

Muratorio, Blanca (1981). "Protestantism, Ethnicity and Class in Chimborazo". In: Whitten, Norman (ed.), *Cultural Transformations and Ethnicity in Modern Ecuador*. Urbana: University of Illinois Press: 506–34.

Roberts, James St. (1980). "Der Alkoholkonsum deutscher Arbeiter im 19. Jahrhundert", *Geschichte und Gesellschaft* 6: 220–42.

Rohr, Elisabeth (1981). *Kollektive Überlebensstrategien und soziale Differenzierungsprozesse in abhängigen Gesellschaften: Das Beispiel der Otavalos in Ecuador*. Diplomarbeit, Universität Frankfurt a.M., Soziologisches Seminar.

Room, Robin (1984). "Alcohol and Ethnography: A Case of Problem Definition?", *Current Anthropology* 25: 169–91.

Salomon, Frank (1980). *Los señores étnicos de Quito en la época de los Incas*. Otavalo: Instituto Otavaleño de Antropologia.

Sanchez-Parga, José (1985). "La bebida en los andes ecuatorianos: ritualidad y control social", *Cultura* 21: 315–38.

Sandoval, Leonidas Rodrigez (1945). "Drinking Motivations among the Indians of the Ecuadorean Sierra", *Primitive Man* 18: 39–49.

Saul, Mahir (1981). "Beer, Sorghum and Women: Production for the Market in Rural Upper Volta", *Africa* 51: 746–64.

Scheffer, Karl-Georg (1981). "Chicha in Südamerika". In: Völger, Gisela and Karin v. Welck (eds.): *Rausch und Realität. Drogen im Kulturvergleich*. Köln: Gesellschaft für Völkerkunde, Ethnologica Neue Folge Bd. 9: 146–51.

Schweizer, Thomas (1981). "Alkohol im interkulturellen Vergleich". In: Völger, Gisela and Karin v. Welck (eds.): *Rausch und Realität. Drogen im Kulturvergleich.* Köln: Gesellschaft für Völkerkunde, Ethnologica Neue Folge Bd. 9: 76–84.

Spode, Hasso (1993). *Die Macht der Trunkenheit: Kultur- und Sozialgeschichte des Alkohols in Deutschland.* Opladen: Leske und Budrich.

Van Onselen, Charles (1982). "Randlords and Rotgut, 1886–1903". In: Van Onselen, Charles, *Studies in the Social and Economic History of the Witwatersrand, 1886–1914.* Vol. 1, Johannesburg: Ravan Press: 44–102.

Vasquez, Mario (1967). "La chicha en los países andinos", *América Indígena* 27: 265–82.

Voltz, Michael (1981). "Hirsebier in Westafrika". In: Völger, Gisela and Karin v. Welck (eds.): *Rausch und Realität. Drogen im Kulturvergleich.* Köln: Gesellschaft für Völkerkunde, Ethnologica Neue Folge Bd. 9: 174–81.

Waddell, Jack O. and Michael W. Everett (eds.) (1980). *Drinking Behaviour among Southwestern Indians: An Anthropological Perspective.* Tucson: University of Arizona Press.

Weismantel, Mary J. (1988). *Food, Gender and Poverty in the Ecuadorian Andes.* Philadelphia: University of Pennsylvania Press.

8. THE PORRIDGE DEBATE: GRAIN, NUTRITION, AND FORGOTTEN FOOD PREPARATION TECHNIQUES

Elisabeth Meyer-Renschhausen
Bülowstr. 74, 1000 Berlin 30,
Germany

For some time now, it has been the height of fashion to eat muesli in the morning. Breakfast porridge, up to ten years ago considered an eccentricity of weird advocates of communal living, has suddenly become common property. Health-food shops, for years on the verge of ruin, have begun to do a lively trade, especially when they also serve snacks, muesli in the morning, and vegetarian roasts at lunchtime. Their customers include by no means only tattered freaks, but primarily young, health-conscious business people like those found at the health-food shops at Berlin's Wittenbergplatz. Even renowned international hotel chains have recently started offering an "alternative" breakfast of porridge oats and fruit. Some years back, a major West German weekly newspaper described the rapid transformation of nutritional habits as the "fastest revolution" of all time.

This recent emphasis on grains and porridge, however, is neither merely a new fashion nor exclusively a matter of healthier nutrition. For many of today's grain eaters, ethical and political considerations also play an important role. Several years back, Frances Moore Lappé called for a "Diet for a Small Planet," that is, for nutritional habits that were not at the expense of the world's poor.[1] She and Joseph Collins, co-authors of the "Myth of Scarcity," demonstrated with numerous examples from various parts of the world that nobody on earth need starve if the rich were prepared to do without their daily steak or roast meat and if the soils of the Third World were cultivated to meet local requirements. Even now enough grain is produced worldwide to enable every human being to receive the daily 3,000 calories a person requires according to calculations of the

World Health Organization (WHO). Fifty percent of the world's population, however, is undernourished, while millions starve. In order to produce one pound of meat a farmer must (depending on the variety of grain and the species of animal) use seven to ten times more grain for feeding purposes (or alternately make available as pasture seven times as much arable land) than would be necessary if the grain were utilized directly for human nutrition. It is a fact that farmers who keep large herds of cattle, including those in West Germany (in North Rhine-Westphalia, for example), use grain, soya, and similar products from the Third World on a large scale for feeding purposes.[2]

Hence, a return to grain-based diets is considered an integral part of the necessary political changes to combat hunger in the Third World. This is not the first time in history, however, that scientists and the urban middle classes have "discovered" the qualities of grain and porridge. A closer look at the history of grain consumption in central Europe and the history of research into the nutritional properties of grain, milling techniques, and consumption habits reveals a long story of spread and recession, esteem and contempt, discovery and neglect. A complete analysis of grain consumption and of how social movements have forced the sciences to reconsider it is beyond the scope of this article. Nevertheless I want to outline important landmarks in the "real" as well as in the "scientific" history of grain and porridge in central Europe, because it is the links between them that are most interesting. So I shall first give a short overview of early social and "ecological" movements and the rising "vegetarian" discourse in the nineteenth and the early twentieth century. I shall then show how the old porridge meal lost the high reputation it had in the Old Society and briefly discuss the most important phases in the more recent history of grain consumption. The main body of this article introduces two members of the first generation of food anthropologists, Adam Maurizio and Anni Gamerith. Their studies focused on food preparation techniques that were almost totally forgotten in Europe around 1900. They showed that these grain preparation techniques brought objectively healthier and tastier food than modern industrialized milling techniques are able to do. A look at the etymology reveals that these techniques were used throughout Eastern Europe. Last but not least I shall discuss reasons for the displacement of traditional grain preparation techniques, despite their benefits in taste and nutrition, and the consequences of this displacement.

THE FIRST WAVE OF VEGETARIANISM

Appeals to return to a simpler, primarily vegetarian form of nutrition are not new, although arguments differ. Throughout the history of mankind leading religious or political figures have called for a return to a simpler, more or less vegetarian diet. Around 1800, Christian Wilhelm Hufeland (1762–1836), doctor to Queen Louise of Prussia, argued that a simpler, more vegetarian diet would prolong life. His appeal won friends and supporters among numerous contemporaries, including Kant and Goethe. In 1809, the members of the Bible Christian Church in England were the first group in modern history to undertake to abstain from eating meat. After the cholera epidemic of 1832 in North America, the Presbyterian preacher Sylvester Graham argued that a return to a "natural" form of nutrition, in particular, to home-baked bread stored over a longer period, was a way of preventing popular epidemics of this kind.[3] In 1847 in Manchester, England, the first secular vegetarian society was founded.[4]

In the second half of the nineteenth century in Germany, the latitudinarian pastor Eduard Baltzer (1814–1887), following the North American doctor Alcott and the German pharmacist Theodor Hahn, demanded for both ethical and health reasons that man adopt a vegetarian diet. He believed that in this way the pressing "social question" of his day, the hunger and malnutrition of the working classes in the large towns, could be solved. He believed that if animals were no longer kept, large estates would disappear, the poor could feed themselves by cultivating their own gardens, and necessary "land reform" could be achieved. In common with the supporters of the humor theory of Galen, which nineteenth-century medical science rejected, Baltzer believed that a diet of meat resulted in aggressiveness, a more powerful sexual drive, and militarism. In 1867 he founded the first vegetarian society in Germany, which, despite its marked sectarian and pseudo-religious character, succeeded in winning numerous supporters, particularly in the last two decades of the century.[5] In 1888 a national vegetarian society emerged in London, and in 1908 an international union of vegetarians was established. So many people from all walks of life responded enthusiastically to vegetarianism, as well as to the movement for medical treatment by natural remedies, the temperance movement, the concept of land reform, and the "garden city movement" in countries such as the United States, Great Britain, the German Empire, France, Holland, Australia, Switzerland, and Austria, that in the last decade of the nineteenth century many doctors changed camps and became supporters of treatment by natural methods and vegetarianism.[6]

It was above all the problems arising from industrialization and capitalist transformation, such as the misery of the masses in the cities and the spread of alcoholism, and the women's movement and its insistence on the social necessity of housework, that led to this widespread interest in nutrition and dietary reform, particularly in the protestant states of northern

Europe. Supporters of this first "alternative" movement, so to speak, were responsible for many innovations, including the American Graham bread (the first wholemeal bread), Swedish crisp breads, Steinmetz's refinement of the grinding process, Lieken's bread, and also the Reform shops. These innovations we still recognise in trade names, even though in some cases the products of the era of so-called pudding vegetarianism have not kept up with the pace of our expanding knowledge.

Both German porridge oats and American cornflakes have their origins in the dietary criticism of that era. "Muesli," developed by the Swiss doctor Max Otto Bircher-Benner was to become particularly well known. From 1891, Bircher-Benner worked as a general practitioner in Zürich. Unable to heal patients by traditional methods, he was encouraged by vegetarian students to experiment with a diet free of meat. In 1897 he opened a dietary clinic and soon became the pioneer of a diet of uncooked food.[7] In its various forms this muesli became in the early years of the present century, as it has become again today, a symbol of the whole, politically very heterogeneous, spectrum of the "alternatives" of the day. In many of the rural communes that sprang up in central Europe from 1900 onward, as well as in the childrens' homes and orphanages founded in the 1920s by social workers involved with the *Jugendbewegung* (youth movement), grain porridge was eaten as a matter of course.[8]

In this way, vegetarianism rehabilitated and reactivated a dish that seemed to be about to disappear forever from the tables of European families. In the towns, grain porridge had in the course of the eighteenth century given way to coffee, bread and butter, and potatoes.[9] By the turn of the last century, grain dishes such as porridge, gruel, or groats were eaten only in residual forms in the countryside, chiefly in the poorer Alpine valleys. But the pomp of the Victorian era on the one hand, and the misery, lack of housing, and malnutrition of the "working classes" on the other, caused members of the "educated classes" to espouse what was in many cases a glorified return to the "primitive power" of "simple (rural) life." Social and political engagement at the local level, particularly among the primary school teachers of the German Empire, who from 1890 on showed an intense interest in social matters, gave rise to a new regionalism. The teachers demanded instruction in local history and culture for their pupils[10]—both from critical social and from reactionary and nationalist motives—and they themselves actively researched and described those rural customs that still existed.[11] During these activities they discovered that some last forms of what had long been believed lost, the country porridge dishes, had indeed survived the urban dietary transformations. But before presenting the biographies and the findings of two of these researchers,

I want to sketch the development of the changing reputation of grain and then give a short outline of the likes and dislikes of consumers with respect to grain and porridge.

PORRIDGE AND ITS REPUTATION

In contrast to some areas of the countryside, from 1770 on the grain dishes porridge and gruel had hardly been eaten in the cities, where they had acquired a bad reputation. For townspeople porridge and gruel had long been a sign of poverty. As early as 1800 Krünitz recommended that millet, "a food difficult to digest and prone to cause constipation," should be left to "the hard-working countryman and common people."[12] In his article about porridge, he warned in particular about its harmful effects on children. Only in England, where the countryside was more dominant in the process of industrialization, could porridge remain.[13]

Already in the early nineteenth century, "barley eater" was a term of abuse for a mean person. Mess officers were scornfully referred to as *Graupenmajor* (barley majors) and prison was known ironically as the *Graupenpalast* (barley palace).[14] In Italy the word "polenta eater" was a term of abuse for a northern Italian. Particularly in the northern parts of central Europe porridge was considered a food solely for children, the sick, and the toothless elderly. The "robust man," in "full possession of his powers," rejected porridge for himself. In Switzerland, bachelors were mockingly referred to as "gruel eaters."[15] Porridge was considered backward, the food of simple peasants and dependents such as household servants and children. Gruel had become a perfect symbol of poverty and monotony, of the limitations of rural life, and even of stupidity.

However, around 1900 middle-class lay researchers of the "simple" rural life, inspired by a critical attitude toward the prevailing cultural values and a desire for a reformed way of life, attempted to counteract this kind of prejudice or "cultural imperialism." Researchers such as the socialist journalist Friedrich Eckstein from Vienna and numerous others before him attempted to show that in the more remote parts of Europe a completely different belief still existed in which—in contrast to the common urban and bourgeois attitudes—porridge played a very special role and was highly esteemed.

At the turn of the last century, for example, household spirits, which had not yet disappeared from the countryside of northern Europe, were principally given porridge with butter or milk (the Tomte in Denmark, the Niss in Sweden, and the Nische Puk in Schleswig-Holstein). In return, they helped harvest the hay. Particularly at yuletide, the Swedish and Norwegian Niss demanded porridge with honey.[16] Until about 1900 in some regions of Sweden "Niss Puge" was given buckwheat gruel with butter every Sunday. But farmers themselves also ate groats at yuletide, because it was supposed to bring luck and happiness. For similar reasons, buckwheat gruel was eaten at Christmas time in Pomerania.[17] In some areas the eating of millet porridge was recommended—for example, in the Ansbach region particularly at Carnival—as a way of preventing people from running short of money.[18] As late as 1900, Russians were still of the opinion that "porridge is our mother," while a Swabian proverb expresses the same idea, as the German scholar and foodhistorian Moritz Heyne discovered.[19]

Interested contemporaries such as Eckstein were particularly fascinated by the fact that both among the Romans and in northern Europe, the food sacrificed to the gods, goblins, and spirits of vegetation consisted mainly of grain porridge.[20] In ancient Greece too, the abundant luxury food of those living in the Underworld was the magic porridge.[21] When it became clear that the central gods of classical times, such as the Greek Demeter or the Roman Ceres, were goddesses of fertility to whom grain in general but especially barley were dedicated, they had to lend their names to the numerous vegetarian restaurants that were established from 1890 on, as well as to "biologically" grown products. In Berlin, the vegetarian restaurant "Ceres" and the "Eden Fruit Cultivation Colony," which was to exist for many decades, were founded. "Demeter" became the brand name of those agricultural products that were grown in accordance with anthroposophical standards, without the help of chemical fertilizers.

Although from 1770 on the new dietary habits, that is, bread and potatoes, sugar, and coffee, were relatively quick to win acceptance, despite the fact that they were said to have all manner of good and bad effects, these kinds of food never held the same significance for country people as the old porridge had had. At the very least farmers considered porridge to be particularly wholesome. Remarkably (or perhaps it is not remarkable at all), it was precisely in "modern" north Germany in 1930 that at Christmas or on New Year's Eve a millet or groats porridge was eaten, although millet had long disappeared and was neither an everyday food nor even widely grown. Nevertheless, in the opinion of the dietician and folklorist Günth Wiegelmann, belief in the salutary effects of porridge eating was an old tradition.[22]

The women of the Kel-Ewey, a Tuareg group of the African Sahel zone, consider their unchanging, daily millet porridge with dates or sour milk to be a particularly tasty and salutary food. They are sorry for Europeans, who in their eyes are tied to absurd variety.[23] As Audrey Richards, an English pioneer in nutrition research in the 1920s and 1930s, discovered for the Bemba in northern Rhodesia, other African peoples regarded their particular kind of grain (in the case of the Bemba it was millet) as the only "real" food in the strictest sense of the word.[24] And indeed, the original meaning of the German word *muos* was not just "porridge," but also "food" in general.[25] Similarly, the word "corn" is not just a general term for grain but is also used to describe the main type of grain found in a particular area, in northern Germany rye, for example; in the southern United States, maize.[26]

Despite the lack of concrete knowledge, for the Kel-Ewey like the Bemba or even the peasants of the Old Society in Europe, we can assume that the simple gruel, the daily food of the "common" people, must previously have consisted of quite a different "stuff," as Bachelard would say.[27]

CHANGING FOOD HABITS

To be sure, the porridge of country dwellers in Europe was not everywhere merely a traditional meal for ritual occasions, a fact that, due to an excess of enthusiasm for the simple and unadulterated, lay researchers such as Eckstein and his contemporaries often overlooked. Porridge still played a central role in the ordinary diet of many poor cottagers and farm laborers, for example, in the German uplands, the north and east, and the Po plain after its early impoverishment. It derived this importance in the course of various developments: the early loss of fishing and hunting rights to the nobility, increasing taxes, liberation of the peasantry, rationalization of agriculture, effects of industrialization, and falling prices for agricultural products.

In the late middle ages and at the beginning of the modern era Europe consumed much more meat than it did in the eighteenth and early nineteenth centuries.[28] It is indeed true, as Marvin Harris neatly summarizes Fernand Braudel, that in a worldwide perspective, late medieval Europe was the center of meat gluttony.[29] From 1550 on, in a process of impoverishment that continued to the middle of the nineteenth century, the standard of living of the common people declined.[30] From this time on, the majority of country dwellers in Germany, France, or other parts of Europe lived for the most part without meat or with very little meat. The pig, slaughtered at the beginning of winter, was mainly a source of winter provisions. It gave preserved meat (smoked or salted) and fat (bacon) and possibly the festive roast. The main source of nutrition for the broad mass of the population was grain, porridge, and, later on, bread. This porridge (*Brei*, or *Mus* to use the older term which today is common only in Switzerland) tended to have a firm consistency like that of polenta or blancmange, a mixture in which a "spoon could stand" and that one could eat with the fingers or with a knife. Alternatively, it was a kind of groat-gruel in which the pieces of corn could be individually recognized. The porridge was eaten either with (usually sour) milk and some fat or as a "sour soup" made by covering the shelled corn with hot water and leaving it to swell and ferment overnight in the oven, in a fashion similar to Russian borscht.[31] The porridge consisted either of one sort of grain (of oats, barley, millet, or rye, later also buckwheat and, increasingly, south of the Alps from the eighteenth century on, of corn) mixed with beans, peas, and other legumes, or of the grain alone. It was eaten with vegetables, especially with preserved sour cabbage, or with beans, and in the south with lettuce, too. For example, we know from the Zürich uplands in the seventeenth and eighteenth centuries that the people ate chiefly a milk and flour soup, porridge with oats, peas, root vegetables, beans, and cabbage.[32]

But the growth of manufacturing and the spread of factories changed things rapidly. With the wide acceptance of new colonial products, above all of coffee, sugar, and potatoes toward the end of the eighteenth century, the old patterns of food consumption gradually disappeared. Porridge was replaced in the first instance by quickly prepared staples such as coffee, bread, and potatoes. From 1800 on, the habit of taking sugar in coffee or tea spread to the masses. Among the poor in England and on the continent, sugared tea and coffee at times replaced complete meals. From 1870 on, bread and jam became a staple food of the English proletariat.[33]

Within this general trend, however, marked regional and social differences existed. Northern Germany, for example, including the rich marshland farmers, was profitably engaged as early as the sixteenth century in the international grain and cattle trade. Thus, the farmers in this region were quite early in adopting urban habits. In the eighteenth century and later, many farm women cooked a stew, a thick soup that consisted mainly of potatoes, meat, and vegetables, while for breakfast they served coffee with bread and butter. At the same time, at around 1820, the peasants of the poor, sandy coastal regions of East Freesia and the cottagers near Bremen continued to eat buttermilk porridge made of rye flour or buckwheat gruel for their morning and evening meal.[34] The peasants of the Lüneburg Heath, another poor, sandy coastal region of northern Germany, still consumed this kind of porridge for breakfast in the mid-1920s.[35]

In the towns themselves, at least among the growing bourgeoisie, the adoption of the court habit of eating with a knife and fork and with individual plates had led to the disappearance of the old porridge dishes in the course of the seventeenth century.[36] By 1770, the dietary transformation in the cities was more or less complete.[37] For Goethe and the young Werther, for example, it was a matter of course in 1772 to have coffee with sugar every day, and they acknowledged that the poor village woman used her porridge pan only to feed the small child.[38]

But despite north Germany's early adoption of the eating habits of the rich, it was not until the middle of the twentieth century that the old porridges disappeared completely from the diet of country dwellers. Up to this point it remained at least as a morning, evening, or quick meal in northern Germany and other areas or even as a festive meal in the "backward" areas of central Europe, such as the poor Alpine valleys, or among the day laborers of Schleswig-Holstein.

It is important to note, however, that the displacement of porridge by coffee, bread, and potatoes was not necessarily and not always a form of imitating the eating habits of the upper classes. It often was a sign of impoverishment: during the time of preindustrialization in the early nineteenth century, some country dwellers, especially in the region of the German uplands (*Mittelgebirge*), and wage earners in the towns were too poor to provide porridge and were therefore left with nothing to eat but potatoes and chicory coffee, if even the latter. Such was the case of the poor inhabitants of the Palatinate, who in 1850 had nothing but potatoes in their skins from a common bowl three times a day, and who, according to Riehl's account, for this reason were scornfully called "potato sacks" by their neighbors.[39] A char and washerwoman from Bremen in the 1850s could barely earn what she needed to provide her school-going child with potatoes (eaten with drippings or vinegar) three times a day.[40] As late as 1930, poverty in some areas—as in the Frankenwald, for example—was such that the people had nothing to eat but potatoes, coffee, and dry bread.[41] For these people grain, porridge, and bread became the expression of luxury.

DISLODGED TECHNIQUES AND THEIR INVESTIGATORS

Not least, the "social question" of the undernourished poor brought a new interest in vegetarianism and *Lebensreform* (life-style reform) and a public discussion of housework, which resulted around 1900 in a boom of research into food habits. While sociologists were debating why disciplines such as economics and sociology had not yet reflected on habits of consumption,[42] other scholars and lay researchers wished to investigate more exactly the history of peasant nutrition. Although they often sought "the whole," the irrational, or "spiritual" as it used to be called, persons engaged in this kind of research were frequently concerned chiefly with those dimensions of the problem that belonged to the natural sciences. Their works, which often involved field studies, are of interest here not only as documents of the early history of food research, but also as meticulous records of the forms of nutrition then prevalent among European country dwellers.

Two researchers who were inspired by the "life-style" reform discourse at the turn of the century were the Swiss botanist Adam Maurizio and the Austrian schoolteacher Anni Gamerith. Both dealt in particular with transformations of the grain-based diet. The great majority of doctors in the nineteenth century were convinced that a human being required a certain amount of animal protein daily and meat in particular. It was against this background that Maurizio and Gamerith both asked how, in contradiction to these assumptions, large sections of the rural population of central Europe survived with very little meat. Although they vehemently opposed a view of the world too narrowly influenced by the natural sciences, they were very receptive to the ideas discussed by early twentieth-century social critics, in whose thought the natural sciences played a key role.

Adam Maurizio (born 1862) worked in Berlin around 1900 at a research institute specializing in milling technology. He was later employed in Zürich as research assistant of the Swiss Institute for Agriculture and Chemistry, before, in 1906, taking the chair of botany and commerce at the imperial and royal Technical University of Lemberg (Lvov). While his first book published in 1903 focused on social hygiene, his main work, *Die Geschichte unserer Pflanzennahrung* (The History of our Vegetable Diet) published in 1927, sharply criticized both the one-sided belief in the value of vitamins and uncooked food held by many reformers and the "dietary imperialism" of richer countries and their industries toward ethnic minorities.[43] A marked feature of his research methodology is that wherever he happened to be, he spoke personally with the peasants, including those of the poor Swiss Bergell valley, his own family home, and of eastern Galicia.[44] In this manner he can be said to have conducted "field research."

Maurizio, who was in the first instance a milling expert, was initially interested in the paradoxical fact that industrially ground flour became increasingly widespread in the course of the nineteenth century, to the point that fine bleached flour became the norm,[45] while popular opinion still held the protein layer of the grain, which was lost in industrial milling, to be particularly valuable.[46] As early as 1903 he pointed out that "the people" were right: he showed that it is precisely this protein layer (or gluten stratum) together with the germ of the kernel attached to it which contains the grain's protein, while the white-flour grain consists only of starch. (The Vitamin B complexes, which also exist in this protein layer, were not discovered until the 1920s.) Thus it became apparent that people with a diet free of meat did indeed obtain proteins, and that they did not suffer any deficiency in not eating meat as long as their consumption was not limited to white flour, which lacked the protein layer.

Maurizio was later fascinated by the fact that around 1900 East Galician peasants still obstinately maintained that their pounded groats tasted much better and sweeter than the modern commercially milled varieties and also kept longer.[47] Maurizio thought that the disappearance of the old techniques of drying the grain could be the reason for this loss of taste and other qualities in industrial milling. In earlier days, the peasants had indeed moistened and then dried and lightly roasted most varieties of grain, in order to help remove the chaff, which could be done relatively easily with a domestic pestle after this process. The heat of the oven set off a process of saccharification, so that compared to the product of the industrial mills, the grains were indeed tastier and more wholesome. As a result of this process, the grain was twice the size, in the same way that barley is larger than the actual barleycorn from which it is made.[48]

Anni Gamerith (1906–1990) continued Maurizio's studies. Until 1990 she was an honorary professor of food anthropology in Graz, greatly respected by her young students. As a young girl she belonged to the "Wandervogel," the main organization of the German and Austrian youth movement in the early twentieth century. Like many of the "Wandervogel"

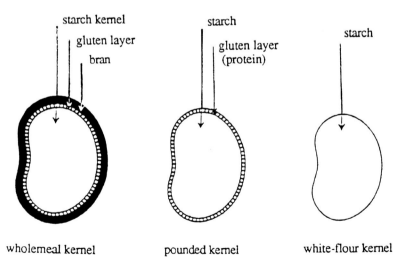

Figure 1   Wholemeal, pounded, and white-flour kernels. From Anni Gamerith, *Ehrfurcht vor Korn und Brot*, 2d ed. (Bad Goisern: Verlag Neues Leben, 1976).

members, she wanted to settle in the countryside. But, instead, she became the sole primary-school teacher in a remote and lonely mountain village on the border of Yugoslavia.[49] Later, she frequently interrupted her teaching service in order to work on lonely farms and learn from anthroposophists. From that time onward she took notes on the peasant diet in Styria and the Enn valley, since the culture of rural women had not yet been investigated by scholars of anthropology. Like Maurizio she also employed methods of "field research," inasmuch as she carried out her search for old techniques of grain preparation through direct contact and conversation with the indigenous population in the course of extended walking tours.

Anni Gamerith was particularly interested in why the mountain peasants in her region, some of whom were extremely poor, seemed to be perfectly satisfied to have as their staple food their simple porridge, which they ate with fat or with sour milk or vinegar. She concluded that the old methods of preparing grain, which by 1950 had almost disappeared without a trace, had probably been underestimated. She discovered that many of the so-called grain mills had not in fact been "mills" in the narrower, modern sense of the word: they did not really grind the grain, but merely removed the chaff, that is, they freed it from its husk and bran layer, without, however, squashing it totally. From older peasants she had heard that the old method of preparing millet, by pounding, resulted in a much tastier food than the modern methods of removing the chaff employed in the industrial mills. The peasants had pointed out to her that millet pounded by traditional methods, in contrast to the new commercial varieties, expanded much more in cooking and at the same time retained its granular texture much better. Above all, when prepared in the traditional way, the millet was much sweeter and also superior in taste, with the result that older people did not like to eat the current commercial varieties.[50]

Although young millers often laughed at Anni Gamerith's questions and although nobody could imagine that she would be able to find anything,[51] she undertook extended walking and cycling tours through eastern Styria until, little by little, she discovered people who were able to explain the lost techniques of preparing millet. In the end they even helped her to find an old peasant mill. This mill contained an old millet mill, a "Gräußstock," and an old grain pound. Even more importantly, it was still used by the miller, who preferred to pound the grain for his family consumption, despite the considerable amount of extra time involved, because it tasted so much better than when it was prepared by modern methods.[52] First, the millet was carefully ground or, more precisely, rolled between two special grindstones. These were made of a special wood or, alternatively, one was made of wood and the other of a soft sandstone.[53] The pieces of corn were

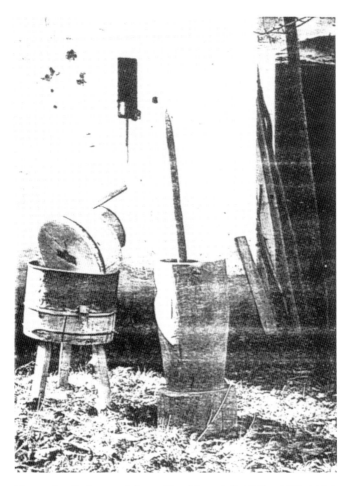

Figure 2 Grain-pound for millet (*Stampf für "Pfennich"*) (right) and groat-grater (*Reibstockl* or *Greissreibn*) (left), from the southern Burgenland, Austria, 1955. Photograph by Anni Gamerith.

rubbed gently against each other to remove the chaff and pounded. This pounding process was done with a pestle and mortar in wooden pounds (Latin *pilae*) and meant that the pieces of grain were rubbed gently against each other so that both the remaining husk and the bran layer were removed, without being lost. The process of separation and pounding was then repeated, the waste product being considered "pig-flour." The work of pounding required experience and skill, so as to prevent damage to the grain. The pestle has to be used in such a way that it sprang back gently after contact with the grain and the grain was pounded only until all the bran had been rubbed off. This process caused the pieces of grain to expand, acquire a floury texture, and exude a slightly sweet smell, the process to saccharification having already begun.

When worked on in this way, cereals lost their bran layer, which is difficult to digest. In contrast, in present-day wholemeal bread the bran is retained, as none of the rationalized methods of grain processing used in the industrial mills is capable of separating the bran from the kernel, without damaging the protein layer. Anni Gamerith's guesswork was confirmed under the microscope. Little or no damage is done to the gluten layer of the kernel when pounded.[54] Consequently, pounded millet could be stored for up to six months. So Anni Gamerith continued Maurizio's work by establishing that it is not merely the drying process that causes fermentation of the corn; rather, the fermentation process continues as a result of the pounding. Moreover, she discovered that the traditional methods of pounding and milling merely removed the husk, while the protein layer remained intact.

In Styria, the most common type of pound was the simple manual pound, made of wood, with a wooden pestle, of the kind known to us today from Africa and India. In some of the poorer valleys of Styria, they could be found on almost every farm as late as the 1920s.[55] Maurizio and another Swiss lay researcher, Moritz Caduff, saw similar old barley pounds in numerous Swiss valleys, albeit some of these were no longer in use.[56] In east Prussia as well, around 1900, one could still find wooden pounds with wooden pestles for barley, buckwheat, oats, and millet.[57] In the Lüneburg Heath Wilhelm Bomann discovered so-called "millet pumps" as late as the 1920s and groat pounds with which buckwheat and other grains could be "separated from the husk by a careful, gentle pumping movement."[58]

In addition to these simple pounds, larger and technically more complicated footpounds existed which were used in Styria almost exclusively for millet and only exceptionally for barley. (Pounds like these are still in use in Asia, for example, at the Salwin River in Indochina—see Figure 12.)

In Styria and in Switzerland, water pounds driven by mountain streams served as stamping mills and were used to process panicled millet, the husk of which—in comparison to Italian millet—could be removed only with difficulty. The peasants brought their millet or barley corn to these water pounds and paid to have the chaff and bran removed. As late as 1900, numerous water-driven pounds still operated in Switzerland.[59]

In order to remove the chaff the grain was, depending on the variety, first moistened or left to soak, then dried, that is, lightly roasted, before being pounded. The husk was then removed, and only at this point, if at all, was the grain ground. The process of moistening, dying, pounding, and separating had to be repeated several times, and the whole procedure was both complicated and time-consuming. Afterwards, however, the grain was almost ready to serve, and in most cases complicated cooking procedures

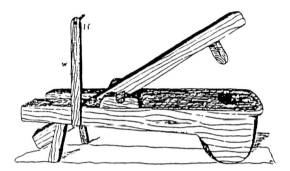

Figure 3   Pound from Western Galicia, Strzelce, for millet, buckwheat, and barley. From Adam Maurizio. *Die Getreide-Nahrung im Wandel der Zeiten* (Zürich: Füssli, 1916).

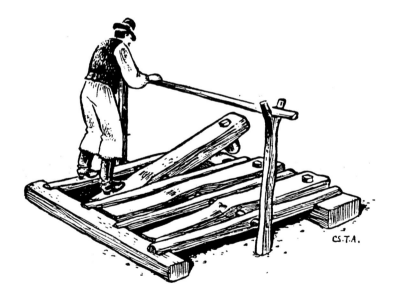

Figure 4   Millet pound from Jászapáti, Komitat Jásznagykunszolnok, Hungary. From Robert Wildhaber, "Gerstenmörser, Gerstenstampfe, Gerstenwalze," *Schweizer Archiv für Volkskunde* 45 (1948): 177–208.

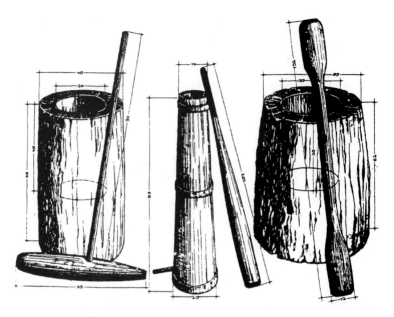

Figure 5 Groat pounds, Lüneburger Heide, northern Germany, early twentieth century. From Wilhelm Bomann, *Bäuerliches Hauswesen und Tagewerk in Niedersachsen* (Weimar: Böhlau, 1927).

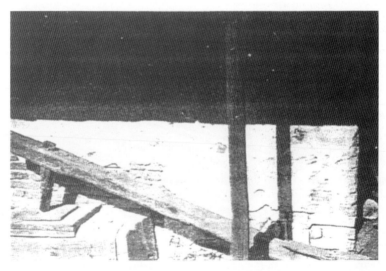

Figure 6 Foot pound for millet, found by Anni Gamerith in Styria, Austria, 1956.

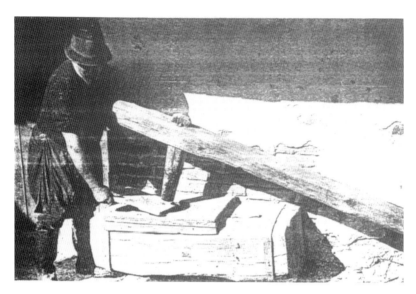

Figure 7–11 Pounding by foot. Photographs by Trummer, courtesy of Anni Gamerith.

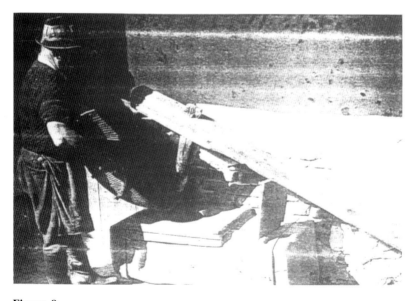

Figure 8

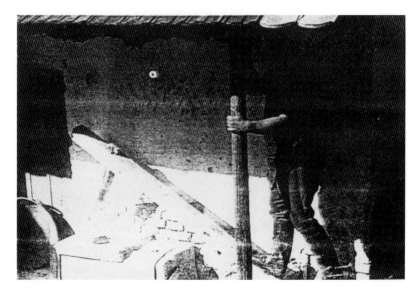

Figure 9

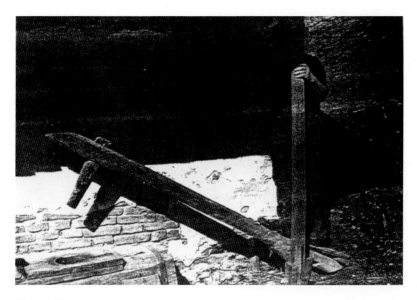

Figure 10

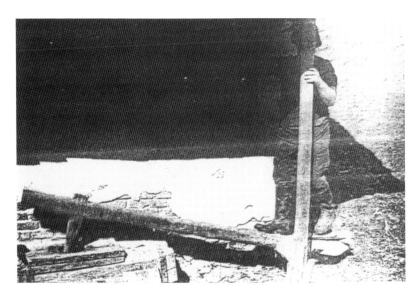

Figure 11

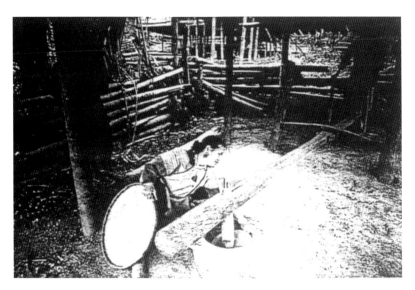

Figure 12 Lisu women, Salwin River, Burma, pounding rice. Postcard from Museum für Völkerkunde Berlin, Staatliche Museen Preussicher Kulturbesitz.

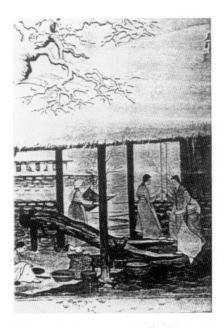

Figure 13 Korean treadmill, nineteenth century. From South Korean postcard, without attribution.

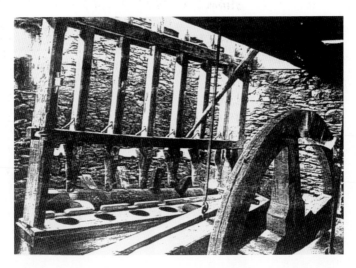

Figure 14 Water or mill pound driven by a mountain stream. (The wheel of an oil press is on the right.) Found by Anni Gamerith in Meisenbach near Birkfeld. Styria, Austria, 1956. Photograph by Hermann Gamerith.

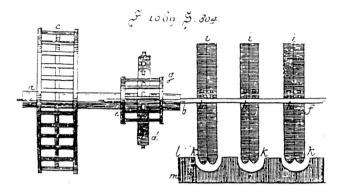

Figure 15 Mill pound, driven by water power, Germany, ca. 1780. From Johann Georg Krünitz, *Oeconomische Encyclopädie*, vol. 19 (Berlin: Pauli 1780).

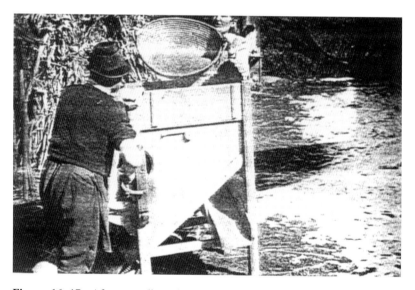

Figure 16–17 After pounding, the millet had to be winnowed to remove the chaff. Photographs by Hermann and Anni Gamerith.

were not necessary. By contrast, the housewife who has to spend half-days in the kitchen was a new phenomenon of bourgeois customs, especially in nineteenth-century cities. In the preparation of "Talggn," an oat dish, for example, the raw grain was first covered with boiling water or boiled; after several hours of soaking (overnight, for example), it was allowed to

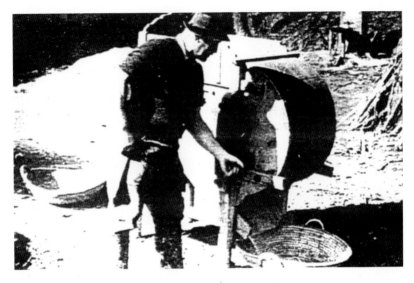

Figure 17

dry in the oven for several days. It was then possible to remove the chaff without difficulty by pounding and to separate it from the grain by allowing it to blow away. Oats prepared in this way could be kept for years and were eaten after soaking in hot water or milk without any other cooking process. Until the turn of the century, the peasants of Styria ate oats processed in this way for lunch, either strewn over sour milk, added to their milk can during harvest time, or served with drippings. In this form they were considered to be particularly invigorating.[60]

ETYMOLOGY

These food preparation techniques, which were mostly forgotten around 1900 and in the early twentieth century, cannot really be considered as exotic. On the contrary a look at the etymology of the terms teaches us that these techniques were very common almost worldwide and throughout history. The pounded but uncooked grain was known in Bavaria and Austria as *Gräuß*, while in northern Germany, from the fifteenth century the word *Grütze*,[61] and from the sixteenth century the word *Graupen*, had become common terms for grain removed from its husk. Prior to this time, the general term was *Grieß*. While in the north, the term *Grieß*, is used today to denote finely ground grain, the Old-High-German *grioz* referred to coarsely ground flour. It is related to the German word *groß*, the original meaning of which is "large grained."[62]

The traditional preparation processes can be seen more clearly in the word *Grütze*. Etymologically, the word originally denoted simply a coarsely uncovered, ground grain; it is related to the Lithuanian *grúdzin*, which means "I pound."[63]

The word *Graupe* (barley) probably has Slavic roots. Related to it is the upper Sorbian word *krupa*, which also denotes barley.[64] The word is also related to the Polish *krupa* and the Czech *kroupa*, both of which denote barley and probably have the same root as *Grütze* (that is, *gruzzi*). Also related are the Latin *grutellum*, "flour," and the Old-French *gruel*, which is also the English word for *Grütze*. The root is *ghreu*, which has the sense of "to rub over it."[65]

Originally, the word *Graupe* was not used exclusively for barley. As late as 1800 according to Krünitz's Encyclopaedia, *Graupen* were made from barley and wheat and also from spelt, either by means of a special process in the mill or at home in a wooden pound made especially for this purpose.[66]

The Italian word *polenta* today denotes a thick mass made of maize flour. In earlier times, this word was used for a similar product made of pounded millet; in Ticino, a poor valley region of Switzerland, the term was used up until the end of the eighteenth century.[67] In the Roman era, the term *polenta* denoted barley pearls.

Whereas today, the words *Gräuß, Grütze, Graupen*, or *Grieß* are used to describe either a cooked dish or a particular form of grain, it is evident that they used to denote a specific process.[68] This special sense of the word disappeared along with the process in question.

MODERN UNDERNOURISHMENT

As the process of rolling barley spread in the mills from 1800 on, the barley was no longer pounded but only sanded, and with the consequent loss of its protein layer, it ceased to have its old nutritious value.[69] Writing about east Prussia, Tolksdorf records that around 1900, the old "country barley" (that is, the barley pounded by the peasants) was greatly preferred to pearl barley from the mills.[70] Although their food was unvaried prior to the emergence of modern forms of diet, the peasants of central Europe were nevertheless sufficiently nourished because their method of pounding, shredding, or grinding retained the protein layer of the grain, rich in proteins and vitamins, which today is lacking in the common varieties of white or fine flour.

As a consequence, the statement of Teuteberg and Wiegelmann that people in central Europe at the end of the nineteenth century were better nourished than had previously been the case because they enjoyed a more varied diet, is true only up to a point.[71] On the one hand, when the natural goodness is removed from foods, a diversified diet has its problems, even for the rich. On the other hand, meal porridge and potatoes (the monotonous diet to which Teuteberg and Wiegelmann refer) constituted a deficient diet only for the urban proletariat who, unable to.grow food for themselves and dependent on the products of large commercial mills, had to use fine flour to make their porridge and meal soup. Also undernourished were those country dwellers who had no access to land or who, due to changing economic circumstances, did not dispose of sufficient time to do their own grinding and pounding and hence had to exchange their grain for industrially milled flour which had already been stored for lengthy periods. In fact, the change to a diet deprived of its natural goodness made the diversification of the modern diet necessary. It must also have been the loss of the old "naturally" sweet grain porridge that brought about the heightened need for sugar, which Sidney Mintz established in English factory workers as early as the late eighteenth century.[72]

If, then, the traditional diet was so much better, why did porridge so quickly lose its place at European tables? It is beyond the scope of this paper to analyze fully the multiple and geographically diverse factors at work, but let me attempt to illustrate the process by taking the case of millet. Millet was particularly popular as a bringer of good luck on feast days, probably because of the extent to which it increased in mass during cooking. It was, moreover, by no means exclusively a meal of the poor, but was also eaten by the nobility. Yet, despite the great significance that millet enjoyed, it was to disappear almost completely as a meal in the course of the nineteenth century, and it did so with almost incredible speed, dislodged by the coffee-and-sugar, bread-and-butter breakfast, as well as by potatoes, rice, and maize. Around 1800 four times as much millet was grown in Germany and Austria as was grown a century later. In 1878 millet was still grown only in southern regions: in the Lausitz region, in Silesia, in the area around Passau, in Styria, in Bohemia, and in parts of Galicia. The main reason for its disappearance was probably the fact that its cultivation was extremely labor intensive. It required repeated weeding and did not allow machine-harvesting, with the result that millet cultivation impeded the process of intensification and rationalization in agriculture.[73] The peasant could no longer afford to grow millet solely for his own use, given the increased tax burden and falling prices for raw produce. Moreover, the "Mühlenzwang" that forced farmers to use the state-licensed mills even for their own products became an important reason for the displacement of home-grown and processed millet by purchased flour. Millet must have disappeared from the peasants' diet at precisely the point where it became cheaper and more convenient to obtain the protein and starch they needed from commercial white bread and meat. The fact that well into the nineteenth century millet was eaten much longer by those who could not afford to buy meat, namely, the rural dwellers of southern Germany and Austria (where, for example, millet did not disappear until the 1890s), seems to support this view.

Another reason for the disappearance of millet was probably the fact that it could be used only for making millet porridge and could not be prepared in any other way, and the eating of porridge enjoyed an increasingly low reputation from the eighteenth century on.[74] In contrast to Africa—as Jack Goody has demonstrated—the development of class differences in diet is characteristic of Europe.[75] The increasing dominance of bourgeois society in the nineteenth century was accompanied by the spread of the bourgeois habit of separated food on separate plates. In Styria, the old porridge of millet barley (*Gräuß*) did not disappear until the great destitution of the First World War.[76] Forced increasingly to produce for the market, the peasants of Styria adopted the urban, bourgeois way of life and style of eating, and the new constraints and conventions were powerful enough to overcome old ideas regarding taste.

For the poor of Europe, the process of industrialization and the change to meals of coffee, sugar, bread, and potatoes meant in some ways a drastic deterioration in the quality of their diet for over a hundred years at least, until they were in a position to participate sufficiently in the mixed diet of the bourgeoisie. Even if, with the introduction of the potato and the railways, the famines that had followed poor harvests disappeared, permanent hunger as a consequence of malnutrition was characteristic of the European proletariat and the lower classes of peasants throughout the nineteenth century. Hunger arose among these groups due to the change in their diet to sugared coffee, white flour, and potatoes. If proteins and vitamins are lost in the grinding of flour, and foods are robbed of their traditional "sense," meat seems to be an alternative.

Vegetarians, life-style reformers, and their sympathizers around the turn of the century cast doubt on the value of the modern meat-dominated mixed diet, seeing it as a burdensome and not particularly wholesome replacement for a grain-based diet. Bircher-muesli, the result of modern, in a sense "sportive," rationalism, was without doubt a pale imitation of the old porridge. The Nazis, who successfully stole important slogans and symbols not just from the workers and womens' movement, but also from the "life-style reformers" and the "Wandervögel," went on to make the "Eintopf" (stew) the "cult meal of the Germans."[77] It is certainly in character that this was not a grain porridge but rather a modern potato and vegetable soup with a little meat too.

What the first researchers of food habits and the life-style reform show is that the old, common porridge was in several respects less profane than the enlightened citizen was willing to accept up to that time.[78] And it becomes possible to understand why porridge was and is even today particularly prone to become the symbol of an "alternative Weltanschauung." We can expect that when "western civilization" attempts to introduce "progress" to the peoples of Africa and Asia and, above all, to their women, doing all in its power to release them from the timeconsuming pounding of rice and millet for more lucrative activities, this is likely to result in a deterioration of the quality of their food, seen in purely physiological terms. We can see that "progress" is ambivalent and that the Third World's poor with their "primitive" food preparation techniques and monotonous" diet should not be regarded just as victims of a "stone-age economy." Their food is an important component of a whole way of life.

NOTES

For assistance and encouragement I want to thank Frau Honorarprofessorin Dr. Anni Gamerith[†]. Dr Claudia Bernardoni. Prof. PhD. Judith van Herrick. Jan Lambertz, and Leah Rosenberg.
1. Frances Moore Lappe, *Die Öko-Diät* (Frankfurt a.M.: Fischer, 1978).
2. For examples. see Joseph Collins and Frances Moore Lappé, *Vom Mythos des Hungers* (Frankfurt a.M.: Fischer), p. 27. (Originally published as *Food First: Beyond the Myth of Scarcity* [San Francisco: Institut for Food and Development Policy, 1977].)
3. Siegfried Giedion, *Die Herrschaft der Mechanisierung*, 2d ed. (Zürich: Buchclub Exklibris, 1982), pp. 103ff. (Originally published as *Mechanization Takes Command* [Oxford: Oxford University Press, 1948].)
4. *Encyclopaedia Britannica*, 1964, vol. 23.
5. Wolfgang Krabbe, *Gesellschaftsveränderug durch Lebensreform* (Göttingem: Vandenhoeck & Ruprecht, 1974), 54ff.
6. *Encyclopaedia Britannica*, 11th ed., 1911, vol. 28; Claudia Huerkamp, "Medizinische Lebensreform im späten 19. Jahrhundert: Die Naturheilbewegung in Deutschland als Protest gegen die naturwissenschaftliche Universitätsmedizin," *Vierteljahresschrift für Wirtschaft und Sozialgeschichte* 73 (1986): 158ff.
7. See Ulrich Linse. ed., *Zurück o Mensch zu Mutter Erde: Landkommunen in Deutschland* (Munich: Deutscher Taschenbuch Verlag. 1983).
8. See, for example, Ulrich Linse, *Ökopax und Anarchie: Eine Geschichte der ökologischen Bewegung in Deutschland* (Munich: Deutscher Taschenbuch Verlag, 1986).

9. Günter Wiegelmann, *Alltags- und Festtagsspeisen: Wandel und gegenwärtige Stellung* (Marburg: Elwert, 1967).

10. See Klaus Bergmann, *Agrarromantik und Großstadtfeindlichkeit* (Meisenheim am Glan: Anton Hain, 1970), p. 101: also Hinrich Wulff, *Geschichte und Gesicht der bremischen Lehrerschaft*, 2 vols. (Bremen: Schünemann, 1950), and Elisabeth Meyer-Renschhausen, *Weibliche Kultur und soziale Arbeit: Eine Geschichte der ersten Frauenbewegung am Beispiel Bremens 1810–1927* (Cologne and Vienna: Böhlau. 1989).

11. See, for instance, Adolf Spamer, "Marie Andree-Eysn zum 80. Geburtstag," *Festschrift zum 80. Geburtstag von Marie Andree-Eysn, Beiträge zur Volks- u. Völkerkunde* (Munich: 1928), p. 2ff.; see also Wolfgang Jacobeit, *Bäuerliche Arbeit und Wirtschaft: Ein Beitrag zur Wissenschaftsgeschichte der deutschen Volkskunde* (East Berlin: Akademie- Verlag, 1965).

12. Johann Georg Krünitz, *Oeconomische Encyclopädie* (1781), 23: 790.

13. See Stephen Mennell, *All Manners of Food: Eating and Taste in England and France from the Middle Ages to the Present*, 2d ed. (New York: Basil Blackwell, 1985).

14. *Deutsches Wörterbuch* von Jacob und Wilhelm Grimm (Leipzig. 1868; reprint, Munich: Deutscher Taschenbuch Verlag, 1984), 8: 2170 (s.v. "Graupe").

15. Adam Maunzio, *Die Getreide-Nahrung im Wandel der Zeiten* (Zürich: Art. Inst. Orell Füssli, 1916), p. 38.

16. *Handwörterbuch des deutschen Aberglaubens*, ed. Hanns Bächtold-Stäubli, 9 vols. (Berlin and Leipzig: Walter deGruyter & Co., 1927–1938/41), 1: 1539 (s.v. "Brei," by Eckstein).

17. Ibid., 3: 1200–1201 (s.v. "Grütze," by Eckstein).

18. Ibid., 1: 1541 (s.v. "Brei").

19. Adam Maurizio, *Getreide, Mehl und Brot; ihre botanischen, chemischen und physikalischen Eigenschaften, hygienisches Verhalten, sowie ihre Beurteilung und Prüfung*. Handbuch zum Gebrauch in Laboratorien und zum Selbstunterricht für Chemiker, Müller, Bäcker, Botaniker und Landwirte (Berlin: Paul Parey, 1903), p. 366; *Trübners Deutsches Wörterbuch* (1939), 1: 424 (s.v. "Brei").

20. *Handwörterbuch des deutschen Aberglaubens*, 1: 1538, 1540 (s.v. "Brei"), and 9: 513ff. (s.v. "Speiseopfer," by Eckstein).

21. Ibid., 8: 222.

22. Günter Wiegelmann, *Alltags- und Festtagsspeisen*, pp. 120–156; see *Atlas der deutschen Volkskunde*, ed. Heinrich Harmjanz and Erich Röhr, 3 vols. (Leipzig, 1938), map 55.

23. Gerd Spittler, "Essen und Moral: Die Nahrung der Kel Ewey im Alltag und in einer Hungerkrise," in *Freiburger Universitätsblätter* 96 (1987): 95–112; Gerd Spittler, "Wie bewältigen die Kel Ewey Tuareg Dürren und Hungerkrisen?" *Journal für Geschichte* 6 (1986): 21–29.

24. Audrey Richards, *Land, Labour and Diet in Northern Rhodesia* (London: Oxford University Press, 1939).

25. Matthias Lexer, *Mittelhochdeutsches Taschenwörterbuch* (Stuttgart, 1981), p. 145; see also Fritz Ruf, "Die Suppe in der Geschichte der Ernährung," in *Essen und Trinken in Mittelalter und Neuzeit*, ed. Irmgard Bitsch, Trude Ehlert, and Xenja von Ertzdorff (Sigmaringen: Jan Thorbecke, 1987), p. 167.

26. See *Atlas der deutschen Volkskunde* (1938); *Deutsches Wörterbuch* (1911), 6: 4453 (s.v. "Korn").

27. Gaston Bachelard, *Die Bildung des wissenschaftlichen Geistes* (Frankfurt a.M.: Suhrkamp, 1987). (Orginally published as *La formation de l'esprit scientifque* [Paris: J. Vrin, 1938].) See also Barbara Duden, *Geschichte unter der Haut* (Stuttgart: Klett-Cotta, 1987), p. 16ff., and Ivan Illich, *H₂O und die Wasser des Vergessens* (Reinbek: Rowohlt, 1987). (Originally published as *H₂O and the Waters of Forgetfulness* [Dallas, Texas: The Dallas Institute of Humanities and Culture, 1985].)

28. Wilhelm Abel, *Massenarmut und Hungerkrisen im vorindustriellen Deutschland* (Göttingen: Vandenhoeck und Ruprecht, 1972). In contrast to Friedrich Engels, Abel stressed that we could find the worst poverty in the century before industrialization. See also Wilhelm Abel, "Die Lage in der deutschen Land- und Ernährungswirtschaft um

1800," in *Die wirtschaftliche Situation in Deutschland und Österreich um die Wende vom 18. und 19. Jahrhunderts*, ed. F. Lütge (Stuttgart, 1964), pp. 238–254; Wilhelm Abel, *Stufen der Ernährung* (Göttingen: Vandenhoeck und Ruprecht, 1981); Wilhelm Abel, "Wandlungen des Fleischverbrauchs und der Fleischversorgung in Deutschland seit dem Mittelalter," in *Berichte über Landwirtschaft* 22, 3 (1937): 411–452.

29. Marvin Harris, *Wohlgeschmack und Widerwillen: Die Rätsel der Nahrungstabus* (Stuttgart: Klett-Cotta, 1988) p. 100. (Originally published as *Good to Eat: Riddles of Food and Culture* [New York: Simon and Schuster, 1985].)

30. Femand Braudel, *Sozialgeschichte des 15–18. Jahrhunderts: Der Alltag* (Munich: Kindler, 1985), p. 201ff.

31. Anni Gamerith, *Speise und Trank im südoststeirischen Bauernland* (Graz: Akademische Druck und Verlagsanstalt, 1988) p. 186ff.

32. Rudolf Braun, *Industrialisierung und Volksleben: Die Veränderungen der Lebensformen in einem ländlichen Industriegebiet vor 1800* (Erlenbach, Zürich, and Stuttgart: Eugen Rentsch, 1960). p. 93.

33. Sidney W. Mintz, *Sweetness and Power: The Place of Sugar in Modern History*, 2d ed. (New York: Penguin, 1986), pp. 114ff., 129ff.

34. Hans J. Teuteberg and Günter Wiegelmann, *Der Wandel der Ernährungsgewohnheiten unter dem Einfluß der Industrialisierung* (Göttingen: Vandenhoeck & Ruprecht, 1972) p. 260; Philipp Heineken. *Die freie Hansestadt Bremen und ihr Gebiet in topographischer, medizinischer und naturhistorischer Hinsicht*, 2 vols. (Bremen, 1836), p. 61ff.: Günter Wiegelmann, "Regionale Unterschiede in den Würzgewohnheiten in Mitteleuropa dargelegt am Beispiel der Würzbrote." in Hans J. Teuteberg and Günter Wiegelmann, *Unsere tägliche Kost: Geschichte und regionale Prägung* (Münster: F. Coppenrath, 1986), pp. 203–216.

35. Wilhelm Bomann, *Bäuerliches Hauswerk in Niedersachsen* (1927), 4th ed. (Weimar: Böhlau, 1941), p. 159.

36. Teuteberg and Wiegelmann, *Wandel*. 40. p. 258ff.

37. Günter Wiegelmann. *Allrags- und Festtagsspeisen*, p. 40ff.

38. Johann Wolfgang Goethe, *Die Leiden des jungen Werthers* (Stuttgart: Reclam, 1986), p. 17 (1st ed., 1774).

39. Wilhelm Heinrich Riehl, *Die Pfälzer*, 4th ed. (Stuttgart: Cotta, 1925), p. 191; Teuteberg and Wiegelmann, *Wandel*, p. 266ff.

40. Dietrich Schäfer, *Mein Leben* (Berlin: Koehler, 1926), p. 28.

41. Alexander Graf Stenbock-Fermor, *Deutschland von unten: Reisen durch die proletarische Provinz* (Stuttgart: Engelhorns, 1931).

42. Teuteberg and Wiegelmann, *Wandel*, p. 51.

43. *Neue Schweizer Biographie* (Basel, 1938); Adam Maurizio, *Die Geschichte der Pflanzennahrung* (Berlin: Paul Parey, 1927; reprint, Wiesbaden: Sändig, 1979). He describes on many pages how the ethnocide of the North American Menomini and others was caused by their loss of traditional food. They protested but without result.

44. Lvov and East Galicia became Polish after World War I and belong today to the Ukraine, USSR.

45. See Giedion, *Mechanisierung*.

46. Adam Maunzio, *Getreide, Mehl und Brot*, p. 355.

47. Adam Maurizio, Getreide-Nahrung, p. 19.

48. Maurizio, *Pflanzennahrung*, p. 44.

49. Anni Gamerith, "Mein Leben," in *Rund um das bäuerliche Essen: Festschrift Dr. Anni Gamerith zum 80. Geburtstag, Feldbacher Beiträge zur Heimatkunde der Südoststeiermark* (1986), pp. 7–13.

50. Anni Gamerith, *Lebendiges Ganzkorn: Neue Sicht zur Getreidefrage* (Bad Goisern: Verlag Neues Leben, 1956), p. 33ff.

51. See also Robert Wildhaber, "Gerstenmörser, Gerstenstampfe, Gerstenwalze," *Schweizer Archiv für Volkskunde* 45 (1948): 177–208.

52. Anni Gamerith, *Ganzkorn*, 36, p. 43ff.

53. The word *mahlen*, "to grind," meant "to rotate" as well as "to grind"; similarly, the Dutch *malen*, also means "to rotate." See Friedrich Kluge, *Etymologisches Wörterbuch*, 20th ed. (West Berlin: deGruyter & Co., 1967–75), s.v. "mahlen." The English word "meal" meant not only food but originally coarse flour, semolina, or barley.

54. Anni Gamerith, *Ehrfurcht vor Korn und Brot*, 2d ed. (Bad Goisern: Verlag Neues Leben, 1976); Prof. Dr. G. Gorbach and Dipl.-Ing. M. Stranger-Johannessen, "Urtümliche Mahlverfahren im steirischen Brauchtum zur Schonung der biologischen Werte der Gerste," in ibid., p. 19.

55. Anni Gamerith, "'Mühlen,' Stampfen und Reiben," *Volkskunst: Zeitschrift für volkstümliche Sachkultur* (1981): 246.

56. Moritz Caduff, "Essen und Trinken im Lugnez," *Schweizer Archiv für Volkskunde* 82 (1986): 223–276.

57. Ulrich Tolksdorf, *Essen und Trinken in Ost- und Westpreußen* (Marburg: Elwert, 1975), p. 115.

58. Wilhelm Bomann, *Bäuerliches Hauswerk*, p. 150.

59. Robert Wildhaber, "Gerstenmörser"; Moritz Caduff, "Essen," p. 227.

60. Anni Gamerith, *Ganzkorn*, p. 13.

61. Moritz Heyne, *Deutsches Wörterbuch*, 2d ed , 3 vols. (Leipzig, 1905; reprit, Hildesheim and New York: Georg Olms Verlag, 1970) p. 1247 (s.v. "Gries").

62. *Duden Herkunftswöterbuch: Etymologie*, ed. Günther Drossowski, 2d ed. (Mannheim, Vienna, and Zürich: Dudenverlag, 1989).

63. Friedrich Kluge, *Etymologisches Wörterbuch*, 20th ed. (West Berlin: deGruyter & Co., 1967–75), p. 270 (s.v. "Grieß"); see also Moritz Heyne, *Deutsches Wörterbuch*, 1: 1271 (s.v. "Grütze").

64. Kluge, p. 269 (s.v. "Graupe").

65. Kluge, p. 276. (s.v. "Grütze").

66. Krünitz, *Oeconomische Encyclopädie* (1780), 19: 797–809.

67. Ottavio Lurati, "Alltags- und Festspeisen im Tessin," *Ethnologica Scandinavica* (1971), pp. 84–90; Piero Camporesi, *Alimentazione—Folklore—Società* (Parma: Pratiche Editrice, 1980), pp. 96, 97.

68. The English word "meal" means not only a dish but also coarse flour, perhaps also groats as well. All of those words are not only words for particular kinds of food but are especially words for grain groats, processed for eating by pounding.

69. Anni Gamerith. *Speise*, p. 245.

70. Ulrich Tolksdorf, *Essen und Trinken*.

71. Teuteberg and Wiegelmann. *Wandel*, p. 92.

72. Sidney W. Mintz, *Sweetness and Power*.

73. See Krünitz. *Encyclopädie* (1789), 23: 779ff (s.v. "Hirse").

74. Günter Wiegelmann, *Alltags- und Festtagsspeisen*, pp. 112–117.

75. Jack Goody, *Cooking, Cuisine and Class: A Study in Comparative Sociology* (Cambridge: Cambridge University Press, 1982).

76. Anni Gamerith, *Speise*, p. 33ff.

77. Konrad Köstlin, "Der Eintopf der Deutschen: Das Zusammengekochte als Kultessen," *Tübinger Beiträge zur Volkskultur* 69 (1986): 220–241 (ed. Utz Jeggle et al.).

78. For the following see also Ivan Illich, *Gender* (New York: Pantheon, 1982); Gerd Spittler, *Handeln in einer Hungerkrise* (Opladen: Westdeutscher Verlag, 1989); Claudia v. Werlhoff et al., *Frauen, die letzte Kolonie* (Reinbek: Rowohlt, 1983).

9. THE RATIONING SYSTEM, FOOD POLICY, AND NUTRITIONAL SCIENCE DURING THE SECOND WORLD WAR: A COMPARATIVE VIEW OF SWITZERLAND

Jakob Tanner
History Department, University of Zurich, CH

Food rationing has expanded steadily since the outbreak of the Second World War, thereby significantly changing the food habits in Switzerland. "Does the national diet, in amount and composition, still meet bodily requirements despite these forced changes?"[1] This question, raised by the Federal Commission for Wartime Nutrition (FCWN) on February 9, 1943, will be examined in this article. The general assumption is, that the features of European wartime food supplies and the different rationing models had a strong political, ideological and psychological impact on society and were advanced by nutritional science which was of decisive importance in the political decision making. As changes in food habits have to be analyzed in the broader framework of cooking skills and practices during the war years, the article tries to connect everyday-life with "big politics". In the long term, there can be observed a tendency toward a "social leveling",[2] which was accelerated by the interaction of food shortages, rationing system and increased agricultural production. In this perspective, the war has to be interpreted as a catalyst for social and cultural changes in the afterwar period.

FOOD SHORTAGES, RATIONING SYSTEM AND NUTRITIONAL SCIENCE

The Second World War was also an economic war, and the more it developed into a "total war", spreading throughout the world, the more effective blockade and counter-blockade became. In addition to it, the destruction of production facilities, infrastructure and stockpiles by the deliberate exercise of military force grew increasingly devastating. At almost every level of the militarized economies, resources procurement became increasingly difficult and was eventually paralyzed. In Europe bottlenecks were most severely felt in relation to food supplies. This situation was not changed by the ending of the war in spring, 1945. On the contrary, in large parts of Europe food shortages and hunger dramatically worsened in the first postwar years.[3] National food policy and above all the rationing of increasingly limited food supplies therefore played an important role until the end of the 1940s.

In a comparative international review of the Second World War, Alan S. Milward made the general observation that "food is a commodity of unique strategic importance".[4] Hunger and public policy exerted a close mutual influence on public opinion. In those countries in which gaps in the food supply became acute after the beginning of the war, the political and economic elites assumed that below a certain critical dietary threshold public health and economic efficiency would suffer and social stability and national unity would be jeopardized. It was the task of food policy to prevent instability or at least to delay it for as long as possible by rationing and price controls. This policy was based on nutritional science, which was to determine a biological and physiological minimum intake as the fundamental criterion for state management of food scarcity and therefore acquired key political importance. The experts task was to integrate the diets of various social groups and strata into an administrative structure and coordinate them with national (military, economic, political and ideological) objectives. Thus, the entire culture of food, from availability of certain food stuffs to cooking techniques and including taste preferences and dietary habits, came under pressure to change both from shortages and from wartime food policy, which was conceived as a response to these shortages.

The Report *"Food, Famine and Relief 1940–1946"*,[5] which was published by the League of Nations in 1946, shows how governments tried to cope with the problem of food. The report pointed to four factors determining wartime food supplies: (1) the level set for the official ration; (2) actual availability of food in the shops; (3) incomes; (4) non-rationed sources of food.[6]

As to the first factor, it was stated that, in order to prevent rationing systems from becoming an empty formality, the wartime authorities were obliged to set ration levels in relation to available food supplies, which in a period of increasing shortage meant constant reductions. A Swiss author established, how painfully limited official rations in some cases were, especially in their protein and vitamin content.[7] However, attempts were made through supplementary production and trade measures to improve the total volume of food available. Since the economic war in Europe was moving towards total protectionism, limiting opportunities for foreign trade and programmes to increase and reshape agricultural production played a central role. In many countries from 1940 onward, agriculture underwent important restructuring; mechanization and land productivity were increased and a new basis laid for the postwar development of this sector.

Beyond the problems of defining an appropriate official ration and of securing a sufficient total food supplies, there is a second factor, which is related to difficulties in the distribution of the available food. "The rationing tables should be used with circumspection" since "legal rations (…) may not have been actually available in the shops".[8] The converse could also occur. Rationing systems do not replace money and market exchange. Buying and selling did not give way to a command economy, in which food was obtained on the basis of warrants for natural products: instead, the state gave the entire population entitlements in the form of ration cards and food tickets exchangeable for the corresponding goods against payment of the actual market price. To obtain food, therefore, the consumer had to have both money and cards. That is, goods might be available in principle but not affordable in terms of purchasing power.

With that, we have identified the third factor. The wartime inflation, i.e. a general rise in prices depressed already low real incomes so greatly that even the minimum standard of living set by the official ration could no longer be achieved by lower income groups. The fact that financial resources as well as food tickets had to be sufficient thus created a dual problem. The First World War had shown that the inflationary financing of rising state expenditure led to a cycle of rising prices which was equivalent to a highly effective system of "rationing" via the loss of purchasing power, which particularly affected lower income groups.

As a fourth factor, we have to take into consideration sources of supply outside the rationing system, including private supplies and the black market. The importance of self-support rose as the number of people working their own land increased and traditions of subsistence economy or new, industrialized forms of private production strengthened. As the registration of goods was "the key point of rationing measures",[9] the introduction of compulsory deliveries was necessary. But this bureaucratic system was far from being perfect. The extensive use of deficiencies and loopholes pushed the peasants towards the black market; in Switzerland objections to food products of this kind were blunted by designating them "grey".

In particular, there were "grey eggs" and "grey butter", but cheese and fish—all containing comparatively expensive, high-value animal protein—also circulated in this intermediate domain.[10] The notion of the black market was reserved for the illegal purchase of goods for money.[11]

According to the logic of rationing the additional procurement of food on the black and "grey" markets functioned on the level of the impoverished, who were unable to purchase independently, and those groups with significant real incomes.[12] In the first case, the black market took the form of trading in ration cards. Members of declining income groups were forced to sell a part of their formal entitlements to the better-off in order to be able to pay for the remaining part of their rations. Goods remained within the administrative system, but its *raison d'être*, the equal distribution of food, was nullified. In the case of the privileged groups, the black market developed directly on the basis of the exchange of money for goods; that it remained liquid was due to the fact that a certain proportion of food output was "set aside" and was consequently distributed outside administrative control at exorbitant prices. The relative size of these black markets varied widely. "In many occupied countries—Belgium was the most notorious—the black market was as active as the official food markets";[13] in Switzerland, conversely, it was "certain" that "black-marketeering ... at no time assumed a scale that even remotely compared with our neighbours".[14] This confidence-building statement was made possible by a broad definition of "private supply" and a narrow understanding of the "black market". But it glossed over the fact that in Switzerland at least six percent of calories, ten percent of fats and ten percent of protein reached the customer via these informal routes, permitting the conclusion that the well-off were in fact more widely involved.[15]

"ANGLO-AMERICAN" VERSUS "GERMAN-TYPE" RATIONING

In 1939, governments were not unprepared for the challenges in food policy with which they were faced. Since the early 1930s it had been understood that the "postwar period" was an "interwar period" and that preparations for war were necessary. The declared aim was to limit the redistribution-effects of inflation to a level that would not damage economic and military objectives. At the same time production and trade measures were to ensure a (still) adequate level of supply and strengthen social cohesion. These efforts were the product of an institutional learning process in the 1920s and 1930s triggered by the experiences of the First World War. The first "total war" had taken root in the collective mind as "the great analogue of war".[16] This war was paid for by increasingly severe material deprivation, which had led to social polarization and growing class conflict. Mass hunger left lasting traces in the popular memory; for the social elites it was directly and symbiotically linked to the revolutionary trauma of 1917–1919, when a graphic example had been given of what not to do in order to preserve dominance.[17]

The system established at the end of the 1930s in response to this problem assumed various institutional forms which were, however, informed less by political principles than by the structural constraints of waging war.[18] In the cited League of Nations report of 1946 two types of food rationing were distinguished: "German-type rationing" and "rationing of the Anglo-American type".[19] The Anglo-American approach was applied in countries able to maintain their world market connections and therefore were only selectively affected by shortages. In this model the state confined itself to rationing goods whose prices were markedly inflated by loss of production or imports and attempted primarily to achieve balanced distribution of scarce food products—in particular meat, fats and sugar—on the basis of fixed *per capita* rations. Staple goods and basic food products, such as bread, cereals and to some extent milk (-products), were not rationed. As "budget regulators" these items gave freedom to consume to large sections of society that could not in any case afford more expensive goods and luxury products. The diet was not changed by comprehensive rationing measures. The available food was familiar, thereby preserving the continuity of dietary and cultural traditions. The limited scope of rationing was paralleled by the modest role of the black market.

Increasing food shortages in continental Europe forced a switch to comprehensive resource management. "The German system represents a development and refinement of rationing as applied during the First World War. This system was adopted, with some modifications, all over the Continent of Europe". This was also true of Switzerland. In most countries rationed foods accounted for 95 percent of the total.[20] The remaining, freely-available food products soon offered too few opportunities to enable differences in needs to be taken into account. "Therefore, in order to avoid inequalities in terms of need, rationing (had) to be made differential. Consumers were divided into broad categories in which each received rations in proportion to alleged needs." The criteria applied in determining the "physiological needs for food" included "sex, age, occupation, etc."[21] A unified, graded system of rationing was created, which endeavoured to link work-related criteria with the requirement for social equality. By the far-reaching distribution of entitlements to receive food the state involved itself massively in the composition of the diet.

The priorities of the war economy and arms production were basic to setting distribution and grading criteria. Since a very high value was attached
to individual work performance, a tension arose between social status
(which was not based on physical effort) and the aimed-for distribution of
food (which rated manual labour highly). This was one of the reasons why,
alongside the official distribution system which, with its differentiation,
was perceived as clumsy and inflexible, a more or less flourishing black
market emerged on the basis of natural exchange, trading in ration cards
and cash payments. The black market introduced flexibility into the rigid
rationing system, above all the better-off population groups or those that
profited from wartime inflation. These groups did not wish to submit
themselves to an egalitarian regime of compulsory distribution and room
was opened up in an irregular, barely controllable way for food procurement via the market mechanism.[22]

In Switzerland, too, a rationing system had been systematically created
since the late 1930s within the framework of a "shadow" organization for
the wartime economy. At the end of August 1939 purchases were curbed;
two months later the first rationing measures came into force, affecting
a population that then exceeded four million. At the beginning of the war
uncertainty dominated, since the forces acting on the country were hardly
calculable. Under these conditions, peoples thinking was mainly in terms
of a "worst-case" scenario, not only among nutritional scientists but also
among the population in general, where fear of hunger was wide-spread.
Alfred Fleisch, director at the Institute of Physiology of the University of
Lausanne and president of the FCWN, explained in November 1940: "The
food plan must be based on the worst-possible case, that is, a prolonged
war with insignificant opportunities for importing food. Just as the army is
trained and shaped for the worst possible case, that of war, so, too, this
food plan must take into account the worst possibility."[23] In the first two
years, it was believed that food rationing could be restricted, according to
the Anglo-American model, to a few food products in short supply. Still
in the spring of 1942, Switzerland was foremost among the countries that
limited the overall proportion of rationed foods: measured against prewar
household bills only 45 percent of food purchases were rationed, compared with 50 percent in the UK, 65 percent in Denmark, 75 percent in
Sweden, more than 80 percent in the Netherlands, Italy and Norway, and
more than 90 percent in Belgium, Germany, Poland and Czechoslovakia.[24]
But in the summer of 1942 Switzerland abruptly moved closer to "German-
type rationing": by June 1942 a unified system of meat rationing had been
introduced, followed in October by bread and in November by milk; apart
from potatoes, vegetables, fruit and a few other, less important food

products all food resources were thus integrated into the wartime system of deficit management. This system of graded rationing was progressively relaxed after the war, but essentially remained in force until the autumn of 1947 (meat) or the spring of 1948 (bread).

Transition to a "unified system of rationing free of loopholes"[25] meant that the basic principle of equal treatment for all had to be abandoned in favour of a system of work-related distribution with a social component. The priority of fairness (the same ration for all) had to give way to the priority of work, which in turn had to be linked to non-egalitarian criteria of fairness. The "community" was thus defined afresh as a dynamic, working collective. It was given an industrial dimension justifying graded distribution to functional categories. "Why should food be distributed in a fair way? In order to enable every inhabitant of Switzerland to maintain his physical and mental efficiency," noted the head of the rationing section of the Federal Office of Wartime Nutrition in 1943.[26] A strict per capita system of rationing, which would have led to "damage to health", was therefore replaced by a system that, as Albert Zeller noted in 1943, had shown "great flexibility with respect to the needs of the individual"[27] and, as Ernst Feisst observed, was based on the new principle of "the most equal distribution possible given equal physiological food requirements".[28] Albert Jung singled out the decisive "influence of work on nutritional requirements": "Diet and efficiency are closely linked. Occupation and the specific associated level of work are therefore decisive".[29] Elsewhere the same author demanded that "every opportunity (should) be used with respect to nutrition in order to (...) produce maximum efficiency (...)".

Authoritative Swiss nutritionists and leading administrators portrayed Switzerland post festum as a paradigm of a socially integrative and progressive solution to "food problems in times of shortage".[30] When the 10 members of FCWN met in September 1946 for its last session, Alfred Fleisch noted with appreciation: "In Switzerland we had the best system of rationing in the world, as all foreign visitors recognized. The Swiss national diet during the war was good and in some respects even excellent".[31] The self-satisfaction paraded by these scientists and officials, who had been responsible for wartime food policy, was, however, principally rooted in the relatively fortunate position of Switzerland as a country that was spared from war but profited from the rearmament of other countries. Although "our country"—as Ernst Feisst stressed as the new head of the Federal Office of Wartime Nutrition—"is largely cut off from its former food suppliers abroad" and "is also in the middle of the European witchs cauldron",[32] supplies remained adequate at first. As late as 1944 Feisst stated: "While destruction, hunger and misery on an unprecedented scale

are the order of the day around us, we still have the advantage of going to
our work in peace and eating our daily bread in peace (...) Swiss stomachs
and the Swiss constitution (will endure) many more deprivations before
there is cause for breast-beating and self-pity".[33] The sense of achievement
of the nutritionists was the expression of a firm national consensus. The
Second World War contrasted favourably with the conflict-ridden atmosphere of the First World War. "Spiritual national defence" threw a huge
ideological arch over the country: trials of strength linked to the class
struggle, such as the national strike of 1918, were no longer to be expected.
Not the least contribution to this inner unity was made in the view of the
political and military leadership by the fact that after 1939 Switzerland
once again succeeded in remaining outside the military conflict, surviving
"in the eye of the hurricane" as a so-called "small, neutral country".

AGRICULTURAL POLICY AND
THE NATIONAL DIET

Food shortages led to a variety of adaptive strategies, the consistent
feature of which was a trend towards increased vegetable consumption.
Figure 1[34] shows that after 1940 a shift towards a vegetable diet occurred
in most countries.[35] These structural shifts represented an effective economization programme. "If, as in Europe, before the war, about seven feed
calories on an average are required to produce one calorie of animal
food, the number of primary calories needed to produce a diet containing
3,000 calories fit for human consumption varies from that number, if the
diet is altogether of vegetable origin, to 21,000 if the diet is altogether of
animal origin."[36] The League of Nations study of 1946 described the
"animal–vegetable ratio" as "perhaps (the) most significant single index of
dietary standards" and estimated that "in certain north-western European
nations or in North America" it was "approximately 40 : 60".[37] According
to this ratio, designated the "modern standard", 10,200 primary calories
are required to supply 3,000 calories in the form of food. However, in
countries in which vegetables accounted for a very high proportion of the
human diet and a significant part of the animal diet consisted of "absolute
feed",[38] thus reducing the competition for food between man and animal,
opportunities for agricultural restructuring aimed at economizing calories
were far more limited. In these countries shortages affected the vegetable
staples most severely, which statistically could produce an increase in the
proportion of the diet accounted for by animal products (for example,
Bulgaria—see Figure 1). Conversely, in industrialized countries, more

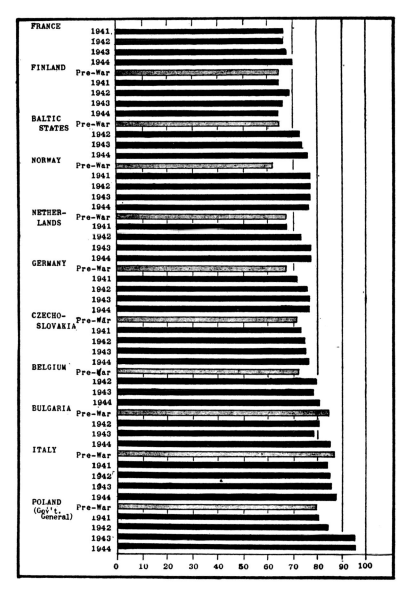

Figure 1 Percentage of vegetable calories in the diet of a typical family, pre-war and during the years 1941–1944 (Calories per consumption unit per diem).

closely integrated into the international division of labour, agricultural land could be turned over directly to crop growing. "The fact of a high animal ratio" implies in these circumstances "the presence of a food buffer of crops that can be diverted to direct human consumption, in addition to the calorie reserve constituted by the livestock itself".[39] The change in consumption that this made possible, reducing the contribution of animal calories by ten percent to a ratio of 30 : 70, produced (in relation to the above data) a considerable saving of 18 percent per person per day. Relatively affluent countries were thus able to counter the threat of shortages by stripping out the calorie-absorbing stages of animal-product processing and switching to plant-based food products; the effect of this measure was that during the transition period, in which animal stocks were reduced, meat remained freely available.

The shift towards a vegetable diet received an ambivalent assessment by nutritionists. The process of industrialization, which produced a long-term increase in real incomes, especially from the end of the 19th century, went hand in hand with a rising proportion of animal calories, fats and protein in the diet.[40] Nutritionists, aware of the value of protein, concluded that for long-term working efficiency about half of protein requirements should be met from animal sources and saw the war as a significant relapse to the dietary standards for carbohydrate intake of the early period of industrialization. However, in light of the latest nutritional research, which was primarily concerned with "protective substances" (vitamins, minerals, trace elements), the deficient diet of wartime also had benefits. For it was not simply latently deficient in calories: at the same time it exhibited a positive return to a healthy, natural diet. The recognition that wide sections of the community had had an excessively fat-rich diet in the interwar years prompted a correspondingly favourable assessment of the changes forced by the war. A diet characterized by shortages harmonized with reformist dietary aspirations and seemed to indicate promising ways of ensuring the quantity and quality of the diet even in face of declining total supply and falling real incomes.[41]

In Switzerland, too, food policies went far beyond rationing: "In our landlocked, resources-poor country an efficient war economy must rest upon three supporting columns".[42] These were the system of differentiated rationing, production measures in agriculture aimed at "expansion of efficient national production", known as "Plan Wahlen", and "expanded stockpiling for the long term". The FCWN had from the outset a clear conception of the close interdependence between supply and demand; in its view rationing and increased production should complement each other. Substantial expansion of cultivated land and more frequent consumption of vegetarian meals were two sides of the same coin.

In its initial phase, therefore, the FCWN concentrated on synchronizing agricultural production (supply) with scientific nutrition (demand): "For the first time in Swiss economic and social policy," wrote the president of FCWN, "the attempt has been made to bring opportunities for food production and human physiological requirements together and to match them".[43] Since the great depression of the 1870s Swiss agriculture had concentrated on animal-based products. The minutes of a conference on the organization and functions of a Federal Wartime Office of Nutrition, held on 22 February 1938, stated that internal production even during the economic crisis of the 1930s had "clearly (been) devoted principally to the creation of animal food values". Under these conditions the goal had to be "to restructure production so that sufficient calories are produced for each and everyone. Rationing should therefore produce a shift in food consumption to those products that offer the greatest calorie yield per hectare".[44] "Plan Wahlen" was launched in November 1940 under the slogan "more farmland–less grassland".[45] It was aimed at activating the "food buffer" latent in a mixed diet by expanding the cultivated area from 200,000 to 500,000 hectares and thereby alleviating the problem of shortages.[46] If the plan for agricultural production had been completely implemented, the "animal–vegetable ratio" would have been reduced to 29 : 71.[47] Until 1943 the successive stages of the plan to increase production were implemented; thereafter restructuring was halted, half-complete, as the war drew to an end, total agricultural land in 1945 reaching about 355,000 hectares. Over the same period dairy and cattle production was substantially cut.[48]

The FCWN was generally positive in its evaluation of these changes with respect to nutrition. It assumed that the intended changes in the production structure were, from the point of view of consumption, not only manageable but also beneficial in terms of the national health and efficiency. This view was based on the recognition that, on the one hand, "the vitamin supply of the population (was) excellent" and "the mineral supply under the dietary plan was significantly larger than the minimum requirement" while, on the other, "the human organism is more adaptable in respect to protein and minimum fat than to the total dietary volume".[49] A scaled reduction in the wartime diet was therefore proposed. Compared to the interwar standard, the minimum "sufficient diet" provided for cuts in the proportions of fat and protein (48 and 38 percent respectively) far deeper than the reduction in the proportion of calories (25 percent).[50] Although this diet was expected to be less satisfying than the relatively high-fat diet of the interwar period, it was nevertheless described as "physiologically superior"[51] by virtue of its high content of micro-nutrients. Figure 2 shows this dietary shift in Switzerland. Consumption of animal products fell

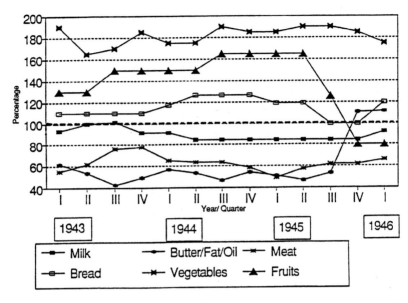

Figure 2 Consumption of foodstuffs 1943–1946. Average-family in %, if 1937/38 = 100.

sharply below that of vegetables. Comparisons between Switzerland and the Anglo-American standard show that daily *per capita* consumption, especially with respect to the extremes of meat and vegetables, diverged widely. Consumption of meat in the USA and Canada was more than double that recorded in Switzerland; conversely "Switzerland broke the record for vegetable consumption" (400 grams daily compared with 116 grams in the USA and 54 grams in Canada).[52]

Food rationing and agricultural expansion were aimed at producing an optimal diet in conditions of increasing shortage. The available reserves could only prove sufficient if the population came to terms with a new diet strongly biased towards vegetables. Publicity, however, focused not on changes on the dinner table but on the "Anbauschlacht" ("battle of cultivation"). There were several reasons for the weight placed on production in the internal politics surrounding the food plan. One was the public relations rule that "to eat less" or "to eat differently" were bad news, while "to produce more" was good news, which meshed very well with the doctrine of "economic national defence". Moreover, presenting a change in dietary habits as the main subject of state propaganda could easily be understood as an illegitimate encroachment upon the private sphere. Opinions, such as those expressed by the Basle professor of physiology S. Edlbacher, that "it is not the business of a free state to involve itself in these private affairs of the population",[53] were not uncontested, but a consensus seems to have prevailed that this kind of interference did not fit well into a state propaganda programme. Matters were quite different in the presentation of increased production. The idea of a nation under arms and victorious on its native soil in collective and heroic struggle against injustice was a message that could be communicated. Ultimately, it was not self-denial, change and adaptation in the kitchen and on the table but the production triumphs of agriculture that were made the keypoint of the food debate. In this narrative, women were replaced and eclipsed by man. The peasants, then fundamental to the Swiss self-image, became the heroes in the successful salvation of the nation.

THE EXPERIENCE OF HUNGER AND THE "VOLKSGEMEINSCHAFT"

Plan Wahlen and rationing system were synchronized in Switzerland from 1940; the extent of agricultural restructuring was directly linked to the expansion of administrative food distribution. The more comprehensive the rationing system, the more closely did the state find itself in direct contact with the population. In particular, through the continental European method of rationing monitoring system was established: the national apparatus which managed food shortages supplied the authorities with important data on the state of health, degree of satisfaction and dietary preferences of various sections of the population. To check the assumptions on diet and food made by their economic authorities, all countries carried out investigations and gathered statistics. Food policy also had an "inspection effect" on the development of wages. It may be stated in general that, both on the basis of an intensive public information programme and diversified secret-service activities and via this kind of information feedback, governments were far better informed of the state of many things than they were before or after the war.

Functioning in reverse, the rationing system acted as a conveyor belt for exhortations to stand firm and calls for discipline from the political leadership to the *Volksgemeinschaft* ("national community"). The introduction of rationing from above was matched by the attempt to create fresh feelings of responsibility and loyalty below, especially in those groups of the population liable to protest. Since social stability, political legitimacy and administrative efficiency were closely interrelated, the rationing system was subject to a self-fulfilling prophecy: constructive cooperation, which could be ensured only on the basis of sufficient trust in government, was in turn a principal condition for the functioning of the distribution system in such a way as to justify these advances of trust *post festum*. "Ensuring an adequate diet is thus an important factor in the internal front" was how the head of the rationing section summarized this insight.[54]

However, "adequacy" was a variable concept that depended on the standards of nutritional science and on the expectations and experiences of the population. "Since rationing began I'm always hungry": this remark, which was discussed in Switzerland by government nutritionists, shows that, among the population generally, the war was closely associated with hunger. That is why successful administrative measures to avoid hunger could themselves evoke hungry thoughts.[55] Far from being a purely physiological response to food shortages, the feeling of hunger was thus also culturally and politically determined. State bodies, conscious that the perception of shortage was institutionally mediated, generated confidence that the socially polarizing effects of hunger could be neutralized by prudent policies or even made to serve social integration. At the end of October 1941 a Zurich doctor, M. Boss, told the members of the FCWN: "Not only have you have been entrusted with maintaining the bodily health of our people, you also possess in the distribution of food an especially effective physiological instrument for maintaining and strengthening or for destroying our national community. If food rationing is successfully implemented with strict fairness and if our people is conscious of firm leadership that can overcome all the special egoims of parties and groupings and does not shy away from unpleasantnesses, then you will certainly be able to go extraordinarily far with material limitation of the food supply, while the people, conscious to a man of the trust of its government, will stand the more united behind you".[56]

The confidence of the people could be utilized above all as a resource for bureaucratic problem solving if the criteria for food distribution matched the generally accepted idea of "fair distribution". The essence of this approach was to use calories as glue to foster social cohesion.[57] If administrative measures could successfully be combined with the morality of the "community", it was also easy to stigmatize criticism of the state as unsocial and even as a threat to its existence. This culturally constructed feeling of social unity was linked to the biologization of politics that traced its origins back to the second half of the 19th century in the tradition of "integral nationalism" and "racial hygiene". In light of the central category of a "healthy people's body", the "degeneration of the people" was interpreted as a form of "social disease".[58] Within this conceptual framework internal opposition and everyday cultural resistance could be reinterpreted as socially pathological phenomena; conversely, it became the task of the "healthy elements" to be aware of the higher interests of society. This analogy promoted the application of pseudobiological models to food policy: under the system of graded rationing "organs" bearing a heavy load were privileged by special rations[59] in order to maintain the full efficiency of the "people's body".[60]

The symbolic representation of the "people" as a united body struggling for its own survival interacted closely with the practical administration of rationing. For this reason "food rationing was introduced in most countries of Europe as an early wartime measure before specific scarcities had had time to develop".[61] Pre-emptive rationing was more than the timely introduction of new shopping and dietary patterns. From the outbreak of war most countries directed political and ideological efforts to identifying the "national interest" with an "ideal of fairness" in order to ensure the governability of the country under difficult conditions. By upgrading food shortage to the status of an integrative principle in the political discourse, it appeared possible to control the feared potential of such a deficit to polarize society and to reverse its social significance: instead of increasing structural disparities and social conflict, shortage would now produce a feeling of national solidarity based on the expectation of a fair distribution of burdens. This campaign was rhetorically orchestrated in the "national community" by the unsparing denunciation of internal enemies. Black-marketeers were described as "a small section of reckless egoists" and there was talk of "the desires of selfish outsiders". The reference to "unsocial individuals (…) who, merely to satisfy their needs for taste, regularly resort to the black market"[62] shows that the criticism referred not only to economic privilege but also to deviant behaviour going far beyond the black market.

WAR AS A "MASS EXPERIMENT IN NUTRITION"

Changes in the agricultural structure and food rationing were two complementary strategies for avoiding malnutrition; both forced a dietary change. In complex problems of this type nutritional science acquired decisive importance. In particular, the more comprehensive "German-type" rationing, which was adopted by Switzerland from 1942, would not have been possible without a scientific basis, since the stricter the dietary standards imposed by the state, the more important nutritional norms, the distribution units calculated from them and a wealth of information on food supply and requirements became. With the establishment in October 1940 of the FCWN, the authorities mobilized the available fund of nutritional knowledge.[63] Scientists, specialists and experts from various institutes, all of whom were medical doctors, were brought together in a "brain trust" and integrated into the economic strategy of the war.

The FCWN was, indeed, confronted by a difficult problem. The Commission repeatedly pointed to the theoretical and practical difficulties that the introduction of a system of graded rationing produced. At the end of 1942 it stated: "On the basis of the enormous amount of scientific work carried out over decades on the relationship between energy requirements and work, the expert today has no difficulty in calculating quite accurately the energy requirement of each individual. But in rationing, which affects the entire population, it is impossible to create a differentiated system that ensures that each person receives precisely the amount of nutrition he needs".[64] The methods of the experts had, therefore, to be perfected, in particular in dealing with large amounts of data and methods of statistics. The difference between the nutritional value of dishes and human nutritional requirements was important here: determination of needs (demand of the body) had to be harmonized with calculations of nutritional value (supply to the body). A method comparing and relating the total supply of food and the aggregated requirement of the population for nutritious substances through nutritional budgeting had also to be developed. At the same time the experts were given the additional, no less important, role of lending scientific legitimacy to the criteria underpinning the grading of food supplies: that is, to provide an aura of incontestability.

The FCWN was thus in a double-bind situation. It had to present a united face to the outside world and by its united and competent approach to build up a basis of trust among the public. According to the minutes of the first session of the commission "the public should be informed (...) that a commission for wartime nutritional problems exists that examines all important questions that may affect the people".[65] Behind closed doors, however, discussions had to be as open and critical as possible because of innumerable uncertainties and problems and in view of the empirically based guidelines. How little agreement there was at first over basic values was shown in particular by the continued revision of the minimum energy requirement, which was first defined as 3,100 calories per head per day, then reduced to 2,400 calories and finally reduced still further.[66]

The successful bridging of the gap between consensus and controversy depended on a close interrelationship between the administration and science. The conditions of war offered a unique opportunity for testing nutritional assumptions and rapidly increasing the stock of knowledge.

Alfred Fleisch characterized food rationing quite frankly as a (in his view successful) "nutritional experiment". He published the most important scientific and political findings of the Commission in 1947 in a report on "Nutritional problems in times of shortage". In the introduction to this study, which contains a wealth of material and facts, the author asks whether it had previously been possible to conduct a scientific, long-term study, carrying with it significant risks, of minimum nutritional standards on 1,000 test subjects; his conclusion was negative. Such a "large-scale nutritional experiment" would be "highly instructive (...) however it is too drastic and prolonged to enable any scientist—*experimenti causa*—to carry it out". But the years after 1939 had forced this experiment "on our country (...) just as nutritionists would have organized it, with the sole difference that owing to wartime economic necessity not 1,000 subjects but an entire people of 4.3 million were subjected to this regime".[67] Switzerland could, therefore, be of international interest since its nutritional level "lay between the luxurious diet of the Anglo-Saxons and the hunger of the occupied European countries and because it declined slowly to the minimum and below". A perfect study arrangement! As a country spared by war, Switzerland was able "to manage (diet) according to scientific nutritional principles and, as a correlate of calculations of the foodstuffs consumed, conduct thorough and continuing investigations of the state of health".[68]

The feasibility and effectiveness of the national "nutrition experiment" were thus a direct function of the food shortage caused by the war; "data on actual requirements" could only be ascertained on this scale because of "the compulsion of shortage".[69] The design of the "nutrition experiment" did not, therefore, exclude a certain paradox: the FCWN had to provide the fundamental information for a rationing system, to prevent malnutrition and acute hunger in the lower income groups and thus to struggle against that very need that was in return crucial to the successful conduct of the experiment. In early 1945 the position, by then critical, was rapidly reversed by favourable external circumstances: measurements made showed that "we (...) have gone below the minimum that is consistent over a period of time with the maintenance of normal efficiency. Fortunately, it was possible to terminate the 'experiment' at that point".[70] As shortages were overcome the experimental design also disappeared and evaluation of the results began.

During the "nutrition experiment" the FCWN accumulated enormous amounts of data on dietary composition, public health and efficiency. The knowledge thus gained was useful in designing the rationing system, which served as an instrument of cultural rationalization in everyday life: that is, a method of introducing modern ideas of "rational diet" to broad sections of the population. Rationing was to reduce the tension that had been increasing since the discovery of vitamins between "taste value" and "nutritional value",[71] bring tradition up to date and rationalize mentalities. However, the scientific observation of diet initially widened the gap between experts and population. In 1943 the nutritionist Albert Jung noted: "The mass of the people is little concerned with the scientifically best diet. They want to fill their stomachs and to eat what tastes good".[72] He expressed the unease that overtook the specialists at precisely the moment when scientific standardization of diet and empirical objectivization of culinary culture could have been consolidated.

The introduction of scientific values directly affected everyday diet through the criteria both of distribution and of evaluation. In particular, the system of differentiated rationing made official the unequal right to food of individual family members. Unequal work conditions and personal differences meant that food requirements differed among individuals. This difference had long been culturally stereotyped, an informal inequality in the distribution of available resources of food within the family having been legitimized in connection with industrialization and paid factory work. Notions such as "heavy work", "the breadwinner" and "a strong man" were combined with the properties ascribed to individual foodstuffs. In particular, "the belief that meat gives strength"[73] made popular a dietary style that came under increasing criticism from science. But for the workers, the taking of snacks to the workplace was a subtle strategy to enforce above-average claims to food within the family: as Erika Rickli, the head of the Domestic Economy Group of the Federal Office for Wartime Nutrition stated in 1943,[74] "household expenditures are also placed under a very heavy burden by food taken to work, consisting for the most part of relatively expensive meat or cheese. The cheapest foods, such as potatoes or flour-based products, are not suited to being taken to the workplace". It was understandable, therefore, that the FCWN, which made preparations for graded rationing from the summer of 1941, proposed in the autumn of that year special cheese rations and, from early 1942, also special meat and fat or oil rations for those performing heavy physical work. At a time when food supplies had begun to decline, what had previously been a (mainly masculine) dietary privilege within the family circle was transformed into a special ration related to work. In this way, manual labour was compensated for by a dietary equivalent in conformity with the wartime economic doctrine of relating reward to performance, while at the same time the other members of the family were also assured of an adequate diet through these special rations.

However, the simple division of all gainfully employed persons in two categories (with/without additional rations for work) did not enable "the demands and above all the feeling of justice of Swiss people (to be) satisfied in the long run",[75] and a differentiation of distribution within the framework of the graded rationing system was imposed. Figure 3[76] shows the approach of the wartime scientific authorities to calorie requirements graded according to age, height, weight and—especially important—work. With respect to the last criterion four categories of beneficiary were distinguished: normal beneficiaries, medium-heavy workers, heavy workers and very heavy workers. By means of a register a "every known and currently practised profession in Switzerland"[77] (a total of 1,030), individual workers were assigned to one of the four categories and placed within the rationing hierarchy. This clear classification founded in nutritional science also prevented endless haggling over special rations for different kinds of work. The general data of the FCWN on the calorific basis of the calculated "nutritional requirement per head of the Swiss population" show that of the 4.2 million nutritional units needed, 2 million were assigned to the male and 1.7 million to the female population. Supplements for pregnant and nursing mothers accounted for 26,000 nutritional units (0.6 percent), whereas 495,000 units (12 percent) were provided for those performing manual labour.[78]

Application of scientific knowledge to diet also led to a proposal to change the established rhythm of meals, a central element in the temporal structure of everyday life and work. Since "filling food with a high protein content and fat (...) has been largely replaced by carbohydrate-rich food with a low satisfaction value", "feelings of hunger arise too soon, (which is) a general and characteristic consequence of the Swiss wartime diet".[79] Since appetite and hunger returned more rapidly, the proposal was made to speed up the sequence of meals. This was based on studies that defined work as a function of the respiratory ratio[80] and showed far better values when a fixed amount of food was distributed among five meals compared with the traditional three-meal cycle.[81] Snacks between meals, the importance of which in maximizing performance and overcoming "industrial fatigue" had been recognized for decades, therefore assumed greater importance in the wartime diet; Albert Jung stated "that efficiency can be improved by at least ten percent if, as well as breakfast, lunch and dinner, a morning and an afternoon snack are also included".[82]

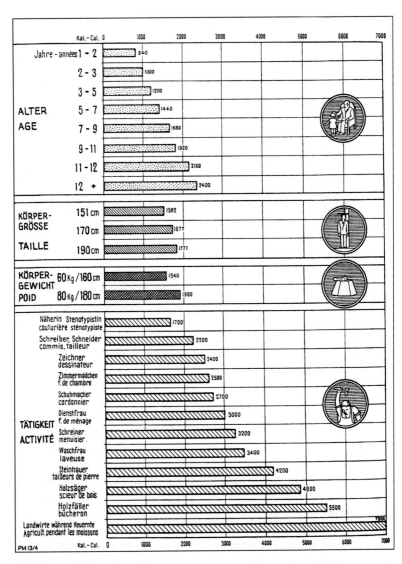

Figure 3   Der Kalorienbedarf nach Alter, Grösse, Gewicht und Tätigkeit (Nach Erhebung der Eidg. Kommission für Kriegsernährung).

THE RATIONING SYSTEM AND DIETARY TRADITIONS

The definition of dietary standards, which form the basis of a rationing system, and the calculation of the respiratory ratio are related to abstract categories. An essential precondition for the functioning of a complex rationing system is the translation of foodstuffs into exchangeable values that can be combined in almost any way to form a diet.[83] However, dietary traditions are by definition opposed to the principle of physiological equivalence. According to culinary culture, lunch is not 1,000 calories, 20 grams of protein, 25 grams of fat and 157 grams of carbohydrates,[84] nor does it consist of nutritional values costing 1 Swiss franc. Instead, it is made up of a selection of specific dishes: for example, a wartime menu might comprise leek soup, potatoes and pasta, kohlrabi, three slices of sausage and a glass of apple juice. To be acceptable, these, to some extent unusual, foods had to be prepared and presented in such a way that they could be assimilated to domestic dietary traditions and acquired conceptions of "good food".

The wartime economic administration repeatedly stated that the introduction of food rationing meant a break in dietary tradition: rationing "largely ignores previous consumption patterns—entitlements are matched as far as possible to recognized needs based on systematic principles".[85] The authorities were well aware of the limited possibilities of food substitution and stipulated that "the more varied consumption patterns and needs are", the more difficult rationing would be. In Switzerland the situation appeared complicated, the head of the rationing department declaring at the end of 1941 that it was "undoubtedly an unsuitable country in which to implement rationing (...) since we are not only at the crossroads of three languages and three cultures, but also at the crossroads of three dietary customs".[86] The problem was addressed by the use of interchangeable coupons and opportunities for exchange: instead of flour and milk the inhabitants of the cantons of Tessin, Uri, Graubünden and Wallis could receive maize, while the people of western Switzerland were entitled to larger quantities of cheese.[87] However, there are good reasons for believing that these regional differences should not be exaggerated and that in Switzerland at the end of the 1930s sociocultural homogenization (taking into account continuing income differences) was already further advanced than federalist and folkloric discussion of cultural diversity suggests. Indications of significant "Americanization" of Swiss consumption patterns are given by a comparison of household budgets in Switzerland and the USA that concluded that "the cost of living in the two countries before the outbreak of war revealed no great differences".[88]

During the war years a contradiction was observed between the levelling of the diet and the polarization of incomes. The aim of rationing did not correspond to the hierarchy of incomes; so far as the privileged position given to manual labour by special rations was concerned, it was directly opposed to it. The slogan "Rich or poor, the ration book makes everyone equal" was unquestionably designed mainly to strengthen national unity. With respect to the deregulation of culinary culture by the ration, however, it hit the mark. Figure 4 shows that rationing was directed at a balanced distribution. The position of the lowest income classes, earning less than 3,000 Francs was improved in every respect (except for bread supplies) by rationing. Since "the lowest income levels had a slightly deficient diet in terms of calorie content even in the prewar period",[89] a productivity-related system could hardly have had a different result.[90] However, the simultaneous decline in real incomes again placed the administratively-planned equalization of food distribution in question. To prevent entitlements being rendered a fiction by the loss of purchasing power, the authorities concerned themselves closely after autumn 1941 with the role of available money in the distribution system. It became clear that in wartime, too, there were families whose consumption "fell below the norm"[91] because of inadequate income. A partial solution was found in

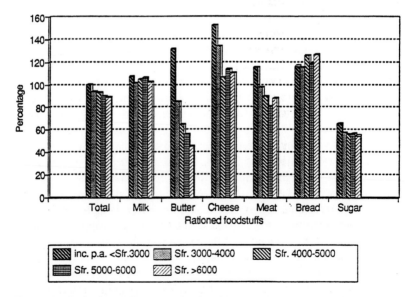

Figure 4   Rationing and consumption levelling calories per income-class. Rations in 1943 (3rd quarter) if pre-war level = 100.

August 1943 with the introduction of the "B-card". Poorer beneficiaries whose income was inadequate were thereby enabled to purchase a selection of cheaper foods that (according to the FCWN calculations) contained the same nutritional values as the "A-card"-norm at a 25 percent reduction in price. The authorities strove to prevent the "B-card" from being stigmatized as a "poor person's card". Since a new policy of cost-of-living bonus and of subsidies on the basic foods, milk and bread, prevented further real wage falls, the purchasing power of the "B-card" was guaranteed and it was a substantial success.

Subsequently, however, rationing coupons regularly remained unused. This was not the result of inadequate means but was mainly due to the resistance expected to changes in the diet. A study conducted at the end of 1942 by the wartime welfare authorities reached the interesting conclusion that failure to claim rations was significantly correlated with "non-requirement" but hardly at all with price levels. Even consumers from the lower social classes could not acquire a taste for millet, pulses, ersatz coffee, synthetic grape honey and egg powder.[92]

FOOD HABITS, THE KITCHEN AND WOMEN'S WORK

Despite such resistant behaviour patterns, the dietary changes brought about by the war had far-reaching effects on the physical state, health and efficiency of the people. The FCWN traced these developments through dietary studies, which produced some surprising findings. A study carried out between autumn 1941 and spring 1946 on the diet of about 700 people from various regions and social strata in Switzerland showed that weight loss was linked to the rate of change rather than to an inadequate supply of calories. In the autumn of 1942, H. R. Hess, the leader of this study, wrote: "It has been established that the declining trend observed since January/February 1942 with respect to bodyweight is continuing. The most recent studies in July (1942) give no evidence of a halt. The degree of loss is not alarming, but is striking".[93] In light of the fact that food supplies were still good at that time, this result produced confusion. "Most complaints about insufficient diet" were received in 1942. "This is odd, because bread and milk were not rationed then and malnutrition was certainly absent." Alfred Fleisch conjectured that "the complaints and the deterioration in the state of public nutrition are probably caused by necessary changes in dietary quality. Before the war our people were used to a highly refined diet containing large quantities of fat, meat and sugar. Rationing has excluded these concentrated foods and replaced them with a cellulose-rich diet, which has resulted in certain disturbances".[94] The fact that bodyweight minima after 1943 were above those of 1942 despite a further cut in the fat ration was consequently attributed to the population's "becoming accustomed to a high-roughage, low-fat wartime diet". "The organism has clearly adapted to the new diet. The metabolism of large quantities of potatoes, fruit and vegetables had improved, so that despite a constant calorie number the initial loss of bodyweight has been transformed into weight gain".[95] As bodyweight rose, so did the number of complaints received by the Wartime Office of Nutrition concerning dietary problems.[96]

However, it is evident that complaints were not directly due to problems in retraining the stomach-guts-canal and thus to difficulties of metabolic adaptation. Coping with "radical changes to the menu"[97] produced by a more vegetable-based diet was equally a matter of culinary preparation techniques and the "new cooking methods" necessitated by the declining fat ration. "Some old and beloved habits had to be abandoned and replaced by untried innovations," Erika Rickli noted in retrospect.[98] And Alfred Fleisch stated after the war: "It is evident that shortages in the food supply had a revolutionary impact on many kitchens, in particular those where the culinary skills of the housewife did not extend much beyond white coffee and bread, instant soup, pasta, sausages and cutlets".[99]

This clearly shows the close link between implementation of the agricultural "economization programme", redirecting production to give the highest possible yields, and adaptation of cooking techniques and food habits, i.e. the entire diet and culinary culture. Not only the availability, composition and importance of dishes, but equally their preparation, the circumstances of their consumption and the recycling of left-overs were affected. In turn, these various changes (with a series of further factors) had an ambivalent effect on gender-specific norms, in particular the social value ascribed to men's and women's work. Wage drops due to the war and the general attrition of real wages by wartime inflation were the main factors eroding the role of the man as breadwinner. Reduced material living standards, expressed in an increase in the proportion of relatively cheap vegetables in the diet, intensified the demands placed on complementary, "informal" work in the household and the family circle. "Housewives have to spend more time in the kitchen than before the war, since food products that take no time to prepare and are quickly cooked, and are also cheap, such as pasta, eggs, milk and bread, are all rationed." In particular, "consumption of vegetables and potatoes increases the burden placed on the housewife".[100] Without innovation and extra work in this sector, which remained "invisible" in terms of national income, that is, without a wealth of invention, the gift of improvisation, a talent for planning, skilful budgetary management and increased work by women in the household, these restrictions and changes would have been unmanageable. Amid wartime shortages a range of almost unnoticed, "updated" traditional cooking skills were revived and turned to culinary "making-do".

The economic authorities recognized the importance of family and house work. They cited US-studies which established "how important it is for the nutrition of a people that the housewife should understand something of cooking and the biological value of the various foods and should, accordingly, spend the available household budget sensibly".[101] Women's skills, in view of the high importance given by governments and military leaderships to an adequate, healthy and, at the same time, tasty diet, won them improved social status and prestige. Women became a central element in official discussions of the national defence and the "national community". The official conclusion of Switzerland's wartime economy, published in 1950, was that "(women's) adaptability, their specialist knowledge and their virtuosity in overcoming limitations by their domestic resourcefulness were largely responsible for the successful management of wartime shortages".[102]

This positive outcome was also ascribed to a systematic educational and information campaign. The household became an even more important focus for propaganda during the war and the housewife was bombarded with information by the state. However, these efforts were not combined to form a national self-assertion campaign comparable with the "battle to expand agriculture". The most important channels of public information were domestic science instructors (who were specially trained), cookery demonstrators, individual consultations, travelling exhibitions, series of talks, brochures, fact sheets, press communiqués, collections of recipes and a "talking menu", which could be consulted by telephone. "What should I do if fats and oil are in short supply?", "The many uses of dried egg powder", "Making flour from jacket potatoes", "Recipes that save meat", "We cook with kohlrabi leaves as well", "Soybeans", "My husband has to take food to work", "Uncooked salads of winter vegetables" and "Tips on using pork fat" were the titles of some of the brochures and fact sheets distributed by the Wartime Office of Nutrition to women at courses and talks.[103] The list also makes it clear that the "price" women paid for their improved position in propaganda and ideology was the strengthening of traditional conceptions of their role. The household was stylized as a genuinely female testing ground on the "internal front". "Housewife" and "mother" were amalgamated to form a compact national stereotype. The identification of "woman-housework-cooking", strengthened by the rationing system and dietary propaganda, retained its force long after the war and began to weaken only during a sustained phase of economic growth. The fact that in Switzerland women were deprived of voting rights on a national level until 1971 was the result in part of this wartime conception of their role.

The changes that affected the quantity, quality and composition of foodstuffs, their preparation and patterns of their consumption placed dietary traditions in question, but should not simply be equated with the transformation of the latter. The war was a transitory crisis that, for a while, compelled people to tighten their belts. However, such "involuntary (...) dietary changes",[104] as a study of nutrition in industry by the International Labour Office termed them, are not the same as a long-term change in dietary traditions: the incalculable effects of the war on everyday life increased willingness to accept measures that in "normal times" would have encountered resistance. Nutritional experts therefore tried to harness short-term measures to their long-term goals. The deficit produced by the war served as a catalyst for a prospective "reshaping" of the diet in harmony with the goals of public health and commerce. But various trends conflicted with the willingness to adapt: despite the demands of the war people were still reluctant in some ways to change. Rangers and Hobsbawm's hypothesis of a compensatory "invention of traditions" is based on the assumption that social collectives would react to abrupt changes by clinging to their customs with especial stubbornness. It is at such times that the "silent routines" of everyday culture (in this case, that of eating and drinking) are transformed into conscious traditions and identity-establishing rituals.[105]

The perception of these culinary traditions was ambivalent. For the social elite, which had acquired new areas of responsibility in health and social policy since the 19th century, it seems to be a matter of irrational mores and practices. In a 1945 report Henri Michel, a rationalization expert at the Institute of Business Management of the Federal Technical University in Zurich, commented on the possibility of rationalizing the household: "Man is a creature of habit. There are good and bad habits; the latter are most numerous and also most tenacious. They are the product of bad models, the environment, relationships, one's own predispositions and lack of self-discipline. They dig a rut, like a wheel on a road that is too soft; the longer and deeper the rut, the more difficult it is to escape. Habits become second nature. One no longer acts consciously but mechanically, unthinkingly".[106] This thesis of persistence, which saw tenacious adherence to inherited conceptions as the main problem, was in direct opposition to the view that public health could be maintained only by the retention of intact dietary traditions. From this point of view it was change that brought ignorance, loss of direction and general deterioration. In particular, the loss of "instinct" was lamented in housewives and cooks, as well as their susceptibility to advertising. In 1947 Alfred Fleisch spoke of "instinct that had become rudimentary" and stated: "In people today the original instinct to choose a balanced and nourishing diet is at least greatly enfeebled by the development of civilization. Modern technology makes it possible to refine natural foods and break them down into their individual components so that only those elements that particularly appeal to the taste organs remain as food. However, these are often not sufficient to meet the biological requirements of the organism".[107]

Both these conclusions presented a challenge to science and politics and were linked to demands for reform. Scientifically-based advice seemed a suitable substitute for lost "instinct", counterbalancing undesirable changes. "All nutritionists confirm that the instinct of people today is no longer sufficient to achieve a sensible choice of diet," Alfred Fleisch observed, concluding the observation quoted above.[108] In the confrontation between "habit" and "thought", a high value was generally attached to scientific information, which should strengthen the willingness to accept beneficial changes. "Rooted habits can be retained only in the absence of thought. As soon as thought commences, bad habits are recognized and the desire is awakened to overcome them. Every normal, educated person inclines towards progress. Where this desire is absent, there is a lack, first and foremost, of education":[109] thus the optimistic credo of Henri Michel. In the same spirit Albert Jung wrote: "We all know the influence that propaganda can have on diet. Propaganda is a form of instruction and the findings of dietary research can be introduced into everyday practice only by untiring instructional efforts".[110]

THE WARTIME DIET AND THE CONSUMER SOCIETY

Despite awareness by nutritionists of these problems, the changes in diet brought about by the war generally received a positive assessment, an increased content of micronutrients and a reduced proportion of fat having previously been regarded as beneficial. The transition to a vegetable-based diet, which was at the heart of the Swiss dietary plan, was seen as both an agropolitical economization programme and a public health programme. At the last meeting of the FCWN Alfred Fleisch summed up the Swiss national diet as "improved compared with the prewar period thanks to the cooperation of science". An optimum diet could now be proposed, but "nutritionists in all countries" would be compelled to conclude that "the customary diet of all 'advanced' countries is far removed from this optimum and therefore fails to produce the standard of public health that would be possible given a suitable diet. During the war our diet could, at least partly, be managed according to the requirements of science for a suitable diet".[111]

In the view of nutritional science, the Second World War marked the culmination of a long period of development during which the captains of industry became aware of the central importance of the human factor in economic growth. In the period of shortage of the Second World War a programme was carried out, achievement of which had been striven for since the end of the 19th century (with very limited success): nutritional science, industrial labour and the national diet were brought together under the banner of "total war" in a national project of self-assertion and modernization guaranteeing public health, military strength and labour productivity while at the same time making possible promising innovations. Yet the war years simultaneously marked a change of paradigms. In practice rationing, with its grading criteria, was still largely determined by the paradigm of the "human motor":[112] work means energy transformation and therefore demands a sufficient intake of nutriment in the form of carbohydrates, proteins, fats and—crucially—calories. This concept, described by Anson Rabinbach as "social Helmholtzianism" and "muscular thermodynamics", became increasingly less plausible as the value placed on the qualitative aspects of diet increased and bodily work and physical strength lost their former importance.[113] The increasing interest in micronutrients that resulted in sophisticated calculations by the wartime authorities of the vitamin, mineral and trace element content of foodstuffs was already guided by another concept of work and health, in which quality had superseded quantity.

The sobering insight soon spread that, for the population, the war had been an exceptional period. The belief that the limitations could be reversed and the desire to return to "normalcy" were still alive. The view expressed in 1950 in the final report on the wartime economy that "the important shifts that have taken place in consumption patterns are probably for the most part transitory in nature"[114] was only confirmed in succeeding decades. There was obviously a striking contradiction between the new nutritional models and the highly varied, fat- and meat-centred consumption pattern of the 1950s and 1960s. The faith in the ability of knowledge to alter consciousness that achieved a late flowering in the early 1940s largely evaporated. The changes forced by the war resulted less in a healthier diet than in a much greater willingness to accept culinary changes and the "delocalization" of food production and distribution.[115] This was in turn a precondition for the far-reaching changes in diet associated with industrialization and Americanization that set in after 1950. In this sense, therefore, the dietary policy of the Second World War had an unintended but important modernizing effect.

NOTES

1. Schweizerisches Bundesarchiv Bern (SBA), 7389/2, No. 10, File "Wartime nutrition and nutritional science".
2. Alfred Fleisch (1947) *Ernährungsprobleme in Mangelzeiten. Die schweizerische Kriegsernährung 1939–1946*, Basel, p. 287.
3. Alan S. Milward (1977) *Der Zweite Weltkrieg*, München, p. 254. For Germany, see Gunther J. Trittel (1990) *Hunger und Politik. Die Ernährungskrise in der Bizone* (1945–49), Frankfurt a.M./New York.
4. Milward, p. 251. The fact that during the war years (in significant contrast to the economic crisis of the 1930s) food supplies were generally inadequate turned the highly productive agriculture of the USA into an Allied strategic factor that continued to be an important political lever in the implementation of US interests worldwide after the war had ended.
5. Geneva, 1946.
6. Ibid., p. 53. See also *Rationnement alimentaire et revitaillement 1943–1944* (1944), ed. Société des Nations, Geneva, p. 57.
7. Josef Rosen (1947) "Die Entwicklung der Kriegsernährung in sieben Europäischen Ländern 1939–1944. Der Verbrauch an Nährstoffen und Vitaminen". In: *Schweizerische Medizinische Wochenschrift*, 31; Fleisch (1947) p. 318ff.
8. *Food, Famine and Relief* (1946) p. 9.
9. Eidgenössisches Volkswirtschaftdepartement (1950) *Die schweizerische Kriegswirtschaft*, Bern, p. 444.
10. Fleisch (1947) p. 274.
11. Ibid.
12. *Wartime Rationing and Consumption* (1942) Ed. League of Nations, Geneva, pp. 14–15; *Rationnement alimentaire* ... (1944) Ed. Société des Nations, Geneva, p. 8.
13. Milward (1977) p. 296.
14. Fleisch (1947) p. 275.
15. Ibid., p. 276ff.
16. Arthur Marwick (1974) *War and Social Change in the Twentieth Century*, London, pp. 223–224.
17. See Alf Lüdtke (1987) "Ihr könnt nun wissen, wie die Glocken eigentlich leuten sollen." Brotration und Arbeiter-(Über)Leben im Sommer 1919—ein Beispiel aus Bochum. In: *Geschichtswerkstatt*, 12, pp. 27–33.
18. For the mechanics of rationing, see *Wartime Rationing* ... (1942).
19. *Food, Famine and Relief* (1946) pp. 1–3.
20. *Rationnement alimentaire* ... (1944) p. 9.
21. Ibid., p. 2.
22. Milward (1977) p. 297.
23. Exposé von Alfred Fleisch (Arbeitsausschuß für kriegswirtschaftliche Ernährungsfragen), 18 November 1940, p. 1; SBA E 7390 (F) No. 31.
24. *Wartime rationing* ... (1942) p. 43.
25. *Die schweizerische Kriegswirtschaft* (1950) p. 426.

26. Arnold Muggli (1943) "Die rationierungstechnischen Grundlagen". In: *Ernährung und Leistungsfähigkeit. Schriften des Zentral-Verbandes schweiz. Arbeitgeber-Organisationen*, p. 30.

27. Albert Zeller, Die Ernährung in der Kriegszeit. Referat Zürich, 23 October 1943, SBA 7389/2, No. 10.

28. Ernst Feisst (1945) p. 31.

29. Jung, Über die Berechnung des Nahrungsbedarfs und die Beurteilung der Ernährungslage, Manus, SBA 7389/2, No. 10.

30. See the title of the book published in 1947 by Alfred Fleisch (Footnote 2).

31. EKKE minutes, 26 September 1946, p. 13; SBA E 7390 (F), No. 36, File 867140 p. 41.

32. Ernst Feisst, 1942/2, p. 26.

33. Alluding to the socio-psychological impetus of "managed hunger", the speaker argued on the basis of the relatively good food supply that there was a possible threat of a "peace psychosis". SBA 7389/1, No. 44, Dossier 0422a, report to a conference of the KZK.

34. *Food, Famine and Relief* (1946) p. 44.

35. Although "in many cases" the "ratio of animal consumption (is) fairly high"; in these countries there was a general shift from meat to the consumption of milk and milk products. Ibid., p. 43.

36. Ibid., p. 41.

37. Ibid., p. 41. The study emphasizes that "this does not mean that satisfactory diets could not be constructed according to a different ratio", but that "according to all indications free consumer choice seems to lead to adequate diets on or about this level".

38. Wilhelm Abel (1981) *Stufen der Ernährung*, Göttingen.

39. *Food, Famine and Relief* (1946) p. 42.

40. Abel (1981).

41. Ultimately such economic change was a prerequisite for non-inflationary financing of the war and the coordination of resource allocation with macroeconomic income distribution. The level of the reserves that could be mobilized for this "food buffer" was thus also dependent on the level of indigenous food supplies; countries with a high proportion of imports had correspondingly less room for manoeuvre.

42. *Die schweizerische Kriegswirtschaft* (1950) p. 158.

43. Fleisch (1947) p. 39.

44. Fleisch (1947) p. 34.

45. See: Peter Maurer (1985), Anbauschlacht. Landwirtschaftspolitik, Plan Wahlen, Anbauwerk 1937–1945, Zürich.

46. Fleisch (1947) p. 42.

47. Ibid., p. 47.

48. Ibid., Table 15, p. 58. See also SBA 7389/1, No. 44, Dossier 0421: Table. Empirical studies have shown, however, that Switzerland's net level of self-supply could have been increased by this programme. According to J. Rosen's calculations the internal contribution of Swiss agricultural production to total calorie demand in 1934/36 was 50.8 percent. The "calculated internal proportion", which relates national production to actual gross consumption, rose to 1944 by more than 30 percent to 82.1 percent. However, if the "real internal proportion", based on the greatly reduced net total calorie consumption, was calculated, the increase was 59 percent (see J. Rosen, "The internal share of Swiss food supply in the war according to nutritional value", in: SZVSt 1946, pp. 151–168). If decapitalization of the land (by running down fertilizer reserves), modernization (mechanization), which is largely import-dependent, and investment for the future (land improvements) are included in the calculation, the increase in autarky was negligible.

49. Fleisch (1947) p. 35.

50. FCWN minutes 5.12.1945, p. 31: response by A. Jung to the "physiological minimum for existence" proposed by the Incomes Survey Commission. SBA E 7390 (F) No. 36 and Fleisch (1947) p. 49.

51. Fleisch (1947) p. 53.

52. Ibid., p. 323.
53. Staatsarchiv Basel-Stadt, report on the plan for a Swiss institute of nutrition, 15 June 1942, p. 1.
54. Arnold Muggli (1943) p. 30.
55. W. R. Hess, director of the Institute of Physiology of the University of Zurich, at the EKKE session of 26 September 1946; EKKE minutes 26 September 1946, SBA E 7390 (F), No. 36, File 86714041.
56. "Nahrungsmittelrationierung und Volkspsychologie". Report to the EKKE, 31.10.1941, SBA 7389/2, No. 10, p. 5.
57. See Alf Lüdtke, "Hunger in der großen Depression. Hungererfahrungen und Hungerpolitik am Ende der Weimarer Republik", in *Archiv für Sozialgeschichte* 27 (1987) pp. 145–176.
58. Stefan Kühl, Die Internationale der Rassisten. Aufstieg und Niedergang der internationalen Bewegung für Eugenik und Rassenhygiene im zwanzigsten Jahrhundert, Frankfurt a.M./New York 1997; Paul Weindling, Health, Race and German Politics Between National Unification and Nazism, 1870–1945, Cambridge et al. 1989; Peter Weingart/Jürgen Kroll/Kurt Bayertz, Rasse, Blut und Gene. Geschichte der Eugenik und der Rassenhygiene in Deutschland, Frankfurt a.M. 1988.
59 In Germany, direct state involvement in nutrition also made it possible in principle to translate racist ideologies into official and informal priorities and to starve minorities to death by selective discrimination. See Rolf-Dieter Müller, "Die Vernichtung", in: Wolfgang Michalka (ed.), Der Zweite Weltkrieg, Munich/Zurich 1989, pp. 240–248. According to the criteria of racial ideology, a "second nutritional pyramid" was distinguished beneath the 'community'" in which a "policy of annihilation through hunger" was conducted (246); this brutal categorization was not present in Switzerland, although there, too, a large number of work camps existed in which living conditions were relatively bad. Categorization in Switzerland was primarily territorial: the Federal Council and the Swiss Army made use of the slogan "the boat is full" and played on fears of hunger and of being swamped by foreigners to barricade Switzerland against refugees and "protect" the "national community" from socio-cultural "undermining".
60. Fleisch (1947) p. 215.
61. *Food, Famine and Relief,* League of Nations, Geneva (1946) p. 1.
62. Fleisch (1947) pp. 275–277.
63. See ibid., p. 21ff.
64. Communication of the EKKE, 15 December 1942, SBA E 7390 (F) No. 36, p. 2.
65. EKKE minutes, 16 December 1940, p. 19; SBA E 7390 (F) No. 36.
66. *Die schweizerische Kriegswirtschaft ...,* p. 163.
67. Fleisch (1947) pp. 17–18.
68. Ibid., p. 18.
69. Alfred Fleisch, "Lohn, Ernährung, Leistung", in: *Schweizerische Zeitschrift für Volkswirtschaft und Statistik (SZVS),* 1947, p. 412, 420.
70. Ibid.
71. *Die schweizerische Kriegswirtschaft* (1950) p. 181.
72. Jung (1943) p. 7.
73. Ibid., p. 20.
74. Erika Rickli (1943) "Betriebsfürsorge im Dienste der Arbeiterernährung", in: *Ernährung und Leistungsfähigkeit. Schriften des Zentralverbandes schweiz. Arbeitgeber-Organisationen,* Zürich, p. 45; the Domestic Economy Group was established in autumn 1942.
75. Jung (1943) p. 33.
76. *Die schweizerische Kriegswirtschaft* (1950) p. 434.
77. Jung (1943) p. 34.
78. Calculations by Albert Jung in: Fleisch (1947) p. 321.
79. Fleisch (1947) p. 353.

80. The respiratory ratio expresses the relationship of carbonic acid output and oxygen intake. In cases of pure carbohydrate metabolism both quantities correspond, giving a respiratory ratio $(RR) = 1$. A fat-rich diet raises oxygen consumption, yielding a RR of about 0.7. In terms of maximum efficiency of oxygen consumption a higher value is better than a lower. In activities (such as industrial work) that are not limited by the input of oxygen and continue for prolonged periods, the absolute level of the RR is less important than the consumption of a balanced combination of carbohydrates, fats, proteins, vitamins, minerals and trace elements. See Atzler/Gunther Lehmann, *Anatomie und Physiologie der Arbeit* (1930) Halle a.S., p. 259ff.

81. For these calculations see Howard W. Haggard/Leon A. Greenberg, *Diet and Physical Efficiency* (1935) New Haven.

82. Jung (1943) p. 26.

83. Milward (1977) p. 255.

84. For calculation factors, see Atzler/Lehmann (1930) p. 250.

85. *Die schweizerische Kriegswirtschaft* (1950) p. 422.

86. Report by A. Muggli on 15.12.1941, SBA 7389/2, No. 11, p. 1.

87. *Die schweizerische Kriegswirtschaft* (1950) p. 442.

88. Walter Kull, "Erhebungen über Haushaltsrechnungen in den Vereinigten Staaten und der Schweiz", in: SZVS 1945, p. 73.

89. Fleisch (1947) p. 302.

90. For the inadequate diet of poorly paid sections of the population in the 1930s, see *L'alimentation des travailleurs et la politique sociale* (1936) Bureau Internationale du Travail, Geneva, p. 181.

91. Fleisch (1947) p. 302.

92. For the results, see Fleisch (1947) p. 410.

93. EKKE minutes, 4 September 1942, p. 16; SBA E 7390 (F), No. 36.

94. EKKE minutes, 24 September 1946, p. 10; SBA E 7390 (F), No. 36.

95. Fleisch (1947) pp. 439–440.

96. Ibid., p. 440.

97. *Die schweizerische Kriegswirtschaft* (1950) p. 178 (author: Erika Rickli).

98. Ibid.

99. Fleisch (1947) p. 425.

100. Erika Rickli (1943) p. 47f.

101. Fleisch (1947) p. 480.

102. *Die schweizerische Kriegswirtschaft* (1950) p. 165.

103. Fleisch (1947) p. 422ff.

104. *Nutrition in Industry* (1946) International Labour Office, Montreal, p. 75.

105. Eric Hobsbawm and Terence Ranger (eds.) (1983) *The Invention of Tradition*, Cambridge.

106. Henri Michel, Bericht über eine Expertise betr. Arbeitsmethoden beim Schweizerischen Verband Volksdienst, 16 October 1945, pp. 12–13; Archiv SVV/Zurich.

107. Fleisch (1947) p. 477.

108. Ibid.

109. Michel (1945) p. 13.

110. Albert Jung (1943) *Ernährung und Leistungsfähigkeit*, Zurich, p. 7.

111. EKKE minutes, 24 September 1946, p. 14; SBA E 7390 (F), No. 36.

112. Anson Rabinbach (1992) *The Human Motor. Energy, Fatigue and the Origins of Modernity*, Berkeley/Los Angeles.

113. Ibid., p. 120ff.

114. *Die schweizerische Kriegswirtschaft* (1950) p. 457.

115. See Gretel Pelto/Perrti Pelto (1983) "Diet and delocalization: dietary changes since 1750", in: *Journal of Interdisciplinary History* 14, pp. 507–528.

10. PLURALITY OF TASTE: FOOD AND CONSUMPTION IN WEST GERMANY DURING THE 1950s

Michael Wildt

"Regarding the desires that should be fulfilled after the war, first of all people want to thoroughly enjoy all the wished-for things they cannot buy nowadays. One wants to smoke a lot, another dreams of butter and fat cheese, women long for coffee, etc."

In this opinion poll which the GfK, the "Gesellschaft für Konsumforschung" (Institute for Consumer Research), took in Germany during 1941, the third year of World War II, food did not hold first place among the wishes people would have after the war. They desired more clothing, shoes, china, and not necessarily more to eat. But if they talked about food, they would spontaneously say:

"I long for something special to eat."—"Sometimes it would be enough," one of the correspondents wrote, "to have a really satisfying meal with rare, delicious things like cream-puffs or something like that—just once. Writing this I can't keep my mouth from watering."[1]

The remembrance of all the former delicacies as expresses here reminds us, that the consumer experience in postwar Germany cannot be separated from the time prior to the war. On the contrary, for a long time following the Second World War people used their memories of the 1930s to measure their consumption in postwar Germany. In the 1950s the "consumer society" had not yet fully developed. However, the necessary practices that supported the "consumer society" can be observed as existing in embryo during this period.

In the following I plan to focus on changes in the practice of consumption in postwar Germany. In the years following the war people who had to rigidly economize their household budgets were by the end of the 1950s able to afford new articles; however, this also involved learning a lot of new skills. Consequently in regarding the development of consumption during the postwar years it is necessary to look at the multifaceted changes in everyday practice. Consumption, in this sense, does not only mean the quantifiable consumption of food or the possession of goods but moreover the "production" of consumption—consumption widely understood as "sensuous human activity, practice" (Karl Marx, Thesen ad Feuerbach), as human agency. Analyzing the practice of consumption therefore does not only mean chronicling the quantitative consumption patterns of working-class families but also illuminating the buying of food, the cooking, the technical changes in the cuisine, and the embedded "production" of cultural meanings, the fabrication of signs and meanings connected with food and consumption.

To begin I will describe the consumer experiences of pre-1950s Germany focusing especially on the war and the late 1940s up to the currency reform in 1948 which marked a deep caesura, both in the history of experience and in the history of consumption in West Germany. Secondly I plan to quantitatively analyze the development of consumption based on empirical household budgets of working-class families kept from 1949 until 1963. The third section deals with the changes in cooking and the appearance of technical equipment in the kitchen, following which I will focus on the new languages which became visible in the rhetoric of the recipes published by the customer magazine "Die kluge Hausfrau" (The Clever Housewife). The new semiotic codes of consumption developed during the 1950s enabled a fundamental change in the selling and buying of food, namely the introduction of "self service". Instead of the personal relations between merchant and customer that had dominated this area and mediated the buying and selling of articles now the goods spoke directly to the customers from the supermarket shelf where they struggled with their "rivals" for space and attention. This fundamental shift as semiotic dimension of consumption symbolizes the new role that consumers had to learn in West Germany during the 1950s. These new practices of consumption in their turn created a new "consumer subject" who perhaps did not became aware of itself at the end of the 1950s, but who gained a powerful social role during the next decades.

SCARCITY, RATIONING AND THE BLACK MARKET: CONSUMERS' EXPERIENCES PRIOR TO THE 1950s

Consumption in West Germany after World War II cannot be fully understood without considering the period prior to the war and the rationing of food between 1939 and 1948. The experience of consumption in Germany following World War I was dominated to a large extent by scarcity and even hunger in everyday life. The insufficient food supply (older people in Germany remember well the so-called "Steckrübenwinter" (turnip winter) of 1916, when turnips were almost the only food available) did not improve in 1919 with the end of the war, but persisted into the early 1920s.[2] 1923, the year of the enormous inflation, forced many households, especially those of workers, to make every effort to feed their families. The Great Depression meant unemployment and distress once more. The brief periods of economic stability between 1924 and 1929 and in the mid 1930s never lasted long enough for people to really lose the feeling of uncertainty and discontinuity.[3]

In September 1939 food was rationed, but for the first months this date did not signify a definitive turning point. The practice of the struggle to survive, the laborious house keeping, the economizing with a small budget were so habitual that the rationing of food did not necessarily mean sudden deprivation. In the years before the war people had been forced to live with scarcity, and now everyone simply tried it again.[4] During the first years of military victories the Nazi regime was able to exploit the occupied countries and so to satisfy the needs of their own "Aryan" people. But once the war had reached the turning point, following the German defeat at Stalingrad in 1943, the conditions of food supply worsened. At the end of the war the rationing system was shattered. The former Reich had been divided into four occupation zones which did not have trade relations with each other. Seeds and artificial fertilizer needed urgently by the farmers were beyond their means. Germans were entirely reliant on imports of wheat from Canada and the United States. The official daily rations were small, and on some days, especially during the winter months, intake declined to less than 1,000 calories per day.[5]

People could only survive if they were able to make use of every possible way to obtain food. Consequently alongside the governmental ration system a second economy grew up: the black market.[6] This illegal market existed everywhere: in the streets and squares, where people bought and sold goods, and in the factories, where most products were exchanged directly to obtain raw materials and to procure additional food for the workers. People who lived in towns travelled out into the country hoping to get some butter, bacon or potatoes in exchange for cigarettes, jewellery and household goods. Last, but not least, the charitable help of British, American or Canadian organizations like CARE provided an indispensable part of the food supply in West Germany during years directly following the war.

The gap between a governmental rationing system, which was unable to feed its people, and the black market economy, which was illegal but offered everything to everyone if they could pay, shaped the important experience that everybody had to rely on himself. This experience taught that a socialistic economy was unable to supply practically everything which was urgently needed, and that the market instead is a hard, but efficient alternative. According to Lutz Niethammer the postwar years were a "school of the market" for the West German people.[7]

As a consequence, the currency reform in June 1948 meant a deep caesura, both in the history of experience and in the history of consumption in West Germany. From one day to the next the shops offered all the goods which had been unobtainable for years before. In the public opinion surveys taken by the US authorities in their occupied zone people claimed that their greatest worries were focused on food, clothing and missing relatives. At the moment of the currency reform, however, all their worries focused on one thing: money.[8] Now that money had had its value restored, after the times of scarcity and hunger, "normality" should return to the households. After the years of the monotony of rations people could now afford long-missed titbits like butter, cream, coffee or white flour.

One of the women I interviewed, Mrs. O., born in 1928 and raised in a working-class neighbourhood in Hamburg, realized at once a long cherished wish:

"1948, after the currency reform, I was not married and worked at my father's office. The first money I got... Nearby the Lastropsweg in Eimsbüttel, there was a confectionary's shop. And there I had purchased a huge heap of biscuits. I remember well the cream-tarts, and we had gorged—awfully, but I loved it."[9]

Immediately after the currency reform the demand for rolls made of wheat meal grew so rapidly that the bakeries had difficulties producing enough bread of normal quality. In autumn 1948 the director of the Food Office of the British and American Occupation Zone, Hans Schlange-Schöningen, warned of the inevitable foreign impression that "the West Germans would have goods in plenty and live on the fat of the land." He urged the people not to eat now "the easter cake and the easter meat" of the next year. Finer qualities vegetables like cauliflower sold much faster than the everyday cabbage. Because of low demand the prices of fish and canned food crashed, whilst meat could be sold with a supplement of 50% to 100%.[10]

CHANGES IN THE FOOD CONSUMPTION OF WORKING-CLASS FAMILIES AFTER 1949

The following years were usually described by terms like "Wirtschafts-wunder" or a succession of consumption waves like the "Freßwelle" (food-wave) or the "Kleidungswelle" (clothing-wave) or the "Urlaubswelle" (travel-wave). Hans Peter Schwarz, among other sociologists and histori-ans, considered the 1950s in West Germany to be a "period of exciting modernization" par excellence,[11] and even for critics like Rolf Sieferle, West Germany displayed "the 'modern' structure in purest form".[12] According to Hans Jürgen Teuteberg there had been a "revolution in nour-ishment" between 1949 und 1965, which had caused the "last break-through to the actual mass prosperity".[13] However, all of these arguments remain locked into a perspective "from above",[14] and what I want to sharpen is the difference, which consumers experienced. Use of the term "Modernization of consumption", as stated by Teuteberg, cannot be under-stood aside from these everyday practices. Therefore, rather than examine society from above I intend to use a micrological examination on the specific development of mass consumption in everyday life.[15]

The development of private consumption in West Germany in the 1950s can be explored by analyzing the daily household budgets of working-class families, who kept records of their income and expenses in order to report to the Federal Statistic Board. From 1949 until now, about 200 working-class households noted their incomes, expenses und consumption every day in a simple, grey exercise book. These books had to be given to the regional Statistic Board. The regional Board then calculated the results and sent the data to the Federal Statistic Board in Wiesbaden. There the statisticians calculated the average consumption of a working house-hold composed of parents and two children, the so-called "4-Personen-Arbeitnehmerhaushalt".[16] I do not intend to stress the representativeness of the selection in what follows—although this type of household accounted for almost 15% of the West German population.[17]

The average income of these households increased from 343 DM monthly in 1950 to 975 DM in 1963 with the greatest increase coming in the early fifties. In general workers' incomes increased exceptionally in the 1950s in comparison to former periods. Supported by the economic boom of the reconstruction and especially by the Korean War, the average worker's income between 1950 and 1954 increased by 40%—a rate that was never again reached in the following years. After subtracting taxes and insurance, the amount of each household's disposable income rose from 305 DM in 1950 to 847 DM in 1963.

Among the total living costs, expenses for food still held the dominant position. In 1950 these households spent 133 DM each month for food, amounting to a proportion of 46%. By 1963 these expenses in absolute figures had risen to 193 DM, and they still made up the largest item in the family budget, accounting for 35% (absolute figures are based on constant prices of 1950 to avoid distortions depending on inflation). The families spent an increasing amount, both in absolute and in relative figures, on so-called "luxury articles" such as coffee, beer and cigarettes. In 1950 the expenditure on "luxury" items amounted to a proportion of 6%, in 1960 10%.

In 1963 these working-class families bought only half of the quantity of flour they had done at the beginning of the fifties. By contrast, the consumption of cakes and biscuits, canned food, honey, sweets and tea had doubled. Tropical fruit, ham and chocolate were eaten quantitatively four times more in 1963 than in 1950, and the consumption of poultry and coffee had also considerably increased. However the record for the highest increase was established by condensed milk: in 1950 the working-class households consumed 205 g a month, as compared to nearly 2,000 g in 1963.

Margarine still continued to be the dominant means of fat intake, however a turning point is discernable in 1956/57, when the consumption rates of margarine declined and those of butter increased. The West German trade company "Edeka", which represented nearly 20% of the total turnover made by the food retail business, analyzed this development in 1957:

> "There is a certain trend to be seen to buy quality food, and the consumers bought more and more butter. Simultaneously the demand for fine qualities of margarine grew in a similar way, whilst the lower qualities remained behind."[18]

The remarkable significance of butter even at a time, when scarcity had definitely ended, was shown by a opinion poll taken in autumn 1953. When asked, which article of food one wanted to eat more of, if the prices were not so high, 74% of the inquired workers (a level that stood 12 percentage points higher than the average!) answered that they would buy more butter.[19] The desire for "good butter" aimed not only at high nutrition value but also at "good taste". Butter was an unmistakable sign of a satisfying, tasteful and pretentious cuisine. In another poll of 1962 butter had been valued as the healthiest fat. It would be much more digestible than even diet margarine.[20]

Connected to the international agro-market and first of all to the European Common Market, West Germany became the most important European importer of fruit and vegetables. Especially fine qualities were imported from the Netherlands, Italy, Spain and other Mediterrean countries, while the domestic farmers concentrated in cultivating cabbages and other lower qualities of produce. The consumption of tomatoes increased at the highest rate of all vegetables consumed during the fifties: in 1950 the working-class households had only eaten 900 g tomatoes a month and in 1963 they consumed nearly 1,300 g. Because of the European Agromarket tomatoes could be sold and consumed all year, and their red color, fresh look and firmness made them perfectly suitable for food decorations, the aesthetic dimension of consumption. The West German "Margarine Union", a subsidiary company of Unilever, made commercials for its product "Sanella" with the slogan: "Modefarbe Tomatenrot auch für unseren Tisch!" ("Dress your table with a fashion color like tomato red"). Since 1958 there was an evident increase in the consumption of fruit, to a large extent of tropical fruit which increased by 20% reaching an amount of more than 5,000 g a month. Oranges and bananas, which had been available as a Christmas treat, were now available during the whole year and became part of the everyday diet.

In the early 1950s meat was not served every day. 1955 the famous "Institut für Demoskopie, Allensbach" explored that 70% of the West German people ate meat three times a week, but only 27% were accustomed to eat meat every day.[21] If you look more closely at the statistics of the working-class households a specific differentiation can be discerned. The consumption of beef increased by only a little but the consumption of pork rose by 41%. In 1963 a single working-class household of four persons consumed 1,476 g of beef and 1,552 g of pork per month. However, the consumption of poultry increased the most, increasing sevenfold between 1950 and 1963. Chicken could be kept frozen since the late fifties in new deep-freezers. In 1955 there were only 2,500 deep-freezers in West German shops, two years later the total increased to 10,000, and by 1964 there were more than 100,000.[22] Chicken accounted for 39% of the turnover made by the frozen food industry, followed by spinach and ice cream. The high demand for chicken could only be satisfied by imports from other European countries and the United States. It may be that besides rock'n roll, American chicken provided one of the lasting elements of the "Americanization" of West German popular culture.[23]

As mentioned above, the expenditure on coffee, tea, beer, liquors and tobacco amounted to a proportion of 6% by 1950, in 1960 10% of the working-class household budget. Among these expenses, preferences changed: In the early fifties households spent most of the money on tobacco, but from 1954 on, beer and liquor made up the largest proportion of the "luxury" items. Coffee remained in the 1950s as a Sunday drink. In 1950 the average coffee consumption per month was 91 g in contrast to 372 g coffee substitute like cichorium or grain coffee consumed. For the first time in 1955 the working-class households drank more coffee than coffee substitute of any sort, but it was not until 1960 that these families consumed more than 500 g coffee a month.

To sum up, the monthly budget of these working-class households obviously remained tight and frugal until the late 1950s. In opposition to commonplace characterizations of the period as "affluent society", these working-class families lived quite modestly, at least during the first half of the decade. In 1962 the trade union institute cautioned against terms such as "Wirtschaftswunder":

> "What was thought to be different consumption waves in West Germany such as the food-wave, or the clothing-wave, the household goods- or the travel-wave was nothing but the expression of a backlog of demand, which could be satisfied successively, in a society which had been deeply shattered and impoverished by the war."[24]

However, the end of the 1950s and the beginning of the 1960s present a distinct hiatus. For instance, from 1956 on the consumption of butter rose continuously, the consumption of poultry increased, and by the late 1950s there was a striking abundance of cold meat and ham in the working-class households. Their consumption of tropical fruit rose remarkably, and the everyday supply of fruit offered a variety that was unknown before— independent of regional and seasonal limitations. Ready-made articles such as canned food became more and more part of daily meals.

Summarizing, West German consumption in the 1950s consists of two different phases: during the first half of the decade, the working-class households tried to satisfy their basic needs, spending a large amount of their incomes on food and to replace things lost or destroyed during the war. By the late 1950s, as incomes rose, people were able to afford new articles. Of course these working-class families still had to economize and follow a budget, but they no longer exhibited a "taste for necessities" (Bourdieu) as was in case in the early postwar years. As Ernest Zahn put it: consumers no longer longed for "scarce goods but for desired ones" (in German this comes across as a play on the words "entbehrt" (missed) and "begehrt" (desired)).

THE TRANSFORMATION OF FOOD PREPARATION PRACTICES

Consumption consists not only of the quantifiable consumption of food but also includes "production." Food had to be supplied, prepared, cooked or fried, and last but not least served. "The inquiry of consumption makes sense only if cooking, eating and suffering hunger will be analyzed as a form of social practice."[25] Therefore I suggest widening the horizon of inquiry to include the cooking, the buying of food, and the "production" of cultural meanings, the fabrication of signs connected with food and consumption. For example, the quantitative consumption of potatoes certainly fell during this decade (as it did in the years since the turn of the century), but at the same time ready-made articles like dehydrated potato-dumblings or potato-pancakes took their place in everyday cuisine, and after the sixties the consumption of pommes frites and potato chips noticeably increased. Or to use another example, although the quantitative figures remained the same, the preparation of rice altered, because it was more and more served with warm meals thus replacing potatoes or cereals, as opposed to being eaten as rice pudding or sweet soup.

A third example: as mentioned above, the working-class households consumed less and less flour but bought more and more biscuits and cookies. Obviously these households did not bake cakes at home as they had done in the years before. This trend was confirmed by the leading West German producer of baking-powder. The marketing board of the Oetker Company stated, that its product "Backin" had experienced continuously declining sales during the 1950s. "The joy of home bakery trickled away", as the sales manager complained.[26] Indeed, the home bakery declined during the 1950s, but it did not vanish. What—presumably male—managers described as "joy" was hard work: one can easily understand that the housewives desired to abandon kneading dough and to prefer buying cakes at the bakery. But they did not give up all home bakery. When in 1950 putting "Tortenguß" (glaze) on the market the Oetker Company was surprised by the success of the new product. "Tortenguß", which was needed for baking fruit cakes, indicated the transformation: instead of old-fashioned stirring cake, the new fruit cakes were the hit of the 1950s. Fruit cakes could be prepared easily and fast, they had a fruity and fresh taste, which was valued as healthy and light. Fruit cakes also gave housewives the assurance that they did not need not to buy all of the family's food in the shops but were still skilled enough to bake on their own.

This opposition between the facilitation of work on the one hand and the competence of cooking on the other also determined the use of electric appliances. The kitchen appeared as the place furnished first with the new durable goods. At the beginning of the 1960s more than 10% of all four-member households in West Germany had an electric kitchen machine. The most sought-after item during the 1950s was the refrigerator. In an opinion poll taken in 1955 only 10% of all households owned a refrigerator, but nearly 50% dreamed of buying one. Even in 1958 the refrigerator still remained at the top of the list of desired goods.[27] The ownership of refrigerators rose between 1958 and 1961 from 19% to 39%, and two years later more than 51% of all West German private households had a refrigerator.[28]

Nevertheless there was a difference between the ownership of such machines and the use of them. Jakob Tanner cited the report of a Swiss housewife about their new electric kitchen machine:

"Crushing food with a rapidity like a flash seems brutal and atrocious to me. I see hard nuts, apples, lemon peels cut to pieces, being transformed into a irrecognizable bulk. Only a few moments later cabbage and carrots, onions and potatoes, bacon and fish could no longe be differentiated. Something inside me rebels against this bringing food into line. (…) I disappointed my husband by my reserve. He has expected me to be heartily delighted over his present because I usually agree with all innovations promising to make the work of housewives easier. Well, he need not wait too long: after some tests I changed my hostility to an honest admiration."[29]

This little story catches our attention. Of course, most of the housewives appreciated any technical innovation that eased their daily work. During the 1950s the working-hours of a house-wife in a household of four to six persons amounted to more than 72 hours a week.[30] With good reason they were proud of their new electric kitchen machines. In several opinion polls taken during the fifties these women said that their work was easier with kitchen machines which would save time and energy. And owning the new machines proved housewives to be modern. Yet on the other hand these answers, as well as the little episode cited above, pointed out that the use of kitchen machines was not at all a matter of course. It was not enough to

read the operating instructions, as the new appliances and their corresponding techniques transformed the way of preparing food fundamentally.

In the beginning of the sixties the "Gesellschaft für Konsumforschung"
discovered that housewives used their electric kitchen machines quite differently from the recommendations of the producers.[31] Exerting work, like
mixing dough or beating eggs, was willingly dealt with by using machines,
but scouring vegetables or peeling potatoes women preferred to do by
hand. "Potatoes have to be peeled plainly", one of the interviewers quoted.
"Peeling potatoes by the kitchen machine lacks accuracy. Therefore most
of the house-wives I have spoken to still peeled potatoes by hand."[32]

Kitchen machines and ready-made food lowered the level of knowledge
previously acquired through experience; personal skills became less
important. On the other hand the machines heightened a formalized understanding of weights, quantities, time and the right handling of machines.
However, such a complex and differentiated practice like the daily "production" of meals cannot be transformed into a purely technical process.
Contrary to the industrial law of efficiency it was still necessary to
"waste" time or energy to improve taste or to discover new ones.

Similarly this ambiguity can be discovered in the simultaneousness of
the use of "modern" industrial products like canned food and traditional
skills such as preserving food and vegetables. In 1953, 76% of all private
households in West Germany canned fruit on their own: households in the
country more so than in towns, households with several members more
frequently than those with only one or two people. Younger housewives
were slightly less used to preserving a little less than elder housewives.[33]
The reason for canning food at home was unequivocal—the women wanted
to save money. In the early 1950s home-made cans were much cheaper
than industrialized canned food. Noticeably more than half of the housewives canned food although they did not have a garden of their own! The
second reason for prefering home-made canned food was the unmistakably good taste. Taste would remain the most important attribute of
homemade canned food, particularly when the rising incomes allowed
consumers to buy more expensive industrial canned food more frequently.

Especially from the mid-fifties onwards the working-class households
consumed more and more canned food. A consideration of the opinion
polls taken by the Allensbach institute reveals the reasons for this increasing consumption:[34] More than half of the house-wives asked estimated
canned food to be comfortable because they were able to prepare a quick
meal at any time. A third of the housewives believed canned food to taste
better and another third held the view that canned food looks fresh and
delicious. Most of the housewives had bought canned food primarily

because the vegetables they wanted to eat were unavailable at this time of the year. Buying canned food obviously meant the attempt to overcome seasonal dependencies. Mainly those women who were employed and also had to do housework, used canned food as it saved time. Yet there was a difference in the consumption of canned fruit. Pineapple slices and tangerines were needed to distinguish dishes on Sunday or feast days. No doubt, canned fruit was a sign of an extraordinary meal.

Above all one tin held the top of the list: condensed milk. The consumption of evaporated milk rose ten times from 1950 until 1963! The market was dominated by four trade marks: "Glücksklee", "Libby's", "Nestlé" und "Bärenmarke" that were run by two Swiss and two US companies.[35] By order of the West German Libby's company the Institut für Demoskopie Allensbach carefully analyzed the consumer behavior during the 1950s.[36] Nearly all consumers used tinned milk for coffee, a third needed it to prepare salad, sauces, puddings or mashed potatoes. When asked which attributes of condensed milk they prefered most of them answered that first of all, evaporated milk tastes creamy, secondly, it goes best of all with coffee, and thirdly, condensed milk is able to colour the coffee in a beautiful way. The traditional advantage of condensed milk—being fresh for a long time—was less and less noted.

This shift of argument from practical reasons to aesthetic ones could also be recognized in the advertisements. In 1950 evaporated milk was praised for its various applications:

> "Libby's milk, ... the creamy one, makes the cake light and tasty, makes the coffee aromatic and the cacao flavorous. It improves the taste of sweet dishes, soups, and many meals. Because Libby's is concentrated milk it contains all of the nutritive aspects that make fresh milk so valuable."

It is notable that besides the indications of taste and aesthetic attributes this advertisement did not lack mentioning the high nutritive content of condensed milk. One year later the praising of variety stood back in comparison to the connection of condensed milk and coffee:

> "Libby's milk ... the creamy one!
> makes the coffee aromatic, flavorous, and full of delight."

The indication of nutritiousness was apparent in the sentence:

> "Libby's milk is concentrated full-cream milk".

The rhetoric shift from the nutritive aspects to aesthetic aspects can be clearly seen. Finally, in 1952, the aesthetic argument dominated:

> "What do you need for the coffee?
> Libby's milk … the creamy one!
> Even the best coffee would be yet more aromatic and flavorous by adding Libby's milk. Only a few drops color it an appetizing brown colour."

This little sequence shows how "intrinsic value" became detached from nutritive value. The sales argument that evaporated milk not only substitutes full-cream milk but is even healthier, stayed in the background. In its place was the continous, subliminal reference to another desired food: cream. Tying together condensed milk and coffee made it possible to initiate an aesthetic discourse about tinned milk. Now the talk was all about the "golden colour of the coffee" and the "creamy flow".

CHANGING DISCOURSES ON FOOD AND THE SPREAD OF "SELF-SERVICE" SHOPS

This shift to semiotic codes and the increasing meaning of signs is one of the most important changes in consumption during the 1950s, and particularly since the late fifties. The new semiotic "languages" consumers had to learn became visible in the rhetoric of the recipes published by the customer magazine "Die kluge Hausfrau".[37] Instead of the anticipated redundance and recurring standardization, the rhetoric of "Die kluge Hausfrau" was exceptionally multifaceted. During the first years after the currency reform in 1948, the recipes the "Kluge Hausfrau" published were rather simple and frugal. For example, there was a macaroni pudding made of minced meat and mushrooms, and beef or butter were seldomly mentioned. Worth noting were not only the pecuniary limits but the lack of international flair or extravagance. The recipes were obviously dominated by the domestic cuisine as it could be found in the former limits of the German Reich. Dishes from Hamburg, Silesia or East Prussia could be found as often as recipes like "the cheap pumpkin" which recommended an economic use of the household budget.

In 1951 the "Kluge Hausfrau" widened its horizons. For a Sunday meal it proposed a pork cutlet prepared à la Milano. Looking at the following recipes which all used the sign "Milano" there was not an uniform way of preparing the food but various ways that only share their connection to the referents cheese and tomatoes. From the mid-fifties the recipes became increasingly international. In 1954 mutton was offered as "Caucasian spit", "Italian mutton", "Mutton cutlets, provencale" or "Viking style". Cabbage was no longer cabbage, but "Swiss cabbage", "Scottish" or "Norman cabbage", even "Cabbage à la Strasbourg". In 1958 the "Kluge Hausfrau" invited its readers to a "culinary journey round the world": "Italy: Fish Milanese", "Portugal: Portuguese spinach roll", "France: Omelette parisienne", "Netherlands: Soup hollandaise"—and "Africa: Banana salad"! It is obvious how strong the Eurocentric mentality was internally fixed. In comparison to the other national states Africa was defined as only one country, and it was moreover presented with a meal of bananas—exactly the white prejudice about what black people in Africa ate. This caricature makes it sharply clear that the international connotations were plain artefacts, fabrications. Just like the "Milano style" had little to do with the authentic cuisine of Northern Italy, all the different international recipes did not represent authentic foreign ways of cooking but the wish for an international reputation, to become a common member of the family of nations again. The rhetoric of the recipes came to symbolize cuisine less as a practice of preparation than a factory of dreams.

In the famous West German periodical "Magnum" Klaus Harpprecht characterized this postwar mentality:

"The Germans long to be part of the 'family of nations'. They get sick of standing apart, being alone, whether in a brillant or in a miserable condition. (...) The wish of being assimilated to the international standard of taste, desires and needs seized their architecture as well as their menus (no architect would dare to build up an office-block in a different style than his colleagues in Louisville, Nagasaki or Lyon. No urban restaurant would relinquish serving Steak à la Hawaii or Nasi Goreng.). The Germans want indeed to have luck with themselves, and the world wants to have finally luck with the Germans. So we are resolved to be happy and mediocre."[38]

Long before West Germans went on their first trip into southern Europe they could taste Mediterranean atmosphere by eating "lamb cutlets á la Murillo", they could prove modernity and an "American life-style" by serving light, low-calorie meals. The early fifties with their frugal recipes, full of references to shortages and the economic use of money, were followed by timid excursions into little peculiarities of everyday cuisine, first attempts to open the rhetoric to little luxury menus or international dishes, the multitude of little snacks, the miniaturization of meals, and finally the new conscience eating healthy and light. The development of this rhetoric showed that these recipes did not stand apart from social reality in

West Germany, but can be read as a text that discloses the development of West German mentality.

Parallel to the discourse in medical magazines the "Kluge Hausfrau" also talked about "healthy nutrition" in a more and more scientific way. In the early fifties the term "healthy nutrition" was connected with an anti-modern way of thinking about and critizising the "sick-making" civilisation. During these years the "Kluge Hausfrau" recommended wholegrain bread and sports, obviously well acquainted with former concepts of "*Volksgesundheit*" (*völkisch* health). In the late fifties the "Kluge Hausfrau" had to take notice of the changing living conditions and became increasingly more realistic. Consequently, the discourse about "healthy nutrition" twisted— now the focus was either on fitness at work, especially for the husbands and the children at school, or on the "slim line". This connection of nutrition to socially-defined standards such as fitness at work or a male dominated, specific imagination of the female body signaled an important change in the discourse about eating during the fifties. The "modern housewife", as "Die kluge Hausfrau" sketched her, knew all about calories, vitamins and other essentials of healthy nutrition, she was busy in rationalizing her household, used gadgets extensively and saved therefore enough time to make herself pretty—the "modern" woman was not only housewife and mother but a clever engineer and an attractive wife, too.

This shift to the increasing importance of semiotic codes was strongly fostered by a new form of selling goods via the self-service store that brought a fundamental change in the way people purchased food. From the 19th century up until the 1950s it was an everyday experience to buy in shops where the shopkeeper stood behind a counter, asked what you wanted, fetched the articles from behind the counter, weighed them or drew them up, wrapped them, added the prices and took the cash. Self-service stores began to spread only from the mid-1950s onwards. Starting with just a few, the numbers then grew rapidly. In 1951 there were still only 39 self-service stores in West Germany, but in 1955 the number had climbed to 203, and only five years later, in 1960, to 17,132. By 1965 West Germany had more than 53,000 self-service stores.[39]

The rupture in experience could hardly have been greater. Not only did the counter disappear, the whole shop was reshaped with respect to the self-service principle. Now all goods were freely available, ready to grasp right at the level of eyes and hands, the arrangement of the articles, colours, light... all was brought into line with the presentation of goods. People who entered a self-service store for the first time were overwhelmed by the wealth of goods on offer. In the grocer's shop there had always been an opportunity to talk with neighbours, to hear local gossip, to "waste" time. The new self-service stores instead represented the modern discourse of the efficient use of time. Time-saving was the argument house-wives quoted most if asked about the advantages of self-service.[40]

The second important experience was the freedom of choice. After their first confusion, most housewives had the feeling of being able to select goods autonomously and without outside influence. For the customers, the mise-en-scéne of a store as a glittering world of goods meant the feeling of individual freedom.[41] Paradoxically, as options increased and as the choice of goods became more and more complicated, the desire of the customers for advice did not increase concomitantly. Instead, the attraction of 'self-service' was being able to choose and purchase individually. In place of the personal relationship between shopkeeper and customer, the goods now spoke directly to the customers and had to compete with their "rivals" on the shelves. This shift from the communicative work of sales clerks (often sales girls) to the semiotic power of goods and their outside appearances amounted to a decisive change in consumption in West Germany from the end of the fifties.

TOWARDS A NEW CONSUMER

The new quality of consumption at the end of the fifties consisted in much more than a further rise in economic growth, a quantitative increase of consumption and the buying of better durable equipment. It was above all a multiplication of options and a diversification of practices. The new world of goods, which West German customers had to deal with, had not yet been fully unfolded. But at the starting point of this development one can clearly see the diversification of practices. Entering a self-service store, buying industrialized food, taking home frozen food for the weekend because the refrigerator held it fresh for two or three days, preparing some snacks for the T.V. dinner in order not to interrupt the T.V. program for a family meal, cooking "light and healthy" so that the "slim line" would not hurt—all of these new skills had to be learned. Consumers, specifically housewives had to perform a multitude of new practices. They had to spell out new languages to decipher the several semiotic codes and had to find their way in a complex, unstable and entangled new world of goods.

The experience of hunger that had been present in the minds of the elder generation during their lifetime had now vanished. The stores full of goods, the abundant window displays of the butcher's shops—they all proved to be not only the transient dream of prosperity but rather permanent affluence. Of course many households still had to economize their budgets, of course they had to watch their pennies, but at the end of the 1950s there was no longer the need to be modest. The structural restrictions and the well-known, traditional limitations of an older way of living passed away. Because of the extension of the "universe of goods" and the variety of consumer options the working-class households took leave of their "proletarian way of living".

The "mass consumption society" was in no case a classless society, as the West German sociologist Helmut Schelsky had expected; social disparity still existed, but instead of traditional consumer hierarchies subtle "fine differences" (Bourdieu) now took their place. Heterodoxy and plurality was the signature of the "mass consumption society" that formed West-Germany since the late fifties onwards. Social inequality was no longer defined by profession and the position in production but by the conditions of work and leisure time, by social security, and chances of individual development—nevertheless gender as a criterion of social inequality still remains.[42]

Observers such as Max Horkheimer had stated that the consumption of food in industrialized societies had lost its "contrasts":

"The process of civilisation can be recognized by the culinary taste. Because of the artificial methods of production in agriculture, butchery and cooperage the strengthening dishes, the contrasts were smoothed off—similar to other fields. As asparagus nowadays tastes like peas, the unambiguous, specific taste of ham, sausage, salad or potatoes is vanishing by the same manipulations. Fermentation of wine is to be interrupted and sulphuric acid is to be added in service of a more rapid, rational and extensive production. As a result the sense of taste flattened, and a carrot of former times would nowadays surely confuse the civilized taste like a bourgois entering one of the garlic-saturated tenements in Lennox Avenue."[43]

Inspite of such global pessimistic views, uniformity of taste did not come to pass, but rather taste itself changed fundamentally. As the number of options increased, the offers of food broadened, and the international agro-market offered fruit and vegetables of all kinds during the whole year, the traditional contrasts of everyday food were disappearing at the same time that contrasts between Sunday and daily dishes, between the seasons and the regions diminished. Indeed, a refinement of traditional taste can be observed, as well as an increase in the multitude of new varieties of tastes. The British historian Stephen Mennell defines this process, although focusing on the 19th century, in fitting terms:

"Underneath the many swirling cross-currents, the main trend has been towards diminishing contrasts and increasing varieties in food habits and culinary taste. One trend, not two: for in spite of the apparent contradiction between diminishing contrasts and increasing varieties, these are both facets of the same process."[44]

By being part of the "consumer society" everyone had, in the words of Pierre Bourdieu, to pay attention "not to differ from the ordinary, but to differ differently."[45] Out of the increasing number of options consumers had to learn choosing and developing their own distinctive style. The previous practice of consumption that for long time meant making much out of little, now transformed into the skill of fabricating individuality out of the multitude.

The practice of consumption that consumers began to get acquainted with since the late 1950s created a "consumer subject" for the future who set a high value on individual freedom of choice. From the point of view of production—the experience of direct, physical work to "produce" food—this subject far removed. The work of preparing food in which a multitude of producers participate, local, regional and international—this relationship can hardly be experienced in a semiotic world of goods. Physical hardship and skill will vanish in the cash nexus. After more than thirty years of living in an "affluent society" furnished with an abundance of goods that no one had dreamt of at the beginning of the fifties, experienced in the usage of signs and semiotic codes, and highly skilled in the freedom of choice this "consumer subject" is nevertheless full of wants because it still mixes up consumption with happiness.

NOTES

1. Der Verbraucher und seine Bedarfslage im Frühjahr 1941. Eine Erhebung der Gesellschaft für Konsumforschung e.V., Berlin 1941 (typescript) (Archiv der GfK, Nürnberg, U 61). All quotations translated from German by the author.
2. Cf. Karin Hartewig, Das unberechenbare Jahrzehnt. Bergarbeiter und ihre Familien im Ruhrgebiet 1914–1924, München 1992.
3. Cf. Alf Lüdtke, Hunger in der Großen Depression, in: Archiv für Sozialgeschichte 27 (1987), p. 145–176.
4. Referring to the living standards of working-class families during the World War II see Wolfgang Franz Werner, "Bleib übrig!" Deutsche Arbeiter in der nationalsozialistischen Kriegswirtschaft, Düsseldorf 1983; generally see Bernd Martin/Alan S.Milward (Ed.), Agriculture and Food Supply in the Second World War. Landwirtschaft und Versorgung im Zweiten Weltkrieg, Ostfildern 1985.
5. Cf. Gabriele Stüber, Der Kampf gegen den Hunger 1945–1950, Neumünster 1984; Günter J.Trittel, Hunger und Politik. Die Ernährungskrise in der Bizone (1945–1949), Frankfurt/New York 1990; and Rainer Gries, Die Rationen-Gesellschaft. Versorgungskampf und Vergleichsmentalität: Leipzig, München und Köln nach dem Kriege, Münster 1991.
6. For a regional study of the black market see Michael Wildt, Der Traum vom Sattwerden. Hunger und Protest, Schwarzmarkt und Selbsthilfe in Hamburg 1945–1948, Hamburg 1986, esp. pp. 101–123.

7. Lutz Niethammer, Privat-Wirtschaft. Fragmente einer anderen Umerziehung, in: L. Niethammer (Ed.), "Hinterher merkt man, daß es richtig war, daß es schiefgegangen ist". Nachkriegserfahrungen im Ruhrgebiet, Berlin/Bonn 1983, p. 17–105. By the way, these oral history studies on life history and social structure in the Ruhr are some of the most widely read books focusing on the history of everyday life in West Germany.

8. A. J. Merritt/R. L. Merritt, Public opinion in occupied Germany, Urbana 1970, p. 16f.

9. Interview with Mrs. O., 9.2.1990, in Hamburg.

10. Cf. Stüber, Kampf gegen den Hunger, p. 384.

11. Hans-Peter Schwarz, Die Ära Adenauer. Gründerjahre der Republik 1949–1957, Stuttgart/Wiesbaden 1981, p. 382.

12. Rolf Peter Sieferle, Fortschrittsfeinde? Opposition gegen Technik und Industrie von der Romantik bis zur Gegenwart, München 1984, p. 226.

13. Hans Jürgen Teuteberg, Zum Problemfeld Urbanisierung und Ernährung im 19.Jahrhundert, in: H. J. Teuteberg (Ed.), Durchbruch zum modernen Massenkonsum, Münster 1987, p. 1–36, cit.: p. 35.

14. Teuteberg explicitly refers to per-caput-data in his analysis of long-time developments; see Hans Jürgen Teuteberg, Der Verzehr von Lebensmitteln in Deutschland pro Kopf und Jahr seit Beginn der Industrialisierung (1850–1975). Versuch einer quantitativen Langzeitanalyse, in: Archiv für Sozialgeschichte 29 (1979), pp. 331–388.

15. The following is based on a larger study of consumption in West Germany during the fifties which was recently published: Michael Wildt, Am Beginn der "Konsumgesellschaft". Studien über Konsum und Essen in Westdeutschland in den fünfziger Jahren, Hamburg 1993.

I owe many thanks to Jennifer Jenkins who has improved the English of this essay with patience and sensitivity.

16. Published by Statistisches Bundesamt Wiesbaden, Fachserie Preise, Löhne, Wirtschaftsrechnungen, Reihe 13 Wirtschaftsrechnungen, Wiesbaden 1949ff.

17. Referring to the discussion about household budgets see Christoph Conrad/Armin Triebel, Family Budgets as a Source for Comparative Social History: Western Europe—USA, 1889–1937, in: Historical Social Research—Historische Sozialforschung 35, 1985, p. 45–66; and Toni Pierenkemper (Ed.), Zur Ökonomik der privaten Haushalte. Haushaltsrechnungen als Quellen historischer Wirtschafts- und Sozialforschung, Frankfurt am Main 1991.

18. Edeka, Annual report 1957, p. 30 (Archiv Edeka, Hamburg)

19. Institut für Demoskopie Allensbach, Die Meinung im Bundesgebiet, 1953 (Bundesarchiv Koblenz B 145/4224-124).

20. Gesellschaft für Konsumforschung, Haushalt und Speisefett. Eine Befragung von 2040 Haushaltungen/Hausfrauen im September 1962, Nürnberg 1962 (typescript), (Archiv der GfK, Nürnberg, U 761 b).

21. Institut für Demoskopie, Allensbach, Die soziale Wirklichkeit, 1955 (Bundesarchiv Koblenz ZSg 132–449).

22. Cf. Wolfgang K. A. Disch, Der Groß- und Einzelhandel in der Bundesrepublik, Köln/Opladen 1966, p. 75; and Unter Null. Kunsteis, Kälte und Kultur. Konzipiert von Hans-Christian Täubrich und Jutta Tschoeke. Herausgegeben vom Centrum Industriekultur Nürnberg und dem Münchener Stadtmuseum, München 1991.

23. One of the first and famous restaurant chains in West Germany founded in the late fifties was the "Wienerwald" which served only roasted chicken in various ways.

24. Strukturveränderungen im privaten Verbrauch, in: Mitteilungen des Wirtschaftswissenschaftlichen Instituts des DGB (WWI), 1962, p. 193.

25. Alf Lüdtke, Hunger, Essens-"Genuß" und Politik bei Fabrikarbeitern und Arbeiterfrauen. Beispiele aus dem rheinisch-westfälischen Industriegebiet, 1910–1940, in: Sozialwissenschaftliche Informationen für Unterricht und Studium (Sowi) 2 (1985), p. 118–126, cit.: p. 120.

26. Jahresberichte der Verkaufsabteilung, 1955ff. (Firmenarchiv Oetker, Bielefeld, P1/431).

27. Institut für Demoskopie, Allensbach, Wunsch und Besitz, 1958 (masch.), (Bundesarchiv Koblenz ZSg 132–707).
28. Statistisches Bundesamt, Fachserie M, Reihe 18: Ausstattung der privaten Haushalte mit ausgewählten langlebigen Gebrauchsgütern 1962/63, Stuttgart/Mainz 1964.
29. Jakob Tanner, Grassroots-History und Fast Food, in: Geschichtswerkstatt 12 (1987), p. 49–54, cit.: p. 52.
30. Ursula Schroth-Pritzel, Der Arbeitszeitaufwand im städtischen Haushalt, in: Hauswirtschaft und Wissenschaft, 6. Jg. 1958, Heft 1, p. 7–22.
31. Gesellschaft für Konsumforschung e.V., Hausfrauenbefragung über Küchenmaschinen, 1962 (typescript), (Archiv der GfK, Nürnberg, U 778).
32. Ibidem.
33. Institut für Demoskopie Allensbach, Das Einmachen. Umfrage 1953/54 (Bundesarchiv Koblenz ZSg 132–284 I/II).
34. Institut für Demoskopie Allensbach, Gemüse- und Obstkonserven. Marktanalyse 1956 (Bundesarchiv Koblenz ZSg 132–544 I).
35. Glücksklee was a product of Glücksklee Milchgesellschaft mbH, Hamburg, which was a subsidiary company of Carnation Co., Los Angeles; Libby's was produced by the German department of Libby's; Nestlé was a subsidiary company of the Swiss company in Vevey, and "Bärenmarke" was produced by the Allgäuer Alpenmilch AG in München, which was also owned by a Swiss company; see Max Eli, Die Nachfragekonzentration im Nahrungsmittelhandel, Berlin/München 1968, p. 30–32.
36. Institut für Demoskopie Allensbach, Verschiedene Untersuchungen zum Dosenmilchverbrauch 1950–1958 (Bundesarchiv Koblenz ZSg 132-88, -165, -280, -392, -465, -630).
37. "Die kluge Hausfrau" was a weekly, free-of-charge consumer magazine of the trade company "Edeka". It was already published before World War II, in 1949 it was put on the market once more, and rose until the end of the fifties to a circulation of more than one million copies. "Die Kluge Hausfrau" was the most widely-read consumer magazine of the food trade and can be compared to famous public magazines like the "Stern", "Quick" or "Constanze".
38. Klaus Harpprecht, Die Lust an der Normalität, in: MAGNUM 29, April 1960, p. 17–19, cit.: S. 18.
39. Wolfgang K. A. Disch, Der Groß- und Einzelhandel in der Bundesrepublik, Köln/Opladen 1966, p. 60.
40. Gesellschaft für Konsumforschung, Einkaufsgewohnheiten in Deutschland, Nürnberg 1953, typescript (Archiv der GfK, Nürnberg, U 183).
41. Ibidem.
42. Cf. Stefan Hradil, Sozialstrukturanalyse in einer fortgeschrittenen Gesellschaft. Von Klassen und Schichten zu Lagen und Milieus, Opladen 1987; also: Wolfgang Zapf, Sozialstruktur und gesellschaftlicher Wandel in der Bundesrepublik Deutschland, in: W. Weidenfeld/H. Zimmermann (Eds.), Deutschland-Handbuch, München 1989, p. 99–124.
43. Max Horkheimer, Bürgerliche Küche, in: M. Horkheimer, Notizen 1950 bis 1969, ed. by Werner Brede, Frankfurt am Main 1974, p. 46–47.
44. Stephen Mennell, All Manners of Food, Oxford 1985, p. 322.
45. Pierre Bourdieu, Klassenstellung und Klassenlage, in: P. Bourdieu., Zur Soziologie der symbolischen Formen, Frankfurt am Main 1975, p. 42–74, cit.: p. 70.

11. MC KEBAP: DÖNER KEBAP AND THE SOCIAL POSITIONING STRUGGLE OF GERMAN TURKS

Ayse S. Çaglar
Free University Berlin

INTRODUCTION

Döner kebap is a fast food introduced and incorporated into the German market by Turkish migrants living in the Federal Republic of Germany (hereafter FRG).[1] Although *döner* (in the form offered in Germany) is itself a new and hybrid product that developed through Turks' migration experience in Germany, it became *the* traditional ethnic food of Turks in the eyes of the Germans. Nothing else is so often quoted as *döner kebap* to refer to the positive effects of Turks' presence in Germany. Indeed it functions as a positive symbol in multiculturalist discourses, more or less like the scarf worn by Turkish girls and women which has become mainly the negative symbol in discourses of the lack of integration of German Turks.

Today around 2 million Turkish migrants live in the FRG. These migrants, recruited within the "guest worker" system designed to serve the labour needs of the host society, came to Germany after the first bilateral agreement signed between Germany and Turkey in 1961. Since then, they have been living there and are economically well integrated into the society. During this 30 year period, these "guest workers" are internally stratified, so that they are now presented in almost all strata of German society. Today German Turks are fully integrated into the German economy. The 35,000 Turkish businesses run by German Turks have an investment figure of 7.2 billion German Marks. Their turnover per annum is around 25 billion German marks (Zentrum für Türkei Studien 1992: 2). As many as 87% of these Turkish businesses are active in food and catering (Şen 1988) and the owners of *döner* Imbisses (small fast food stalls or "restaurants" offering *döner*) compose their big majority.

Berlin, with its 150,000 Turkish residents has the largest Turkish population of any German city. It is often called the largest Turkish city outside Turkey. Moreover, it has a very active and lively Turkish business life with more than 6000 Turkish businessplaces. Today, due to *döner Imbisses* (over 1300) abounding in its streets and to 40–50 Tons of daily *döner* production, Berlin came to be known as the "*döner* centre", *döner* metropole" or "*döner* paradise" in Germany.[2]

Döner means revolving (Redhouse 1984: 311) and *kebap* which is an Arabic word, is a generic term used for roasted or broiled meat. Thus, *doner kebap* means "meat roasted on a revolving vertical spit" (ibid.: 311). *Döner kebap* in Germany, referred to shortly as *döner* or interchangeably *kebap* is a "sandwich" of roasted spicy meat slices prepared in a quarter or one fifth of a Turkish flat bread (*pide*) garnished, depending on taste, with a combination of different sorts of salad (lettuce, tomatoes, cucumbers, red cabbage, onions) and topped with a choice of garlic yoghurt or hot ketchup like dressing.

Döner was introduced to Germany by Turkish migrants. However, although produced and sold mostly by Turks, and known as a Turkish food in Germany, *döner kebap* in the above mentioned form is not available in Turkey. In Turkey, until the 60s, *döner* was offered only as a main dish in restaurants (especially, in specialized restaurants known as *kebapci*). With the rapid urbanization and the spread of fast food in the 60s, *döner* sandwich appeared in the major cities of Turkey on the market as a fast food variety. The roasted meat slices, garnished with a pickle and sometimes with ketchup would be sold in a sandwich bread or in a quarter of a loaf of bread. However, in this form, it never became and still is not a very popular fast food in Turkey as *döner kebap* is in Germany.

Since its appearance in the German fast food market, *döner* consumption in Germany and particularly in Berlin has showed a steady increase. Today, *döner kebap* is firmly established in the German fast food market. In 1992, the daily *döner* production—estimated by the producers—to be a minimum of 40 Tons for Berlin and of 70 Tons for Germany. Given that each *döner kebap* contains 80–90 gr. of *döner* meat, this figure means production and consumption of daily 7,800,000 portions of *döner kebap*. Interestingly, this gradual incorporation of *döner kebap* into the fast food diet of Germans was never accompanied by advertisement campaigns aiming German customers.[3] Other than one or two advertisements (in German) in public places, *döner* trade is still running without advertisements.[4]

In the beginning of 1990s the market for *döner kebap* was expanding and *döner* as an ethnic fast food it was on its haydays. However, there appeared signs of a change in the marketing strategy of *döner kebap*. More and more Turkish *döner Imbisses* started to offer their "regular" ordinary *döner kebap*s under names such as "*Mc Kebap*", "*Keb'up*", "*Mac's Döner*", etc. In its marketing, an effort to underplay *Döner*'s ethnic connotations became apparent. It is difficult to explain this change solely in reference to the market forces, because by the time of this change *döner* was selling better than ever as an ethnic fast food.

With its introduction into German society, this new food item took on new meanings in its new context, went through and is still going through some changes. Embedded into the social relations and set of meanings surrounding it, *döner* became an integral part of Turkish migrants' relations with the Germans and of their identities in Germany.

The uses of goods are social and goods carry social meanings. They have communicative value due to their symbolic and expressive functions (Douglas and Isherwood 1979: 12). Moreover, they act as markers. Thus, objects that have acquired intimate associations with a social group are integral to the development of the group identity and social relations of this group. In a similar way, food and food consumption have symbolic and constitutive functions in inter group relations. "What people eat expresses who and what they are to themselves and to others" (Mintz 1985: 13). Like other goods, food acts as a marker and especially in cases in which particular food items are associated with ethnically and culturally differentiated groups, these items more often function as ethnic signifiers. *Döner* functions in German society as such. In exploring the way its meanings and images are manipulated and transformed in Germany, one also needs to examine the web of social relations German Turks are embedded in Germany and the transformations of these relations. This article focuses on the changes in *döner*'s marketing strategy and aims to explore the dynamics behind these in a broader context of the social positioning struggle of German Turks in German society.

A BRIEF HISTORY OF *DÖNER KABAP'S* INCORPORATION INTO THE BERLIN MARKET

As stated, *döner kebap* was introduced to Germany by Turkish migrants who were recruited as guest workers. Following the oil crisis and the consequent economic stagnation, the German government, like other European governments of migration countries officially banned the entry of non-EEC workers to Germany in 1973. However, although the number of foreign workers decreased in the post-recruitment period, the foreign population in Germany has continued to grow because of the implementation in 1974 of the policy allowing migrant families to be brought to Germany. The number of Turkish migrants increased from 910,500 in 1973 to 1,268,300 in 1979 in the FRG (Statistisches Bundesamt) as a whole and from 79,468 in 1973 to 100,217 in 1979 in Berlin (Statistisches Landesamt). The ratio of workers among foreign residents has continually decreased with this development.

Unemployment among foreigners rose from 0.7 in 1972 to 6.8 in 1976 (Castles, Heather and Wallace 1984: 185). Thus the rise of unemployment, arrival of new family members of Turkish migrants seeking for jobs, and some Turkish migrants' readiness to invest their savings in Germany paved the way to the self-employment of Turkish migrants (mostly as grocery store and *Imbiss* owners) and to *döner* production in Germany. According to one *döner* producer in Berlin, this link was very direct and crude. He said: "the time unemployment appeared among Turks was the time Turks started *döner* business in Germany".[5] In fact the very first *döner Imbiss*es appeared around the central train station (Bahnhof Zoo) in Berlin in 1975 when unemployment was increasing among Turks.[6] The number of *döner Imbiss*es increased rapidly in the late 70s, but they gained real momentum in the 80s reaching their haydays when the Berlin Wall fell in 1989.

From the very beginning, *döner kebap* was marketed as a Turkish speciality and targeted Germans as its consumers. Still today, according to *Imbiss* owners, 95% of *döner* consumers are German. This orientation on German customers however, should not be interpreted as *Imbiss* owners' desire to extricate themselves from the fellow countrymen. It was based on economic considerations. German customers simply meant a greater market for *döner*. For this reason, in marketing *döner* in its new form, the "German taste" was the primary concern of Turkish *Imbiss* owners. This "German taste" had a substantial impact in orienting the changes in the composition and the taste of *döner kebap* until it reached its more or less standardized taste in Germany. This is not to say that Turkish migrants did not and do not consume *döner*. They did and still do, but their percentage in its overall consumption was and is still very low. Since the second half of the 80s, *döner* has been firmly incorporated, at least in Berlin, into the daily fast food scene of *"Hamburger"*, *"Curry Wurst"*, *"Bockwurst"*, *"Bulette"*, and french fries.

DÖNER AND *PIDE*: A SYMBIOTIC SUCCESS

The introduction and popularity of *döner kebap* was not without effect on the consumption and production of some other food items on the market. Moreover, it gave rise to new forms. The most important change of *döner* on its journey from Turkey to Germany is the substitution of the sandwich bun or the quarter of a regular loaf of Turkish bread by *pide* (Turkish flat bread). In Turkey *pide* is <u>not</u>, unlike in Germany, a kind of ordinary bread on the market all around the year. Although there are various forms of *pide* in Turkey, the *pide* sold in Germany all the year round (mostly in Turkish stores and bakers) is in Turkey available only during the Ramadan, the fasting month in Islam.

Imbiss owners give the following reasons behind their preference of *pide* for *döner kebap*: its practicality to serve as a bread pocket thick and curved enough (1/4 or 1/5 of the round flat bread) to hold the roasted meat, the salad and the dressing; the smooth texture of its crust; most importantly its quality of being more filling than a sandwich bun, but less than a Turkish loaf of bread—which is believed to be too much for the "German taste".

Döner's major effect on *pide* was to increase *pide* production drastically in Germany, especially in Berlin. *Döner* increased the demand for *pide*, thus consequently, its production. For this reason, the success of *pide* covaried with the success of *döner kebap*.

"When I started the business in 1975, there were five, six small Turkish bakeries. But, I am the first to bake and sell *pide* [wholesale] in Berlin. *dönerImbisses* of that time baked their own *pide* for their *dönerkebap* in their own shops, in their small ovens. Today, there are over 70 Turkish bakeries producing *pide* in Berlin. How to say, it is *döner* which brought *pide* to this level".

The figures of *pide* production also confirm the words of the owner of this Turkish bakery. Today, daily *pide* production is estimated to be around 200,000 in Berlin and over 500,000 in Germany. Most importantly, it is estimated that at least 70% of this figure is consumed by *döner Imbisses*.

Although unintended, using *pide* for *döner kebap*, changed the meaning and the connotations of *pide*. Among Turkish migrants in Germany it lost its association with Ramadan. The fact that Turkish bakers in Berlin now produce a different kind of *pide* as *ramazan pidesi* (*pide* for the Ramadan) whose form is slightly different (more of an elipse) though its dough is the same, points to this decontextualization of the regular *pide* in Germany. The *ramazan pidesi* weighs a little more than a regular *pide*, has more sesam and black cumin on its surface, and is more expensive. Now, except one Turkish baker, all Turkish bakers in Berlin produce this new type of *pide* only during the Ramadan. People que for this *pide* in Turkish bakeries in Ramadan, although what would be a *ramazan pidesi* in Turkey, but not considered as such in Germany, remain unnoticed on the shelves. When asked for the reasons behind the introduction of this new *pide* as *ramazan pidesi* in Berlin, one baker answered *"döner* business finished up the *pide*. It had nothing left to do with the Ramadan"*. It is also noteworthy that all the *Imbiss* owners and the *pide* bakers I interviewed use *pide* and "bread" interchangeably and most often refer to *pide* as "the bread" (*ekmek*). This is also a further sign of *pide*'s recontextualization as a regular type of bread.[7] Now, in some *Imbiss*es, *pide* found its way to *"Wurst"* (sausages—mostly pork—) and some *Imbiss*es sell sausages within a slice of *pide*. Although most of these *Imbiss*es are owned by Germans, there are some Turkish *Imbiss*es that also sell sausages in this fashion.

Döner kebap not only determined the scale of the production and consumption of *pide* to a large extent, it also paved the way to *pide*'s incorporation into the fast food market in Germany. Now, the latter is also established in this market, but *döner* dominates its symbolic field. It is noteworthy that *pide* finds its way as *Döner—Brot* (*döner bread*) to the other fast food products such as to falafel (see *Zitty* May 1994: 19).

Pide has a share in the success of *döner* as much as *döner* has in *pide*'s popularity, because *pide* played a very important role in *döner*'s competition with more familiar fast food items in the market. Starting from the end of 70s, *döner* is portrayed in the German media in strong competition with other fast food types in the German market, namely with *"hamburger"*, *"Bockwurst"* and the Berliner novelty, *"Curry Wurst"* (*Bild* Berlin 4 August 1982; *Der Tagesspiegel* 15 February 1983; *Berliner Morgen Post* 30 October 1988). The mini surveys of the newspapers showed that among the consumers who were asked to compare these fast food types and voice their preference, the proportion of those who preferred *döner* to other fast food varieties was steadily increasing in Berlin.

Döner producers, *Imbiss* owners, and consumers more or less agree on the factors behind *döner*'s success. First of all, compared to *"Curry Wurst"* or *"Bockwurst"*, *döner*, with its substantial amount of "bread", spicy meat, variety of salad and dressing, is a meal in itself that would still one's hunger. "It is not appropriate to compare *döner* to *"Curry Wurst"*, they are not comparable" said one *Imbiss* owner who owns 22 *Imbiss*es in Berlin (in the Eastern section of the city)

"one is a meal and the other is not. With a portion of *"Curry Wurst"* you could still your hunger only for a while, for that moment, but with one *döner kebap* you have your meal. It is settled. Instead of spending DM 2 or DM 2.50 on *"Curry Wurst"*, one buys a *döner* and it is all done"

Pide plays an important part in this filling quality of *döner kebap* which consumers always underline. It is more filling than a sandwich bun, but not as much as a quarter of an ordinary loaf of bread. When this quality of *dön*er and its nature of being a meal in itself are taken into account, then it is apparent that *döner*—oscillating between DM 3 ($1.8) and DM 4 ($2.4)—is relatively a cheap and practical fast food meal.

There are also other factors pointed out for *döner*'s success. These are: its attractiveness in terms of its ingredients and its aesthetical attractivity. Here, the attractiveness of *döner* in regards to its ingredients *vis-à-vis* *"Curry Wurst"* or *"Hamburger"* needs to be contextualized within the healthy nourishment discourse which became popular especially in the second half of 80s. First of all, *döner* meat is mostly veal or beef and in contrast to pork in *"Curry Wurst"* or *"Bockwurst"* leaner, thus more in line with the low-fat diet discourse of the late 80s.[8] The salad in *döner kebap*, a mixture of lettuce, red cabbage, onions, cucumbers and tomatos, topped with a yoghurt dressing is also apparently attractive to those whose consciousness of healthy nourishment is basically shaped by the discourse on a diet of fresh vegetables, salad and yoghurt. Moreover, all the ingredients of *döner* are fresh. *Döner* meat on the spit is supposed to be and mostly is consumed daily, thus it is fresh.[9] Being free from chemical ingredients, especially in comparison to *"Curry Wurst"* or *"Bockwurst"*, *döner* has a clear advantage over the former. On the basis of these qualities, *döner* fits into the discourse on healthy nourishment of the late 80s.[10] The aesthetical attractiveness of the colorful salad in *döner kebap* topped with yoghurt dressing which the consumers never fail to point out should also be understood within the context of these discourses.

All these factors, combined with German's increasing desire, since World War II, for international and exotic food (Wildt 1993), established the ground for *döner kebap*'s success in Germany. *Döner* was gradually incorporated, at least in Berlin, into the fast food diet of Germans and with the fall of Berlin Wall, it became the number one fast food of the East Germans.

MARKETING *DÖNER KEBAP*

In terms of German Turks' marketing strategies of *döner kebap* in the German fast food market in Berlin, it is possible to differentiate two

periods: the period from its introduction in the mid 70s to the standardization of the composition and taste of *döner* meat in Berlin in 1989 by
German authorities and the period after the fall of the Berlin Wall.

The first stage covers the period from the introduction of *döner* in the
mid 70s to the standardization of the composition and taste of *döner* meat
in Berlin in 1989 by German authorities (Berliner Verkehrsauffassung für
das Fleischerzeugnis *"döner kebap"*) and is characterized by small scale
individual production of *döner* in apartment basements or at Turkish
restaurants or *Imbiss*es. At this stage, the taste and the composition of
döner meat, as well as its price varied considerably. Although the meat of
döner kebap in Turkey does not entail minced meat, this was and still is
the basis of the *döner* produced in Germany. However its ratio varied
strongly. Consequently, the production costs of *döner* showed a considerable variation depending on the ratio of the minced meat (sometimes
reaching to 80–90%) and on the other binding ingredients. It is noteworthy
that this period is marked by fierce price wars among *döner Imbiss*es. The
price, even in the late 80s, fluctuated between DM 1.80 and DM 3.50 for
one *döner*.

In order to keep the quality of *döner* meat standard and to avoid *Imbiss*
owners using high rates of minced meat and of binding or chemical ingredients in their fierce battle to cut down the cost, German authorities in
Berlin officially defined in 30 October 1989 the ingredients of *döner* meat
(veal, beef or lamb) and the ratios of these ingredients, (fat, spices, % of
minced meat). In 1991, the same regulation was adopted for Germany.[11]
Under this regulation, only those *döner*s in line with the specified ingredients and ratios of ingredients are entitled to be sold as *döner kebap*. This
regulation standardized the taste of *döner* meat to a great extent.

This setting of product norms for *döner* was initiated by some German
Turks who were in *döner* trade. They urged the authorities to take measures
against the detoriating quality of *döner* meat in severe competition. Most
of them looked upon the new regulations very positively as the fierce price
wars was putting them under pressure to cut down the production costs by
all means.

Moreover, this setting up product norms was also seen as a kind of official recognition and admission of *döner kebap* into the German market.
When explaining these product norms, one *döner* producer said

"today *döner* is firm in Germany. Even the authorities have recognized this
fact. They understood and appreciated its value and set regulations on its ingredients. *Döner* business is not like a jungle any more. There are standards. It is
a serious business. You can not put whatever you want and sell it as *döner!*"

Thus, this act was not considered as an unwanted interference of the German authorities in German Turks' affairs.

In the period until the standardization, the composition of *döner* meat varied, but the form of the *döner kebap* was pretty standard during this period. Slices of spicy *döner* meat within a quarter of *pide* garnished with a combination of salad and topped with the garlic yoghurt dressing is the *döner kebap* of this period. There was not a product differentiation. There was basically one type of *döner* with a varying quality of *döner* meat.

The presentation and marketing of the *döner kebap* of this period was embedded in a folkloric discourse of Turkishness. *Döner Imbisses* offered this "Turkish" speciality in a highly accentuated oriental and folkloric atmosphere. Touristic Turkey posters, several types of souvenir from Turkey and colorful lights dominated the interior decoration of *döner Imbisses* of this period. The ethnic and exotic associations of *döner kebap* was at the fore front. In marketing *döner*, the *Imbiss* owners' strategy was to promote its Turkishness and exoticness. They exploited its ethnic associations.

DÖNER KEBAP AFTER THE FALL OF THE BERLIN WALL

Setting up product norms for *döner kebap* by the German authorities coincided with the fall of the Berlin Wall in 1989 (9 November). A focus on the period starting from this date reveals that, starting in 1990, both the production of *döner* and its marketing went through and are still going through some important changes. The most striking characteristics of this period is a substantial increase in *döner* production, introduction of new *döner* varieties, that is product differentiation and an image renewal.

After the fall of the Berlin Wall and the reunification of the former German Democratic Republic (GDR) and the FRG, the number of firms producing wholesale *döner* increased rapidly in Germany, and particularly in Berlin. Although the exact number of these *döner* meat "factories" are not available, they are believed to number between 25 and 30 in Berlin now. However, other than four or five of them, these are still small size family firms. As stated before, the daily *döner* production is estimated to be a minimum of 30–40 tons for Berlin and of 70 Tons for Germany. This amount is evaluated to be the saturation point for West Germany, but the previous GDR is seen as an expanding and promising market for increased production. Consequently, Turkish migrants in *döner* business are investing rapidly in this part of Germany. In 1992, from the 115 Turkish firms active in the Eastern section Berlin, 80 of them were restaurants and *Imbiss*es offering *döner*. (Blaschke and Ersöz 1992, Supplement 1). With a complete incorporation of the former GDR market, daily *döner* production is anticipated to reach to 200 Tons in Germany.

It is again during this period *döner kebap* is integrated into German language. In 1991, *döner kebap* made its way into the authoritative German dictionary *"Duden"* as *der döner kebap*.

By 1991 we see new varieties of *döner kebap* in the market. There is an apparent attempt at product differentiation by changing the composition of *döner* meat within the allowed limits, or by changing the garnishings of *döner kebap*. Different varieties of *döner* meat with no minced meat at all or solely beef or veal or a mixture of beef, veal and lamb *döner* are marketed as new varieties of *döner kebap* under such names as *"efendi döner"*, *"oba döner"*, *"bey döner"*, *"tosun döner"*, *"döner light"*, *"tava döneri"*, etc. The other new varieties of *döner* are made simply by adding feta cheese, fried egg plants or pieces of french fries to the *döner kebap*. Here, it is important to note that all these changes are accompanied with price differentiation, and the prices increase by each new variety.

Today in Berlin *döner* or *kebap* serve as generic terms for all fast food types prepared in *pide* like *döner kebap* with different types of salad and dressing such as "vegetarian *döner*", "zucchini *döner*", "chicken *döner*" or "turkey *döner*". The most recent example of these new products is the "Korean *döner*" offered by Koreans. A piece of *pide* is filled with some pieces of meat (not *dön*er meat), cooked soja sprouts topped with "Korean hot souce". It is noteworthy that in all these new forms offered as different types of *döner*, *pide*, not the *dön*er meat, is the only common ingredient and all have the quality of being a meal in themselves. These new varieties, however, except "chicken *döner*", are not yet widespread.

However, the most important change taking place in the marketing of *döner* is at the symbolic level. Both *döner* producers and *Imbiss* owners try to give *döner kebap* a new image with a different field of connotations.

While *dön*er was becoming almost a generic name for fast food served in *pide* in a fashion similar to *döner kebap*, and new varieties of *döner* made their way to the fast food market in Berlin, another kind of practice gained momentum. Today, more and more Turkish *döner Imbiss*es offer their "regular" ordinary *döner kebap* under names such as *"Mckebap"*, *"Keb'up"*, *"Mac's döner"*, *"Mister kebap"*, *"McKing"*, *"Dönerburger"*, etc. But, the *döner kebap*s offered under these names are *not actually different* from ordinary *kebap*s. There are no alterations, neither to the *döner* meat, nor to the garnishings and it is important not to confuse this development with the above mentioned product differentiation.[12] Interestingly, all these adopted names are in English. Although the Turkish owners of these *Imbisses* do not speak English, the names they choose for their products are in English not in German. In all these names, except *"McKing"*, either *döner* or *kebap* is used in combination with an English word or suffix.

Mckebap Imbiss chain has five stores, (two of them in the former East Berlin), all called *Mckebap*. The allusion of this name is clearly to "McDonald's". The other chain, also with 5 stores, two of them in the eastern section of the city is called *"Keb'up"*. However, the *"Keb'up"* chain is more ambitious than the *"Mckebap"* chain. The staff working in each branch are all dressed in white T-shirts with red aprons and red caps, with Keb'up prints all over their clothes. "Keb'up" stores offer three types of *döner*: "Mini *döner*", *"döner"* and "Big *döner"*. All are wrapped in *"Keb'up"* imprinted paper pockets. Again the model of presentation and the labelling of their products is clear: the fast food chains of "McDonald's" or Burger King. In fact, McDonald's and its place in German society orient the major *döner* producing firms and the owners of *Imbiss* chains considerably in their attempt to transform the image and the place of *döner* in German society. I will return to this point.

"Mister kebap" on the other hand is an *Imbiss* chain of 22 *Imbisses* in "East" Berlin. Each *Imbiss* has the emblem of *Mister kebap* that appears between Coca-cola stickers. This emblem is particularly interesting (see below Figure 1). The script *Mister kebap* takes the form of a crescent and apparently alludes to the Turkish flag. The owner also explained the

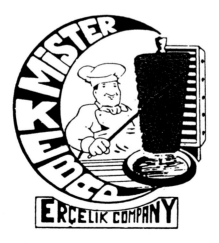

Figure 1 The logo of *Mister Kebap*.

emblem in this way. According to him the Turkishness of the food is symbolized by the crescent.

Interestingly, everything on this logo, including the name of the company (although it is based in Berlin and operates only in Germany) is written in English. Neither symbolically nor linguistically is there any reference to Germany. This absence is noteworthy. When I asked the owner of *Mister Kebap* cahin why he chose a name particularly in English, given that he was established in Germany, he answered

> "you know here in Germany, everything American has a better value. How can I say. They have high esteem. That is the reason for example why some friends [he refers to other *Imbiss* owners] chose names like *Mc Döner* or *Mc Kebap*. Now there is this phenomen Mc Donald's. I think they wanted to imitate it [Mc Donald's]. So we thought ours should also be international. We combined English with something from us. We said, 'let's take one from you and one from us'"

THE SYMBOLIC FIELD OF *DÖNER KEBAP*

In our contemporary world, identities and belongingnesses are more and more asserted by life styles, which in turn are encoded in the images of consumer goods that act as markers (Featherstone 1987). Thus, material objects are more than ever a pivot around which social identities are constructed and asserted (Miller 1987: 124). In this context, goods associated with a particular life style easily become a social arena for the social positioning struggle of various groups as well as an arena in which belongingness is formulated and asserted. Thus, the analysis of the way the meanings and images of goods are manipulated and transformed is important to explore the processes by which identities and social relations are constituted.

Thus, in order to disclose the factors behind Turkish migrants' attempts to redefine their image and place in the society by manipulating the image of *döner* in Berlin, we need to disclose the web of meanings and social relations in which *döner kebap* is embedded in Berlin, and for that matter in German society.

In Germany and Berlin, *döner kebap* is strongly associated with Turks. It became the traditional ethnic food of Turks.[13] In this way it symbolizes Turks and things thought to be Turkish. This strong association, almost an identity, is observable at different levels in a wide spectrum of practices ranging from children's books to official international evenings.[14]

Döner, by means of its strong association to an ethnic group in Germany found its way into the folklorism of multiculturalist policies. Not rarely, it is used to refer to the multicultural quality of Germany (see Tageszeitung, 15 February 1989), and of Berlin. The name of the widely announced youth get together organized for Turkish and German youth in Berlin in 1987: "Disco *döner*" is only one example of how *döner* is used to refer to Turks in Germany within the context of multiculturalism.

Due to this association, *döner* became integrated into the discourse on the "Ausländerfrage" (the foreigners question) in Germany. "Kein *döner* ohne Ausländer!" ("No *döner* without the foreigners") "Kein *döner* ohne Türken!" (No *döner* without Turks!"), "Kein *döner* ohne Wir!" (No *döner* without us!") were the banners of the biggest pro-foreigners demonstrations of the eighties in Berlin. Given the fact that "Ausländer" and "Turks" were almost synonymous at that time, again a direct association between *döner* and Turks was manifest. This association reaches such dimensions that a young German man, asked to comment on the attacks on the foreigners and the increasing enmity against the foreigners on TV in 1991 (after the brutal attacks raged by the Neo-Nazis in 1991 Fall) answered a little surprised, as if his opinion on this subject was very obvious by saying "I have nothing to do with these, I am not against the foreigners, I eat my *döner*". It is noteworthy that although the attacks were not raged on Turks but on other foreigner groups in the former GDR, he voiced his opinion by means of his relationship to *döner*. Thus *döner*, due to the strong association it acquired with Turks and consequently with foreigners, functions as an arena in which hostilities against and solidarity with Turks and foreigners are asserted.

This associaton between Turks and *döner kebap* in Germany is manifest at different levels in the society. An article titled "*kebap* Kapitalisten" (the "*kebap* capitalists") in *Die Zeit Magazine* in 1992 (28 August) on successful Turkish businessmen in Germany illustrates this in an interesting way. Although it is titled "the *kebap* capitalists", the article is on successful Turkish businessmen/women in Germany and ironically, none of the Turkish businessmen/women portrayed in the article has or had anything to do with *döner* business, but all are active in areas different than *döner* related ones. The *kebap* in the title is simply used to substitute the adjective Turkish. Sometimes *kebap* simply substituted the Orient and Islam. An intereseting example of such use is the title of a symposium organized by the "Evangelische Akademie Iselohn" on 19–21 November 1993 in Iserlohn. The title is "Kebab oder west-östlicher Diwan" ("Kebab or West Ost Diwan). Interestingly, none of the topics on the program has anything to do with *Kebap*, but deal with the issues related to Islam and Orient-Europe relations.[15]

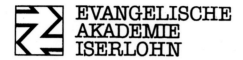

**EVANGELISCHE
AKADEMIE
ISERLOHN**

Kebab oder west-östlicher Diwan?

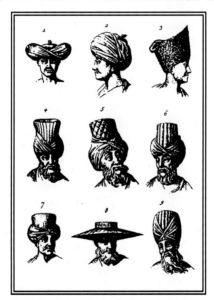

**Die Erfahrungen der Kulturorganisationen und
Institutionen der Entwicklungszusammenarbeit
im Umgang mit den islamischen Ländern**

Tagung

121   **19. - 21. November 1993**

Figure 2

German Turks in *döner* trade would get rid of the above mentioned association of *döner kebap* with Turkishness, whereas in the past their strategy was to accentuate the Turkishness or exoticness of their product. Now they prefer to distract their customers' attention from their ethnicity. In adopting new names for *döner*, Turkish *döner Imbiss* owners try to pluck *döner* out from its articulation and rearticulate it with a different set of connotations. They seek to get hold of the language and the image of modern technologies to dissociate *döner* from the web of connotations it is embedded in. It is not simply a matter of adopting new names for their products and the *Imbiss*es, it is also of changing marketing, presentation, and the image. Today in Berlin more and more Turkish *Imbiss*es seek to downplay their previous folkloric and oriental "Turkish" atmosphere in their new decorations.

In 1992, a new *döner Imbiss* (called *"Efendi"*) was opened at the site of an old Turkish *döner Imbiss "Topkapi"* in downtown Berlin. The modern decoration of the former with no allusion to Turkey and Turkishness at all, is in strong contrast to the heavy oriental atmosphere the latter had. Interestingly, the owner remained the same. When asked for the reasons behind this drastic change, he said:

"Before, there was a place called "Topkapi" here. A place with our [Turkish] atmosphere. But I thought, in the midst of Europe, on Ku'damm I want to realize something close to McDonald's. I want to show that Turks are also capable of setting up good business and running it. The problem is to change the atmosphere, to offer a Turkish speciality without our atmosphere, to present it in a modern way. I want *döner* to go further. We changed it. Believe it, even the nature of customers changed"

It is clear that the adoption of American names is part of the new marketing strategies of the *döner Imbiss*es.[16] McDonald's, representing the highest level of modern western technology plays an important role in orienting their endeavour to renew the image of *döner*, and to give it a character in which the hold of Turkishness has partly evaporated. The tendency is to dislocate *döner kebap* from the particular set of connotations it is woven into in German society, and to present it within a context in which its ethnic and folkloric associations are downplayed, but never totally eroded. From this point, the transformations *döner kebap* goes through manifest the new ways of articulation and negotiation between the local and the global.

Here, it will be misleading to expect that Turkish *Imbiss* owners' most important motive for imitating McDonald's is that they just want to appeal to a wider public, including people who are not attracted by "exoticness". Turkish *Imbiss* owners' desire to become upscale might seem to contradict their efforts to model themselves after McDonald's. However, this is a contradiction only when we assume that McDonald's signify the same thing to everyone in different parts of the world. Although McDonald's caters to a broad public and does not have a high prestige in North America, German Turks have a different image of McDonald's. It is identified with high technology, good business and with something advanced, modern, clean and efficient. As the owner of Mister kebap expressed it, it represents something American that is of high value.

MARKETING STRATEGIES OF *DÖNER KEBAP* AND SOCIAL MOBILITY

The confusing thing in *döner kebap*'s story in German fast food market is that a new strategy of its promotion and image came in the beginning of 1990s, when *döner kebap* was selling better than ever. There seemed to be no need for an image renewal. The market for *döner* grew significantly by the reunification of Germany and *döner kebap*, as a cheap and exotic fast food meal in itself had something to offer to the former East Germans. Ironically, Turkish *Imbiss* owners started to downplay the ethnic connotations of *döner kebap* when the demand for exotic and "ethnic" food was increasing. Thus it is not possible to explore the dynamics of this change from within a framework which only takes into account the market forces. *Döner kebap*'s story has to be placed into a broader context of German Turks' social exclusion and quest for social mobility in Germany.

THE SOCIAL SPACE GERMAN TURKS OCCUPY IN GERMAN SOCIETY

The social space German Turks occupy in German society show some anomalies. Social space refers to the space of social positions, as defined by objective social structures that shape the subjects' social beings (Bourdieu 1990: 123–130). In this view, the position of a given agent is identified on the basis of his or her position in different fields and of his or her different kinds of capital, namely economic, cultural, social and symbolic (Bourdieu 1985: 724). Economic capital refers to all goods that are immediately and directly convertible into money (Bourdieu 1986: 243).

By cultural capital, the ensemble of embodied dispositions such as learnable skills is understood. This usually refers to educational qualifications (ibid.). Social capital is composed of resources based on connections and group membership (Baourdieu 1987: 4). Symbolic capital is simply the "form which is assumed by different forms of capital when they are perceived and recognized as legitimate" (Bourdieu 1990: 128). The structure of social space is given by the volume and composition of the overall capital the individual has (Bourdieu 1974: 114). Moreover, these four forms of capital are, under certain conditions, convertible into one another. Thus, within this framework, social mobility not only refers to changes in the volume of capital, but also covers changes in the distribution of total capital among its different kinds (Bourdieu 1974: 115–142).

A focus on the social space German Turks occupy in German society discloses that in terms of economic capital there are no significant differences between Turkish and German workers. Moreover, there is an increasing trend towards stratification among German Turks and the growing number of Turkish firms and employees indicate an upward economic mobility achieved by some German Turks (Blaschke end Ersöz 1992; Sen 1993).

Although German Turks have a clear deficit in cultural capital in comparison to Germans, their educational qualifications are gradually increasing that they started to occupy also different positions in respect to this dimension. However, with regard to distinct forms of capital they have a real deficiency in their symbolic capital. The distinctive quality of symbolic capital is that "while the other forms of capital have an independent objectification, be it as money, titles or behavioral attitudes and dispositions", this form of capital "only exists in the eyes of the others"(Joppke 1986: 60). Thus it is nothing more than economic or cultural capital which is acknowledged and recognized (Bourdieu 1990: 135).

The derogatory jokes about Turks, the increasing antipathy towards foreigners, the attacks and insults directed towards Turks all indicate that German Turks have a very negative image in German society. There is a severe deficiency in their social recognition and German Turks are aware that this lack of social recognition negates the success they have achieved in different areas such as business and education. Other types of capital that they manage to acquire lose their value because of this deficiency.

In short, the social space German Turks occupy in German society is characterized by a deficiency in symbolic capital. Volumes of economic and cultural capitals vary within the stratified German Turks in Germany, but this deficit in symbolic capital affects all of them. For those German Turks who moved up economically, especially for Turkish businessmen in

Germany, this discrepancy between their economic and symbolic is more drastic and it hinders their full *social* mobility.

This anomaly is the consequence of the social exclusion German Turks face in Germany. Turkish businessmen and those in *döner* business who compose their majority are particularly affected. In the beginning, *döner* trade was not a simple way of earning their living in Germany, but was one of the most important ways of becoming self-employed, that is becoming one's own boss. It symbolized breaking from being a worker in Germany. In that sense, *döner* trade which functioned as a symbol of economic and consequently social success for German Turks, was a prestigious line of business in their eyes in the late 70s and 80s. It was a symbol of their economic integration. However, their lack of social recognition and the discrepancy between their upward economic and social mobility became more apparant when they started to increase their economic capital significantly, especially after the fall of the Berlin Wall. Due to *döner kebap*'s aforementioned strong association with Turkishness and Turks' negative image in Germany, this group of German Turks suffered from lack of social recognition as businessmen *per se*. Their reluctance to exploit "Turkishness" and "exoticness" of *döner* in its marketing can be evaluated in this context of social exclusion and anomalies of their social space in Germany.

The change in German Turks' marketing strategy of *döner* in Germany is part of German Turks' efforts to re-work the connotations of *döner kebap* to make *döner* and consequently themselves respectable. Changes in *döner kebap*, and especially those regarding its image are part of Turkish migrants' efforts and desire to cut across national boundaries to create a new local identification. As such, it could be seen as a part of "new ways of articulating the particularistic and the universalistic aspect of identity" (Hall 1992: 304). Thus, what is taking place around *döner* is symptomatic of the production of Turkish migrants' new identities in Germany and of their desired place and image in German society.

In all the changes *döner kebap* is going through in Germany, different efforts and strategies to open up *döner*'s way up in society are evident. After having established itself among the lay public, it is trying to find its way up in German society.

Döner producers and *döner Imbiss* owners agree that *döner* does not have the place in society it deserves, and for that matter, it has a fair way to go. "First of all, its price should go up" says a manager and immediately adds that its form should be altered so that it could be mass produced. Most importantly, according to him, *pide* and the salad should be eliminated from *döner kebap*. A bun should substitute the *pide* and a leaf of lettuce, or a pickle should replace the rich and colorful salad in *döner kebap*. "The consumers, their taste and habits are changing" he says

> "slim-line, diet, freshness, minimality [*öz* in Turkish], etc. These are important. The taste of the meat is more prominent in a sandwich bun. Everything is more aesthetical. Then *döner* would be attractive to other "tastes". High society German will also eat it. Someone from the upper class will also eat it."

It is ironical that what made *döner* attractive among the lay public, namely the filling quality of *pide* and the combination of different sorts of salad are seen by the Turkish businessmen to be the very factors hindering *döner*'s move up in the society. Now, targeting a different group of consumers in German society, they seek to incorporate *döner* into the consumption patterns and discourses of different social groups.

In this endeavor, there are also Turkish *Imbiss* owners who prefer to dissociate themselves from *döner kebap* completely in their effort to become upscale in the food and catering sector. Those German Turks who used to be in *döner* trade and owned *Imbiss* chains and are now moving gradually into restaurant business catering Italian food belong to this category.[17]

Döner, by having played an important role in the economic success biography of several Turkish businessmen in Germany, contributed to their economic empowerment there. Faced with social exclusion, such German Turks employ certain strategies to convert their economic capital into symbolic capital to achieve the social mobility they desire. Thus, the changes in the marketing strategy of *döner kebap* and German Turks' efforts to re-fashion its set of ethnic connotations are part of German Turks' social positioning struggle in Germany. For this reason their efforts to move up in German society would not only depend on their ability to transform *döner* to fit to the "taste" of the social groups targeted or on its success in renewing its image, but also on the power relations Turkish migrants are embedded in in German society.

NOTES

1. I would like to thank Garry Bamossey, Georg Elwert and Carola Lentz for their comments on an earlier version of this article. Of course the final responsibility for the contents of the present work is mine alone.
2. In the former West Berlin municipalities, the percentage of Turkish *döner* Imbisses, grocery stores and restaurants offering *döner kebap* as fast food in all Turkish stores vary between 56.3% and 83.3%. In the areas densely populated by Turks, although the number of such stores is higher than it is in the areas where Turks are not populous,

their share in all Turkish stores alltogether are smaller than their share in the latter. From 129 Turkish stores in Kreuzberg 75 of them offer *döner kebap*. (Zentrum für Entwicklungsländer-Forschung FU Berlin 1990).

3. There are commercials of *döner* producers or wholesale meat retailers on Turkish cable TV in Turkish. These aim Turkish *Imbiss* owners. In the European editions of Turkish newspapers there were always and still are *döner* producers' advertisements targeting *Imbiss* owners. But all these are in Turkish and do not aim German consumers.

4. In Berlin, the first serious *döner kebap* advertisements (in German) apppeared in subway stations in 1992.

5. All data about the introduction and development of *döner*, and about its consumption in Germany and in Berlin are based on the interviews the author conducted with owners and managers of *döner* producing firms and *Imbiss*es in January–February 1992 and September 1993.

6. The first *döner* Imbiss, as many informants recalled was located around the central train station (Bahnhof Zoo)

7. *Pide* is not the only type of Turkish bread produced and consumed by German Turks. There is also Turkish loaf of bread. It is noteworthy that the former type enjoys the status of "bread" in Germany, while in Turkish cities this term is reserved for the latter.

8. This is one of *döner*'s major advantages over Gyros produced and marketed by Greek migrants in Germany. The latter contains pork.

9. In fact, on the basis of a regulation enacted in 1989, to use *döner* meat in *döner* kebap from a day before is prohibited. Fines could be charged in such cases.

10. Of course *döner*, as a fast food type with a considerable meat input, is not in line with the vegetarian nourishment discourses. However, its exoticness and low fat content still have something to offer to those young Germans and students who are relatively health price conscious.

11. According to this regulation, for example, no binding substances and chemicals are allowed and the rate of minced meat can not be higher than 60%. For a detailed definition of the ingredients of *döner kebap* see Berliner Verkehrsauffassung für das Fleischerzeugnis "*döner kebap*".

12. In the *Imbiss*es offering new varieties of *döner kebap*s, there is a sign of *döner kebap* somewhere on the shop window, but the real emphasis is on the adopted new names. These names are printed on the aprons of the workers, on the napkins, and on the waxed paper pockets for *döner*.

13. In Germany, Istanbul has somehow the repuation of being the homeland of *döner* (see *Der Tagesspiegel*, 15 January 1992). A recent notice in a Turkish newspaper illustrates this connection in an interesting way: according to the newspaper, two officials in Berlin were sent to court on charges of insulting foreigners. In the receipt of the parking bill sent to a Turk, these officials are acuused of altering the place of birth of this person (Istanbul) as "*döner* town" (*Hürriyet*, 2 April 1993).

14. See for example R. Meier *Achmed und Stefan*. Düsseldorf: Schwann Verlag, 1982.

15. I am thankful to Lale Yalcin-Heckmann in bringing this document to my attention.

16. Although this practice of adopting American names is mostly observable in *döner* business, it is not limited to this branch. This is becoming a general trend in the catering business run by Turks. The catering company called "picnic" run by two German Turks which offers "picnic döner kebap" and "picnic fried chicken" (*Hürriyet* Mayis 31, 1994) is a stiking example of such companies.

17. *Döner Imbiss* owners are now opening pizzerias especially in the former GDR. Pizzeria owners give the following reasons for their decision: low production costs and high profit rate of Italian food in comparison to *döner* and Turkish food; the unsaturated market for Italian food in the former GDR and the former East Germans' eagerness to adopt "West-German" life styles; the increasing hostility against foreigners, especially to Turks and Turkish businessplaces in the former GDR; and last but not the least, the prestige involved in running a "proper" restaurant.

REFERENCES

Berliner Morgen Post (1989). Döner Kebap macht der Curry Wurst immer mehr Konkurrenz. 30 October.

Berliner Verkehrsauffassung für das Fleischerzeugnis "Döner (1989). Kebap", Senatsverwaltung für Gesundheit. Ges IV C 3.

Bild Berlin (1982). Döner Kebap. Ende unserer Curry Wurst. 4 August

Bourdieu, P. (1974). *Distinction: A Social Critique of the Judgement of Taste.* Malbourne and Henley: Routledge and Kegan Paul.

———. (1977). (reprinted in 1985) *Outline of a Theory of Practice.* Cambridge: Cambridge University Press.

———. (1985). The Social Space and the Genesis of Groups. *Theory and Society* 14: 723–724.

———. (1986). The Forms of Capital. In J. G. Richardson, ed., *Handbook of Theory and Research for the Sociology of Education.* Pp. 241–258. New York/Connecticur/London: Greenwood Press.

———. (1990). Social Space and Symbolic Power. In P. Bourdieu, ed., *In other Words Essays Towards a Reflexive Sociology.* Pp. 123–139. Cambridge: Polity Press.

Blaschke, J. and A. Ersöz (1992). *Bitte sehr!—Buyurun—Türkische Unternehmer in Berlin* Berlin: Edition Parabolis.

Castles, S., B. Heather and T. Wallace (1984). *Here for Goog: Westren Europe's New Ethnic Minorities.* London: Pluto Press.

Douglas, M., Isherwood, B. (1979). *The World of Goods.* New York. Basic Books Publishing Inc.

Featherstone, M. (1987a). Consumer culture, symbolic power and universalism. In *Mass Culture, Popular Culture and Social Life in the Middle East.* G. Stauth and S. Zubaida, eds. Frankfurt am Main: Campus Verlag

———. (1987b). Life style and consumer culture. In *Theory Culture and Society* 4: 55–70.

Hall, S. (1992). The Question of Cultural Identity. In S. Hall, D. Held and T. McGrew eds. *Modernity and Its Futures.* Cambridge: Polity Press.

Meier, R. (1982). *Achmed und Stefan.* Düsseldorf: Schwann Verlag.

Miller, D. (1987). *Material Culture and Mass Consumption.* Oxford: Basil Blackwell.

Mintz, S. (1985). *Sweetness and Power.* New York: Elisabeth Sifton Books.

Redhouse Turkish—English Dictionary (new) 1984 Istanbul: Redhouse Yayinevi.

Sen, F. (1988). The Turkish Enterprises in the Federal Republic of Germany. Report. Türkei Zentrum.

———. (1993). 1961 bis 1993: Eine kurze Geschichte der Türken in Deutschland. In C. Leggewie and Z. Senocak eds., *Deutsche Türken—Türk Almanlar.* Hamburg: Rowohlt.

Tageszeitung (1989). Das Image des Döner Kebab ins Rotieren gekommen. 15 February.

Volksblatt Berlin (1987). Weg vom Döner-Kebab und Bauchtanz-Image. 14 April.

Wildt, M. (forthcoming) Plurality of Taste. Food Consumption in West Germany during the 1950s. Bremen: Edition Con.

Zentrum für Entwicklungsländer-Forschung (FU Berlin) (1990). Die Raumliche Ausbreitung türkischer Wirtschaftsaktivitäten in Berlin (West)—Dichte der türkischen Wohnbevölkerung—Gesamtzahl der türkischen Läden-Prozentualer Anteil der einzelnen Branchen.

Zentrum für Turkeistudien (1992). Konsumgewohnheiten und wirtschaftliche Situation der türkischen Bevölkerunf in der Bundesrepublik deutschland. Essen. Ms.

Zitty (1994). Die Bohnen-Bulette. May. Berlin.

INDEX